OXFORD MEDICAL PUBLICATIONS

Fetal Medicine

OXFORD MONOGRAPHS ON MEDICAL GENETICS

General Editors

ARNO G. MOTULSKY
MARTIN BOBROW
PETER S. HARPER
CHARLES SCRIVER

Former Editors

J. A. FRASER ROBERTS
C. O. CARTER

Fetal Medicine

Prenatal Diagnosis and Management

Edited by

ANDRÉ BOUÉ

Translated by

MICHEL VEKEMANS *and* LOLA CARTIER

Oxford   New York   Toronto   Tokyo
OXFORD UNIVERSITY PRESS
1995

This book has been printed digitally and produced to a standard design
in order to ensure its continuing availability

OXFORD
UNIVERSITY PRESS

Great Clarendon Street, Oxford OX2 6DP

Oxford University Press is a department of the University of Oxford.
It furthers the University's objective of excellence in research, scholarship,
and education by publishing worldwide in

Oxford New York

Auckland Bangkok Buenos Aires Cape Town Chennai
Dar es Salaam Delhi Hong Kong Istanbul Karachi Kolkata
Kuala Lumpur Madrid Melbourne Mexico City Mumbai Nairobi
São Paulo Shanghai Singapore Taipei Tokyo Toronto

with an associated company in Berlin

Oxford is a registered trade mark of Oxford University Press
in the UK and in certain other countries

Published in the United States
by Oxford University Press Inc., New York

First published in French, 1989, by Flammarion Médecine- Sciences, © Flammarion, 1989
© This edition, Oxford University Press and M. Vekemans and L. Cartier, 1995

The moral rights of the author have been asserted
Database right Oxford University Press (maker)

Reprinted 2002

A catalogue record for this book is available from the British Library

Library of Congress Cataloging in Publication Data
Fetal medicine: Prenatal diagnosis and management / edited by André Boué;
translated by Michel Vekemans and Lola Cartier.
p. cm.—(Oxford medical publications)(Oxford monographs on medical genetics; 26)
Includes bibliographical references.
1. Fetus—Diseases. 2. Fetus—Abnormalities. 3. Prenatal diagnosis.
I. Boué, André. II. Title. III. Series. IV. Series.
Oxford monographs on medical genetics; no. 26.
[DNLM: 1. Prenatal Diagnosis—methods. 2. Fetal diseases. 3. Pregnancy complication.
WQ 09 M488 1994a]
RG626. M42513 1994 618.3'2—dc20 93- 39528

ISBN 0- 19- 261904- 7

Preface

In the early 1970s a new medical activity evolved: prenatal, or fetal, medicine. In addition, from 1980 onwards progress in the investigation of the fetus *in utero* has grown exponentially and the variety of indications for such testing has broadened.

Visualization procedures, of which ultrasonography is the most important, have transformed the examination of the fetus and guided fetal sampling, allowing development of a new area of biology: the clinical biology of the fetus. We felt that a monograph on this new biology had become essential for practising doctors.

Certain questions always arise when one undertakes the compilation of a book describing medical techniques: for whom is it written, and why? The clinical biology of the fetus is different from other branches of clinical medicine. It is unique because, as we shall see, the patient we want to examine is not independent: he or she is in the mother's womb. Biological parameters that are normal for a child, a newborn baby, or even a premature baby cannot be applied to the fetus, even by extrapolation.

Fetal medicine can lead to serious decisions. The results of laboratory tests can leave doctors and parents facing a dramatic choice: to continue or terminate a pregnancy. The situation is rarely so acute in paediatrics or adult medicine.

Most practising doctors have been taught little about fetal biology in the course of their medical studies. The information they need is often widely scattered throughout the specialist literature, because these techniques are still in the research domain and there has been little attempt to make them more accessible. However, there is considerable public interest in the subject. The demand from the families involved is pressing: after 'quantitative' birth control, some kind of 'quality control' is required.

This book is intended for doctors — general practitioners, obstetricians, or paediatricians — in the hope that it will help them to answer the questions that are asked of them by the families in their care.

The other question that arises is whether this is the appropriate moment to write such a book. Progress in this field is rapid, and a book is out of date even before it is published.

This book is based on the experience of biologists who have been specializing in the field of fetal medicine for ten or twenty years. We have the impression that the extraordinary progress of recent years is slowing down, at least in certain areas. Present techniques are applicable to a very wide range of anomalies, and there are few diseases justifying prenatal diagnosis for which a test is not available even though the benefits may be limited. Also, the application and use of the commonest techniques is becoming more standardized.

For the authors, producing a book is a chance to pause for breath rather than be swept away by the headlong rush for progress; to take stock of what has been accomplished and consider where further research efforts should be directed.

One of the major objectives in the clinical biology of the fetus is a better definition of those pregnancies in which the use of the techniques at our disposal is justified. For example, with autosomal recessive diseases, how can we find out which couples are at risk before the birth of a first affected child? For cystic fibrosis, how can we screen for heterozygous parents? In particular, where chromosomal anomalies are concerned, how can we pick out the pregnant women who have an increased risk of giving birth to an affected child? In these areas we welcome progress that would make the present book out of date as soon as possible!

This book is really an essay, as defined in Robert's dictionary: 'a prose work, free in nature, not exhausting all the possibilities of a subject, or made up of several contributions'. It certainly does not exhaust the subject — some aspects of prenatal biology are not covered; for example, isoimmunization. The contributions of which it is made up have one thing in common: they have been written by doctors and biologists who have been working together for several years and who, with their colleagues, have had to face the day-to-day problems of this area of biology. They have also benefited from regular collaboration with many clinicians.

Finally, the production of this book would not have been possible without the patience and good will of our secretaries.

Boulogne   A. B.
1989

Contents

Contributors

ANDRÉ BOUÉ, Université Paris-Ouest; Hôpital Ambroise Paré, Boulogne; INSERM Unité 73, Château de Longchamp.

JOËLLE BOUÉ, INSERM, Unité 73, Château de Longchamp.

SOPHIE COIGNARD, Université Paris-Ouest; Hôpital Ambroise Paré, Boulogne.

JEAN DUNAND, Université Paris-Ouest; Hôpital Ambroise Paré, Boulogne.

MICHEL GOOSSENS, Université de Paris-Val-de-Marne; Hôpital Henri-Mondor, Créteil; INSERM, Unité 91.

CLAUDINE JUNIEN, Université Paris-Ouest; Hôpital Ambroise Paré, Boulogne; INSERM, Unité 73, Château de Longchamps.

CLAIRE MALBRUNOT, Université Paris-Ouest; Hôpital Ambroise Paré, Boulogne.

FRANÇOISE MULLER, Université Paris-Ouest; Hôpital Ambroise Paré, Boulogne.

JEAN-FRANÇOIS OURY, Hôpital Robert Debre, Paris.

LIVIA POENARU, Université de Paris Faculté Cochin-Port-Royal; Hôpital Cochin; INSERM, Unité 127.

MICHEL VIDAUD, Université de Paris-Val-de-Marne; Hôpital Henri-Mondor, Créteil: INSERM, Unité 91.

PART I FETAL INVESTIGATIVE TECHNIQUES

Introduction

Recent developments in ultrasound have improved the clinical assessment of the fetus. Not only can the external anatomy be examined in search of malformations such as anencephaly or limb defects, but the internal morphology can also be examined for malformations of the brain, heart, kidney, gut, and spine. Real-time ultrasound permits the examination of fetal movement and an assessment of the development of the central nervous system. Finally, ultrasound guidance techniques permit fetal sampling, thus opening the door to prenatal diagnosis.

The following chapters will address on the one hand, fetal sampling techniques, invasive procedures which must be performed by well-trained teams to minimize risks to mother and fetus; and, on the other hand, the most commonly used laboratory analyses.

Laboratory analyses specific to certain diagnoses (enzymopathy, virology, etc.) will be covered in the chapters addressing the particular diagnosis.

1 The fetus as patient

Twenty years ago, *in utero* fetal examination was done by tape measure and wooden stethoscope. Ultrasound, introduced by Ian Donald, was, at that time, a technology of mediocre quality and was little used. In 1972, Campbell *et al.* made the first ultrasound diagnosis: anencephaly. In 1967–68 the first prenatal diagnoses using laboratory techniques had been achieved: diagnosis of chromosomal anomalies using cells from amniotic fluid, diagnosis of inborn errors of metabolism, and diagnosis of primary rubella virus infection by measurement of IgM-specific antibodies in maternal blood. (See for example Jacobson and Barter, 1967; Vesikan and Vaheri, 1968.)

Today, thanks to enormous technical progress, ultrasound and laboratory methods together form the foundations of a new branch of medicine: prenatal medicine.

How important is laboratory testing? In France alone, in 1989, more than 25 000 chromosomal analyses of amniotic fluid were performed; added to this are biochemical analyses (approximately 1500) and molecular studies (approximately 500).

Diagnosis of fetal anomalies can present itself in two ways: diagnosis in pregnancies where a risk of anomaly has been predicted; and diagnosis in pregnancies where a risk could not have been predicted.

Prenatal diagnosis when there is a predictable risk of anomaly

The risks involved are, above all, genetic risks: chromosomal anomalies and single-gene disorders. Genetic counselling prior to prenatal testing (or better, prior to a pregnancy in which prenatal testing is indicated) will establish the risk, and the appropriate method of sampling can be chosen.

The diagnosis of all *chromosomal anomalies* relies on the same methodology: the analysis of chromosomes in metaphase, and karyotyping using different staining techniques. This method allows the detection of change in chromosome number and/or structure.

In contrast, the diagnosis of single-gene disorders relies on specific techniques for each disorder. These methods work by analysis of the expression of the gene mutation, by looking directly at the mutant protein, or indirectly, by studying the biochemical expression of the disorder. They also rely on analysis of the gene itself using the techniques of molecular biology.

Prenatal diagnosis when there is no predictable risk of anomaly

The risk of fetal anomaly can be related to maternal disease, infectious disease, or medication prescribed to the mother.

In practice, most of the time, it is an abnormal ultrasound finding that leads to prenatal diagnosis. With few exceptions (anencephaly or dominantly inherited limb defects), laboratory studies are an essential complement to medical intervention:

– in establishing a diagnosis: for example in demonstrating the presence of a chromosomal anomaly or in confirming the diagnosis of a neural tube defect by measuring acetylcholinesterase;

– in establishing a prognosis: for a continuing pregnancy, laboratory tests allow a measure of the severity of the disorder (for example in kidney disease, a measure of renal function), and most of all provide a recurrence risk for future pregnancies (for example in the finding of a chromosomal translocation).

As we have seen, chromosomal analysis relies on one technique, whereas for other laboratory analyses one can choose between different techniques applicable to different kinds of samples. Rarely are we dealing with a qualitative measure of a substance that is normally absent; rather, most laboratory analyses are a quantitative measure of a normal substance. These quantitative tests can only be used for diagnosis once careful study has established the normal physiological variation of the substance in question. Indeed, the fetus is rapidly developing within, and non-independently of, its mother. Moreover, some samples, such as chorionic villi and particularly amniotic fluid, are not derived from the embryo proper. A knowledge of fetal development and physiology is essential for the interpretation of laboratory findings. Acquiring knowledge of the normal human embryo–fetal development has been difficult, for obvious ethical reasons, and many unknowns remain. We will address certain of the more important aspects of the more common diagnoses encountered.

The fetus as an evolving organism

Evolution at the molecular level

Haemoglobin   Haemoglobin is a tetramer made up of either four identical chains or two pairs of different chains. Figure 1.1 shows the evolution of haemoglobin chains during ontogenesis. The ε chain appears during the early weeks of gestation and disappears prior to twelve weeks, while the γ chain is synthesized at the beginning of the tenth week, decreasing before birth to disappear completely between 6 months and one year after birth. The β chain is synthesized in low amounts early in embryonic life and then in greater amounts after birth. The α chain begins production early in gestation and continues throughout life.

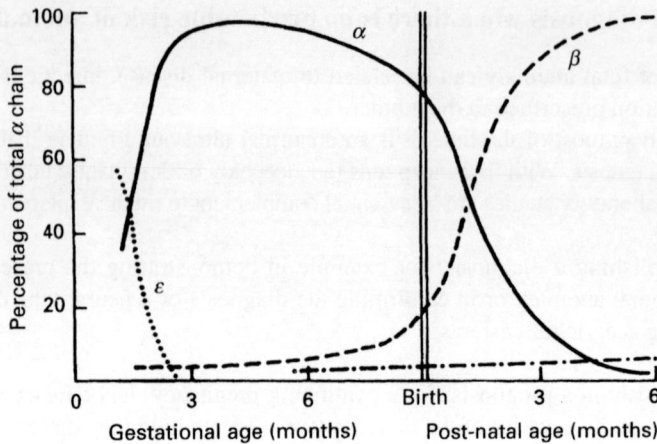

Fig. 1.1 Development of non-α haemoglobin chains during fetal life, at term, and after delivery. From Bernard *et al.* (1976).

The embryo produces two forms of haemoglobin, Gower I and Gower II. Gower I is a tetramer of four ϵ chains and Gower II is a $\epsilon_2\alpha_2$ tetramer. The fetus synthesizes haemoglobin F and the $\alpha_2\gamma_2$ tetramers. Haemoglobin's affinity for oxygen is regulated by the presence of 2,3 diphosphoglycerate (2-3 DPG) which binds to deoxyhaemoglobin but not to oxyhaemoglobin. The 2-3 DPG and oxygen bonds are mutually exclusive. Fetal haemoglobin F has less affinity for 2-3 DPG than does maternal haemoglobin A, and therefore has a greater affinity for oxygen.

Acetylcholinesterase   Acetylcholinesterase, an enzyme which hydrolyses the acetylcholine neurotransmitter, exists in a number of molecular forms: globular forms, G, and asymmetric forms, A. During rat development, a change in the proportion of the tetrameric form and the monomeric form have been observed. The tetrameric form, G_4, represents 10 per cent of total activity in a ten-day embryo, 50 per cent of activity at birth, and 90 per cent of activity in the adult rat. A similar change in the molecular forms of acetylcholinesterase has been observed in the human. In brain tissue of a seven-week-old embryo the monomeric form G_1 is observed, whereas in the eleven-week embryo, as in the adult, it is the G_4 form which predominates.

Therefore, while in the rat the maturation of the molecular form of acetylcholinesterase covers the fetal and neonatal period, in humans the same evolution takes place between the seventh and eleventh weeks of embryonic life. These stages of maturation are a general phenomenon, as the morphological and biochemical differentiation of nerve cells in culture is also associated with a change in the G_4 forms of acetylcholinesterase.

These two examples clearly demonstrate that such changes must be taken into consideration when a diagnosis rests on this product.

Evolution at the cellular level

Ontogeny of the immune response The ontogeny of the immune system has mostly been studied in animal models; mice for T lymphocytes, birds for B lymphocytes, and sheep for immune response. In humans, examination of fetal tissue after pregnancy termination (thymus) or study of fetal blood (for example, sampled at testing done for advanced maternal age) has provided normal reference values, and (sampled at the time of infection), measurement of pathological response.

Our understanding so far rests either on studies of human fetuses or on experimental data derived from animal models and consistent with observations made on the human fetus.

Immune response begins early in embryonic life. Appearance of cell membrane markers which precedes acquisition of an immune response is detected in T cells around the eleventh week of gestation by the rosette assay. The antigen-specific helper T cells can appear even before the fetus is able to produce antibodies to that particular antigen. The first stage of B cell differentiation, associated with the presence of intracytoplasmic IgM (without any surface Ig) is recognized around the eighth week.

The humoral response comes later. The B cells with membrane immunoglobulins (IgG, IgA, IgM) appear at the eleventh week, rapidly increase, and at the fourteenth week reach a level equivalent to that observed at term. These cells, however, cannot differentiate into lymphocytes and are not able to secrete immunoglobulin.

Only after the seventeenth week can we detect a low level of IgM in the fetal serum, and this level will be maintained until there is antigenic stimulation. The fetus also produces IgG, but at low levels; most of the IgG present is therefore of maternal origin. Figure 1.2 demonstrates the sequence of development of the immunoglobulins.

Development of the immune response occurs in stages as a function of the antigen. Animal studies, of sheep in particular, have demonstrated that for each antigen there is a particular time before which there is no response and after which there is always a good response. The appearance of this immune competence is species-specific and is not related to the physical and chemical characteristics of the antigen.

At the time of antigen stimulation the fetal immune response is qualitatively (in the sequence IgM, IgG1, IgG2) and quantitatively, with few exceptions, well established. The antigenic environment may induce premature development of the immune system. Certain antigens, by crossing the placenta, may sensitize the lymphocytes to these antigens, which explains why the newborn baby may give a positive skin test (tuberculosis bacillus, *Escherichia coli*). We shall sub-

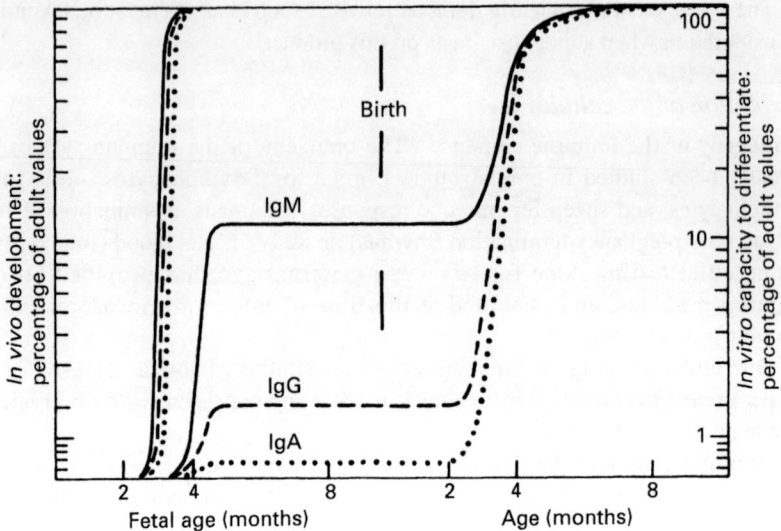

Fig. 1.2 Ontogenesis of the immune response. On the left, ontogenesis of B lymphocytes, carrying IgM (solid line), IgG (dashed line), or IgA (dotted line). At 15 weeks the three classes have reached proportions equal to those observed in adults (left scale). The right scale represents the B lymphocytes' ability to produce immunoglobulins after stimulation *in vitro* by pokeweed mitogen; values are expressed as a percentage of adult values. From Alford *et al.* (1975).

sequently see (p. 000) the importance of these sequence of events in the newborn.

It follows then that study of the fetus' humoral response, to a viral infection for example, can only be carried out with certainty after the twentieth week of gestation.

Evolution during organogenesis

The nervous system   The anlagen of the nervous system (the spinal cord and brain) or neuroblast appears at around the seventeenth day of fetal development. The neuroblast is derived from the ectoblast located in the dorsomedian region of the embryo.

Neurulation starts on the seventeenth day, is completed by the twenty-eighth day, and occurs in three consecutive steps: the neural plate corresponding to differentiation and thickening of the ectoblast above the notochord, the neural groove formed by invagination of the neural plate, and finally the neural tube formed by fusion of the folds surrounding the neural groove.

At a particular time, in any particular embryo, looking at different locations of the neural tube, one can observe these three steps simultaneously. At around the twenty-first day, the closing of the neural tube starts at the median part of the

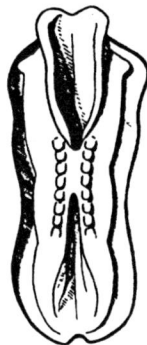

Fig. 1.3 Human embryo 22 days old. From Auroux and Haegel (1974).

embryo and progresses in a zipper-like fashion towards each end of the embryo. This middle region, midway between the cephalic and caudal points, will eventually form the cervical region of the embryo (Fig. 1.3). For a relatively short time the tube remains open at either end, and these areas are known as the posterior and anterior neuropores. The anterior pore closes at around the twenty-fourth day and the posterior pore at around the twenty-eighth day (i.e. 6 weeks after the mother's last menstrual period). This developmental sequence explains neural tube closure defects:

1. *Anencephaly*, resulting from closure defect of the anterior neural tube:
2. *Cranium bifidum*, corresponding to localized closure defects of the anterior neural tube, cranium bifidum occulta, cerebral meningocoele, and meningo-encephalocoeles:
3. *Spina bifida*. Formation of the neural tube induces the formation of the posterior arc of the vertebrae, consequently any neural tube defect may result in a spine defect, spina bifida. There are several forms:
   - *myelomeningocoele*: nervous tissue is either continuous with the skin or within a meningeal sac which protrudes through the musculoaponephrotic wall defect;
   - *meningocoele*: accumulation of cerebral spinal fluid in meningeal spaces producing a meningeal cyst containing only cerebrospinal fluid.

Spina bifida is usually limited to the lumbosacral region.

The urinary tract   During embryo–fetal development the kidney develops in three successive steps, from the cephalic towards the caudal region: pronephros, mesonephros, and the metanephros.

1. Embryonic period. The pronephros, or cephalic kidney, differentiates at the third week and regresses at the fourth week. The excretory canal reaches the cloaca at the end of the fourth week and forms the Wolffian tube. This tube

induces differentiation of the first mesonephros at around the twenty-fourth or twenty-fifth day. Their differentiation resembles that of the metanephros. Whereas differentiation progresses caudally, the first mesonephros formed begin to degenerate between the 6th and 9th week. At the 11th week regression of the mesonephros is complete.

Differentiation of the metanephros or the kidneys proper starts at around the fifth week, when the mesonephros is still functional, and continues into the eighth month. The metanephros results from the interaction of the urethral bud and the metanephrogenic blastema. The urethral bud is derived from the cloacal end of the Wolffian tube and moves up toward the nephrogenic blastema, at around the fifth to eighth week of development, to form the collecting system.

The metanephrogenic blastema, of mesoblastic origin, differentiates into glomerular and tubular epithelial cells. The endothelial cells are derived from the blood vessels which infiltrate the kidney. Some of the cells of the blastema will become the interstitial cells.

2. Fetal period. Mature nephrons become functional around the ninth and tenth week, and urine is present in the bladder around the thirteenth to fifteenth week.

At the ends of the arboring urethral bud an accumulation of mesoblastic cells can be observed. The urethral bulb bends, whereas the mesoblastic cells form into a hollow ball (stage I). That ball then takes on an S shape (stage II). The distal portion of the urethral bulb forms the Bowman's capsule and the glomerular chamber. Simultaneously, a small vessel penetrates the concave area of the S, and the other extremity of the S narrows and opens into the bulb. The cellular differentiation of the proximal tubule precedes that of the distal tubule (stage III). Stage IV corresponds to development of function (Fig. 1.4). Nephrons continue to develop until the thirty-sixth week. Between the thirty-fourth and thirty-sixth week nephrogenesis is complete. The oldest glomeruli are the deepest and the biggest.

In utero, the kidney serves no function in fetal homeostasis: this function is fully ensured by the mother through the placenta. The fetus can be considered to be in continuous dialysis. This is why the study of a maternal urine sample at a given time is a good reflection of fetal renal function. This is not the case after birth, when renal function is affected by digestive and respiratory function. Fetal serum, being in equilibrium with maternal serum, is not a good measure of fetal renal function.

Digestive system   In the cephalic region the digestive tube is covered by the buccopharyngeal membrane, and in the caudal region it is covered by the cloaca. At the sixth week, the buccopharyngeal membrane disappears and in so doing allows free communication between the digestive tube and the amniotic cavity. Swallowing begins around the fourteenth week. The cloacal membrane opens at the end of the eleventh week. The rotation of the primitive gut and its insertion into the abdomen ends at the twelfth week. At the fourteenth week of gestation

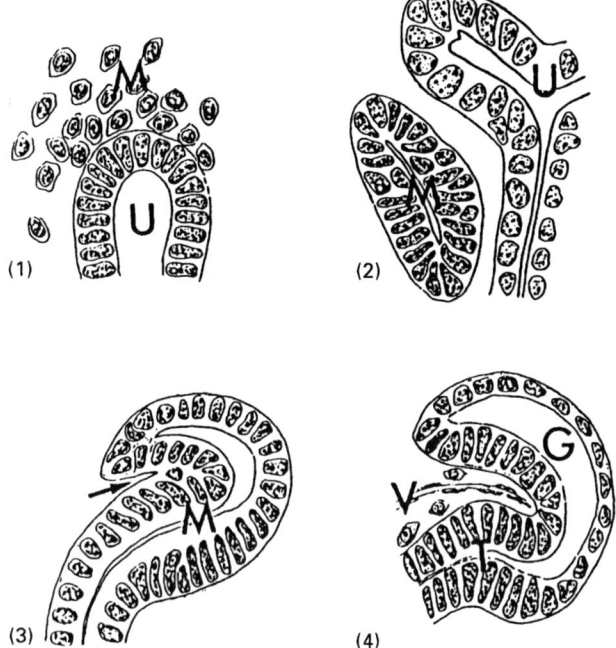

Fig. 1.4 Formation of the nephron. 1. The urethral bud (U) is covered with metane-phrogenic mesoblastic cells (M). 2. The cells migrate to form a vesicle. 3. The metanephrogenic vesicle (M) lengthens and becomes S-shaped. Nephron differentiation continues: the future glomerulus is indented by formation of a vessel (V). 4. The nephron's tubular pole (T) is connected to a collecting tube derived from the urethral bud. From Osathanondh and Potter (1963).

the intestinal villi begin to secrete digestive enzymes which, through the anal canal, reach the amniotic fluid.

The appearance of digestive enzymes in the amniotic fluid occurs soon after the development of the fetal gut: Fig. 1.5 shows that the digestive enzymes are absent from amniotic fluid prior to twelve weeks but suddenly present at thirteen weeks once the anal membrane opens. The concentration of these enzymes in the amniotic fluid decreases slowly around the twentieth week when the anal sphincter becomes active. A quantitative analysis of the concentration of intes-tinal enzymes between the thirteenth and twentieth weeks demonstrates a decrease or disproportion in their concentrations. After the twentieth week, it is mostly abnormally high levels of these enzymes which can be shown.

Evolution in growth

The fetal growth curve demonstrates continual growth even after birth (Fig. 1.6). The rate of growth is variable during development. Figure 1.7 shows a steep

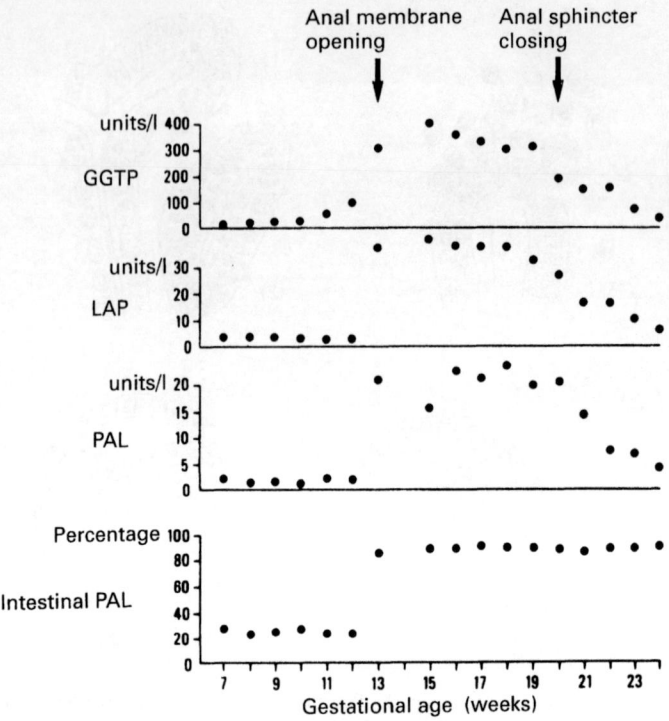

Fig. 1.5 Digestive enzymes found in amniotic fluid during development. Digestive enzymes are present in the fluid only after opening of the anal membrane at 13 weeks. Prior to this, there are traces of alkaline phosphatase, but only the kidney-liver-bone type; the intestinal form appears only at 13 weeks. Starting at 20 weeks, digestive enzyme levels decrease. This decrease corresponds to the amount of amniotic fluid swallowed by the fetus. Abbreviations: GGTP, gammaglutamyl transpeptidase; LAP, leucine aminopeptidase; PAL, total alkaline phosphatase; intestinal PAL; percentage of intestinal-type alkaline phosphatase. From Muller *et al.* (1988).

increase in fetal length until the fifth month, decreasing in the second half of the pregnancy. It is at the time when most prenatal tests are done that growth is at its peak, and it follows that results from these tests should be made available rapidly so that any decision to terminate can still be made.

We may use alphafetoprotein as an example. It is synthesized by the yolk sac until the twelfth week, and by the liver from the twenty-ninth day. The total concentration of alphafetoprotein in maternal serum therefore increases rapidly until the twelfth to fourteenth week, plateaus until the thirtieth to thirty-second week, and then decreases rapidly.

The concentration of serum alphafetoprotein in a seven-week fetus is 0.67 mg/L, increasing rapidly to reach 20 mg/L at nine weeks and 30 mg/L from ten to thirteen weeks. From fourteen to thirty weeks the concentration of

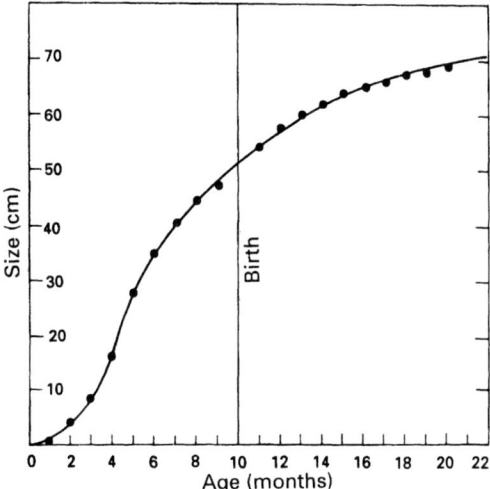

Fig. 1.6 Growth curve (in centimetres) before and after birth. From Harrison (1978).

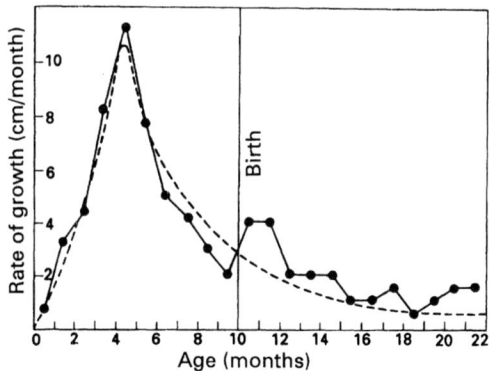

Fig. 1.7 Monthly growth in length before and after birth. From Harrison (1978).

alphafetoprotein decreases exponentially, with a half-life of thirty-two days. This decrease is due to a rate of fetal growth which surpasses the rate of synthesis during that period. At term, the range of normal values for alphafetoprotein is wide, being between 14 mg/L and 1.8 mg/L. At birth the serum alphafetoprotein concentration decreases rapidly with a half-life of three and a half days, and finally reaches a level of 0.1 µg/L (Fig. 1.8).

The fetus is not independent

The fetus is within the maternal organism, with which it has permanent exchanges through the placenta and through the amniochorionic membranes.

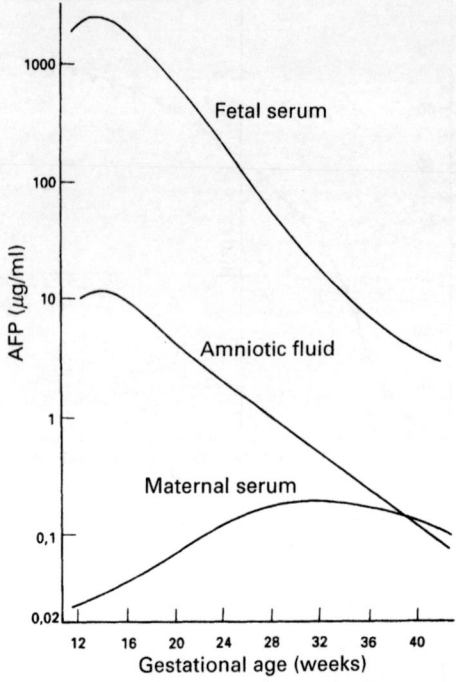

Fig. 1.8 Median value for alphafetoprotein in fetal serum, amniotic fluid, and maternal serum, according to gestational age. From Seppala (1977).

The placenta is an important temporary organ permitting an exchange between maternal and fetal blood. Morphologically, it stems in part from the fetus (the trophoblast) and in part from the mother (by transformation of the uterine lining into decidua basilis).

The trophoblast is visible as of the fifth day and at the sixth or seventh day, by its proteolytic action, allows for implantation of the egg into the uterine lining. At the thirteenth day, villi appear. At about the fifteenth day, the trophoblastic cells develop and invade the maternal blood vessels, resulting in the spreading of maternal blood into the intervillous spaces. This is the beginning of the maternal–placental circulation.

Around the eighteenth day the villi are formed, with a mesenchymal core surrounded by a cytotrophoblastic layer and a syncytiotrophoblastic layer. At the middle of the mesenchymal core, blood vessel precursors appear (Fig. 1.9), beginning fetal circulation. In the intervillous spaces there is an intense maternal circulation. At the twenty-first day there is anastomosis of the intravillous - vascular network with the umbilical–allantois vessels, becoming the fetal–placental circulation.

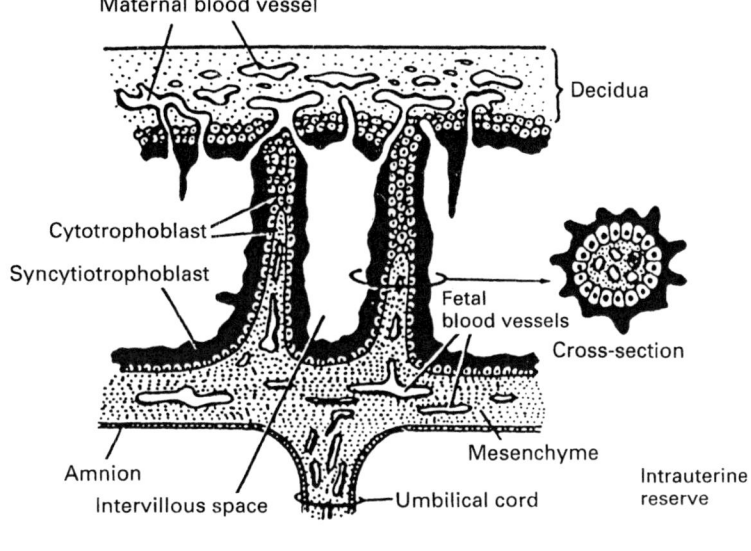

Maternal blood vessel

Decidua

Cytotrophoblast

Syncytiotrophoblast

Fetal blood vessels

Cross-section

Amnion

Mesenchyme

Intrauterine reserve

Intervillous space

Umbilical cord

18-day embryo

Fig. 1.9 Placental villi of an 18-day embryo. From Pansky (1986).

The placenta is of the hemochorial type, as the fetal tissue is in direct contact with maternal blood. The membrane consists of three layers, the syncytiotrophoblast, the conjunctive tissue, and the fetal vascular endothelium (Fig. 1.10). At four months, the tissue is heavily vascularized. The branching of the villi is an important factor in providing a large area for fetal–maternal exchange. At term, this placental area is 10 m^2. Three functions characterize the placenta: an exchange role, a metabolic role, and an endocrine role.

Exchange

Four mechanisms are involved in maternal–fetal and fetal–maternal exchange:

1. Diffusion, until equilibrium between the two compartments is reached. This involves small molecules (urea, creatinine, water, etc.), some electrolytes, gases, and unconjugated steroid hormones.
2. Exchange, using a protein carrier but without energy expenditure, for example glucose.
3. Active exchange, energy-dependent, able to go against a concentration gradient, for example amino acids, iron, calciums.
4. Pinocytosis, which plays a role in the exchange of certain macromolecules such as IgG and fatty acids.

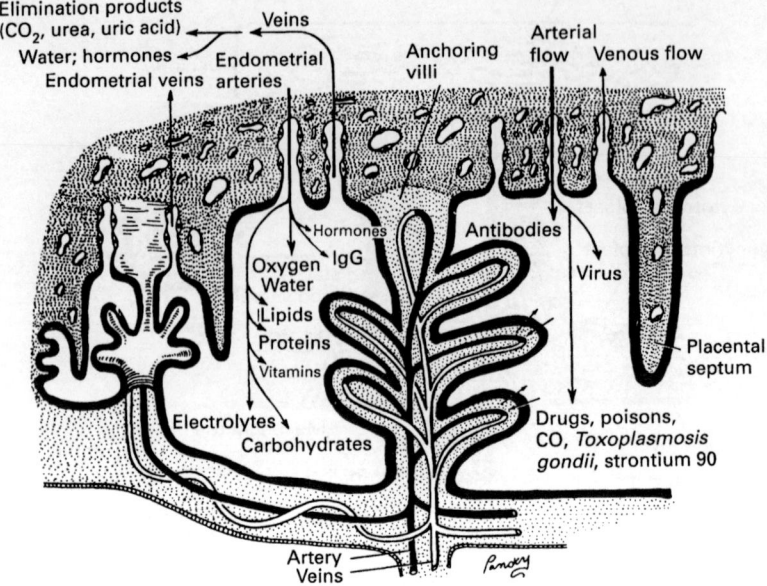

Fig. 1.10 Placental blood circulation. From Pansky (1986).

The consequences of these exchanges occurring simultaneously are:

1. The passage to the fetus of maternal metabolites having a primordial role in its protection (IgG), or its nutrition: gas, water, glucose, amino acids, vitamins, lactic acid, essential fatty acids, ketones:
2. The passage to the fetus of toxic substances, present abnormally in the mother; drugs, maternal antibodies (lupus, rhesus disease), metabolites of maternal phenylketonuria, excessive glucose in maternal diabetes.
3. The passage to the mother of catabolites formed during fetal metabolism; urea creatinine, lactic acid, bilirubin, which serve a purification function.
4. The passage to the mother of fetal substances, not synthesized by the mother; alphafetoprotein, carcinoembryonic antigen, and fetal cells.
5. The passage to the mother of substances synthesized by the placenta; placental hormones (βhCG is essentially secreted in maternal circulation and very little is found in fetal circulation).

Endocrine secretions

The placenta is characterized by its ability to synthesize different types of steroid or protein hormones. It produces homologues to hypophysial hormones. It plays a role in maintaining gestation, in the growth and development of the fetus, and in the induction of delivery at term.

The chorionic gonadotropic hormone (βhCG) is secreted by the egg from the time of fertilization and it can be detected in maternal serum at the time of implantation, allowing an early diagnosis of pregnancy. The measurement of this hormone in maternal serum, between fifteen and nineteen weeks after the last menstrual period, to screen for pregnancies at increased risk for trisomy 21, will be discussed in Chapter 9.

The measurement of pregnancy hormones was more often used in the 1970s and 1980s than it is today to oversee the development of the fetus. This is true in the case of placental lactogen hormone (HPL), now called HCS, and of plasma estriol for screening of intrauterine growth retardation. Study of placental proteins, pregnancy-specific β 1-glycoprotein (SPI), pregnancy-associated plasma protein-A (PAPP-A), and placenta protein 12 (PP12) does not permit a better surveillance of the pregnancy.

Tissues and fluids usually sampled are not embryonic

Chorionic villi

The chorionic villi, once freed of maternal decidua, are a tissue of zygotic origin. They are thus an excellent source of fetal DNA, and very often an excellent tissue for the measurement of enzymes involved in inborn errors of metabolism. One must ensure that the enzymes to be measured are normally expressed at a sufficiently high level; this is the case for the 'housekeeping' enzymes found in all cell types. Some enzymes, however, have a specialized function and are expressed only in differentiated cells or after cell culture.

Experience with direct cytogenetic analysis of chorionic villi has demonstrated that in 1–2 per cent of cases there is discordance between the karyotype obtained from villi and the embryo karyotype (see p. 152 ed. p. 165).

Different cell types make up the villi. The cells making up the trophoblast layer are in active proliferation, and these mitoses can be analysed directly. The syncytiotrophoblast layer does not undergo mitosis, and will not grow *in vitro*. Both layers are of trophoblastic origin (Fig. 1.11). It is the fibroblast-like cells of the villi which will grow *in vitro* (see p. 48), those which are derived from the inner cell mass. This should be kept in mind when interpreting results.

Amniotic fluid

The amniotic fluid is an ever-changing, complex medium, which shows large variation in its composition throughout pregnancy. Briefly, one can distinguish the period before 20 weeks from the period after that date.

Before 20 weeks   The volume of amniotic fluid, which reaches 30–50 mL at around eleven weeks of gestation, increases by about 25 mL/week until the fourteenth week, and by 50 mL/week after the fiteenth week. There is a parallel

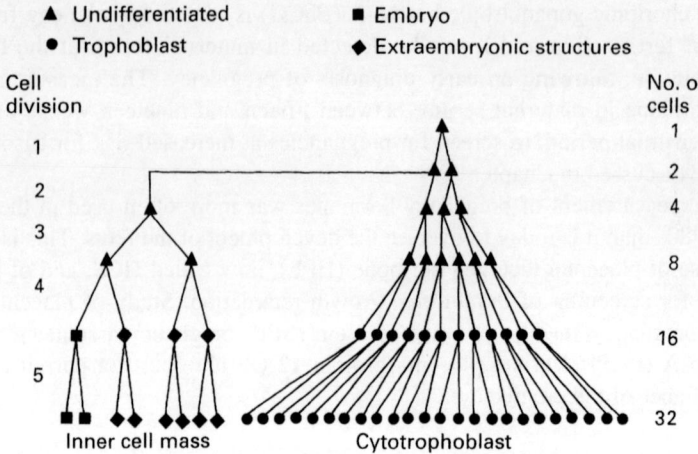

Fig. 1.11 Normal embryogenesis through the first five cell divisions (32-cell morula). The majority of cells are destined to form cytotrophoblast. Of eight cells within the inner cell mass, only two will form the embryo *per se*, with all other cells destined to form extra-embryonic structures (yolk sac, amnion, chorion, mesodermal core of chorionic villi). From Crane and Cheung (1988).

between the increase in volume of amniotic fluid and growth of the fetus. During the first period fluid is isotonic to the fetal and maternal plasmas.

Fetal exchanges occur through fetal skin, and maternal exchanges occur through the chorioamniotic membrane. Until the twentieth week of gestation, small intercellular channels in fetal skin allows permeability to water and to sodium and chloride ions. The amniochorionic membrane with its porous structure is also permeable.

During this period, another means of circulation exists, namely the digestive tract. It is around the thirteenth week that the anal membrane opens, allowing access to the amniotic fluid. The digestive tube is open until the anal sphincter becomes innervated at the twentieth to twenty-second week of gestation. The circulation of amniotic fluid swallowed by the fetus and excreted by the anal canal is well illustrated by the levels of digestive enzymes in the amniotic fluid. Exchange through the umbilical cord and contribution to the fluid by fetal urination is negligible.

During this first period amniotic fluid renewal is rapid, the fluid being replaced within 3 hours. This explains how amniotic fluid sampling for diagnostic purposes has no consequences for the fetus.

After the twentieth week   The great modification in amniotic fluid exchange, occurring around the twentieth week of gestation, explains how some fetal malformations have an impact on its volume. With keratinization, the exchange via the skin stops; the sebaceous glands will appear only later.

The volume that the fetus swallows increases, being 10 mL/day at twenty weeks and 450 mL/day close to term. This explains the observed increase in volume of amniotic fluid in syndromes associated with obstruction of the upper digestive tract. Under normal conditions elimination through the digestive tract would not be possible as the anal sphincter is operational, but some duodenal atresias are associated with regurgitation, as the presence of enzymes in the fluid shows.

Simultaneously, the urine volume increases, being about 10 mL/h at 30 weeks and 30 mL/h at term. This significant contribution of urine to the fluid explains why oligohydramnios or even anamnios is observed in cases of urinary tract obstruction.

Also, during this period the lungs contribute to the contents of amniotic fluid as can be shown by studies of fetal pulmonary distress and measurement of surfactant.

In practical terms one can consider that the biochemical content of the amniotic fluid is a reflection of fetal serum, through permeability of fetal skin, and from 13 weeks onwards, also reflects the contents of the digestive tract. Therefore, steroid concentrations in amniotic fluid are a direct reflection of fetal and not maternal serum.

After 20 weeks, fetal urine contribution dominates. It is not yet known whether regulating mechanisms exist in amniotic fluid.

There is an apparent contradiction in clinical observations: the oligo-hydramnios associated with renal obstruction and polyhydramnios associated with duodenal obstruction. Also, how can one explain the oligohydramnios in a normal fetus produced by endometacin prescribed to the mother, while there is evidence (often outdated) showing the importance of the exchange of water in the three compartments (10–12 L/day), independent of the existing volume of amniotic fluid. At this stage of pregnancy, the fetus therefore, has an important role in the regulation of fluid volume. However, the chorioamniotic membranes appear unaffected to any variation in amniotic fluid volume.

References and further reading

Alford, C. A., Wu Fly, Blanco, A., *et al.* (1975). Development humoral immunity and congenital infections in man. In *The immune system and infectious diseases* (ed. E. Neter and E. Milgrom), pp. 42–58, Karger, Basel.

Auroux, M. and Haegel, P. (1974). Embryologie, organogenèse. In *Embryologie* (ed. M. Auroux and P. Haegel), p. 23, Masson, Paris.

Bernard, J., Levy, J.-P., and Varet, B. (1976). Embryologie et evolution de l'érythropoïèse. In *Hématologie* (ed. J. Bernard, J.-P. Levy, and B. Varet), p. 34. Flammarion Médecine Sciences, Paris.

Boué, A., Henrion, R., and David, G. (1980). *Développement prénatal normal et pathologique*. Flammarion Médecine Sciences, Paris.

Campbell, S., Johnstone, F. D., Holt, E. M. T., *et al.*. (1972). Anencephaly: early ultrasound diagnosis and active management. *Lancet* ii, 1226.

Codaccioni, X. and Delecour, M. (1980). Physiologie du liquide amniotique. In *Développment prénatal normal et pathologique* (ed. A. Boué, R. Henrion, and G. David), pp. 393–426, Flammarion Médicine Sciences, Paris.

Crane, J. P. and Cheung, S. W. (1988). An embryonic model to explain cytogenetic inconsistencies observed in chorionic villus versus fetal tissue. *Prenat. Diagn.*, **2**, 119–29

Harrison, R. G. (1978), *Clinical embryology*. Academic Press, London.

Jacobson, C. and Barter, R. (1967). Intrauterine diagnosis and management of genetic defects. *Am. J. Obst. Gynecol.*, **99**, 769.

Mohr, J. (1968). Foetal genetic diagnosis: development of techniques for early sampling of foetal cells. *Acta Pathol. Microbiol. Scand.*, **73**, 73.

Muller, F., Oury, J.-F., Dumez, Y., *et al.* (1988). Microvillar enzyme assays in amniotic fluid and fetal tissues at different stages of development. *Prenat. Diagn.*, **8**, 189–98.

Nadler, H. L. and Messina, A. M. (1969). In utero detection of type II glycogenosis (Pompe's disease). *Lancet*, **ii**, 1277.

Osathanondh, V. and Potter, E. L. (1963). Development of human kidney as shown by microdissection. *Arch. Path.*, **76**, 271–302.

Pansky, B. (1986). *Embryologie humaine*, pp. 97–103. Marketing, Paris.

Papiernik, M. and Bach, J.-F. (1980). *Développement du système immunitaire*. In Développement prénatal normal et pathologique (ed. A. Boué, R. Henrion, and G. David), pp. 305–26. Flammarion Médecine Sciences, Paris.

Seppala, M. (1977). Alpha-foetoprotein in the amniotic fluid in relation to neural tube defects and other congenital genetic disorders of the fetus. In *Amniotic fluid*, 2nd edn. Eskes TKAB, Amsterdam.

Van Bogaert, E., Robyn, C., and Vekemans, M. (1984). Physiopathologie du placenta In *Encycl. Med. Chir. Obstétrique, Paris*, 5005, A 10.

Vesikari, T. and Vaheri, A. (1968). Rubella: a method for rapid diagnosis of a recent infection by demonstration of the IgM antibodies. *Br. Med. J.* 221–3.

2   Prenatal diagnosis techniques

There are many techniques for prenatal diagnosis: sampling of chorionic villi, amniotic fluid, fetal blood, urine. The method used is dependent on the anomaly being looked for and gestational age. Collaboration between geneticist, obstetrician, and laboratory is essential to ensure appropriate testing, taking into consideration the diagnosis sought for any one case.

Recent developments in ultrasound have dramatically improved old sampling techniques such as amniocentesis, increasing its precision and decreasing associated morbidity. In particular, they have made possible the introduction of new techniques (chorionic villus sampling and fetal blood sampling). Prenatal sampling should be performed under continual ultrasound guidance by a team trained in these procedures.

Early amniocentesis

Amniotic fluid sampling is technically possible at an early stage in pregnancy. The disappearance of the external coelom by fusion of amniotic and chorionic membrane occurs at about 13 weeks' gestation. Ultrasound guidance and the choosing of an area for sampling must be precise. Ultrasound-guided puncture of the amniotic membrane must be firm in order to avoid a tenting effect which pushes away the membrane, rendering sampling dangerous and resulting in a failed sampling. Contraindications to early amniocentesis are maternal obesity and the presence of fibroids on the needle's trajectory, both of which can interfere with ultrasound guidance.

Early amniocentesis can be done from 10 weeks after the last menstrual period, generally transabdominally. Some teams have sampled transvaginally, but apparently infections are not rare in these cases.

The amount of fluid sampled is determined by the gestational age and the types of analyses required. Only small quantities of amniotic fluid (2–5 mL) are required for hormone measurements (diagnosis of 21-hydroxylase deficiency) or for the diagnosis of enzyme deficiencies (methyl malonic acidemia, arginosuccinuria, proprionic acidaemia, mucolipidosis type II, citrullinemia).

Although sampling is possible as early as 10 weeks, it seems reasonable to wait until 12 weeks for cytogenetic analysis to ensure a good quantity of fluid (10 mL) in good and safe sampling conditions. Under these conditions, culturing success and the waiting period for results (10–21 days) are identical to those of mid-trimester amniocentesis.

Acetylcholinesterase electrophoresis for the detection of neural tube defects can be done on amniotic fluid as early as 12 weeks' gestation.

More data are necessary to evaluate risk to the pregnancy with certainty, but it appears to be about 1–1.5 per cent for fetal loss — not significantly different from the risk in chorionic villus sampling. Spontaneous abortions are always preceded by some bleeding or some amniotic fluid loss shortly after sampling. There does not appear to be an increase in pulmonary or orthopaedic problems in children born after early amniocentesis.

It is therefore now possible to move the time for amniocentesis forward in order to obtain a result 3 or 4 weeks earlier. The psychological and medical advantages are obvious, should pregnancy termination be required.

Amniotic fluid sampling

This is the oldest sampling technique, and the most commonly used. The first amniocenteses, carried out in the 1960s were performed blind and were associated with considerable fetal–maternal complication and maternal blood contamination of amniotic fluid.

Current amniocentesis technique

Second trimester amniocentesis   The appropriate gestational age and indication are decided in collaboration with clinical staff and the laboratory that will perform the analyses, and the appointment is made at a time convenient to the laboratory.

The risks and advantages of the prenatal procedure, as well as the decision to be made should there be a diagnosis of abnormality, are discussed with the couple. Testing may be less worthwhile if the couple have already decided not to terminate the pregnancy.

Sampling is usually done between 16 and 19 weeks of gestation, but specific indications or findings can be reasons for earlier or later sampling.

Prior to sampling, it is important to check the following:

- expected date of delivery (LMP, cycle regularity),
- the absence of threatened abortion (metrorrhagia, uterine contractions),
- the size of the body and fundus of uterus ensuring a minimum height of 12 cm.

Sampling is done after emptying of the bladder. Ultrasound is indispensable, to ensure fetal viability (fetal heartbeat and fetal movement) and appropriate gestational age by comparing date of the LMP with fetal measurements. It also determines the presence of twins and the possible presence of fetal malformations or uterine anomalies. The placenta is localized and the sampling site is determined, preferably away from both placenta and fetus, in a pocket of liquid whose depth is measured in relation to the abdominal wall.

Sampling procedure All sampling requires a thorough washing of the hands, and use of sterile gloves; preparation of instruments on a sterilely-draped table; disinfection of the maternal abdomen, and sterile draping around the sampling site. The ultrasound probe is shielded by a sterile cover and the puncture site is identified, ensuring proper distance from the fetus; a local anaesthetic is not required.

A 20–22-gauge (0.9–0.7 mm) and 9–13 cm long needle is introduced into the maternal abdominal wall guided by ultrasound ensuring continual visualization of the full length of the needle and its movement into the amniotic cavity to minimize risk of fetal injury (the needle should be within the cross-section of the ultrasound and not perpendicular to it, otherwise it is possible to misjudge the depth that the needle has reached).

The needle's obturator is removed, a 20 mL syringe is attached to flexible tubing, and a gentle, steady suction is applied permitting the rise of the usually clear yellow fluid into the syringe. Continual ultrasound guidance allows visualization of the tip of the needle and avoidance of fetal injury. After withdrawal of 10–20 ml of amniotic fluid, the needle is removed and ultrasound is used to check for the absence of bleeding and uterine contractions, and for the presence of a fetal heart beat. The fluid is placed (with sterile precautions) into a carefully labelled falcon-type tissue culture flask. Instructions are given to the patient in case of bleeding, amniotic fluid leakage, or uterine contractions: a few days off work, and the possibility of an anti-spasmodic being prescribed. Anti-D immunoglobulin is injected intravenously, 400 μg/IVD, if the patient is Rhesus negative. The fluid can be taken to the laboratory by the patient herself.

Special cases

1. *The obese patient.* The thickness of the maternal abdominal wall limits ultrasound study of the fetus and renders the choice of a sampling site more difficult. After evaluating the distance between the probe and the amniotic cavity, one can decide on the appropriate sampling needle; it should be of the same (20–22) gauge, but of a length varying from 12 to 17 cm.

2. *The patient with fibroids.* These benign lesions are quite frequent and are easily seen on ultrasound, changing the configuration of the uterine wall. To avoid the risk of haemorrhaging and necrosis and difficulty in sampling, it is best to avoid them by sampling at some distance. The presence of fibroids should not be confused with localized uterine contractions, which on careful and prolonged visualization will be observed to disappear.

3. *The patient with an anterior placenta.* As ultrasound allows precise sampling, it is rare that a window cannot be found through which sampling can be performed beyond the placental insertion. One must not hesitate to do transplacental sampling if no alternative exists, and it is wise to advise the laboratory of this. In these cases, bloody samples are more common.

4. *Multiple pregnancy*. Twins can be bichorionic biamniotic, monochorionic biamniotic, or monochorionic monoamniotic. Dizygotic twins (70 per cent) are always bichorionic biamniotic. Monozygotic twins, which are from one egg, can have any of the above characteristics depending on the stage of cleavage of the egg. Distinguishing by ultrasound which of the above characteristics exist is essential to obtaining amniotic fluid from each amniotic cavity. It may be useful to have a schematic diagram of the fetus, the placenta, and the membranes with their respective orientations.

A technical trick is to insert Congo Red into one cavity in order to dye the fluid and ensure sampling of the other cavity. However, this practice has been associated with infection and an increased risk of pregnancy loss. It is important to label each fluid sample with respect to the localization of each fetus. Biochemical analysis can confirm the different origin of the two fluid samples.

Pregnancy loss after amniocentesis is more frequent, 1.5–2.5 per cent, and special precautions should be taken such as time off work and an antispasmodic; at times, even hospitalization for 48 h should be considered.

First trimester amniocentesis   In certain circumstances, amniocentesis is possible after 10–11 weeks: for example, when hormonal or biological substances in the amniotic fluid have to be measured (e.g. congenital adrenal hyperplasia, see p. 133). However, the cavity is much smaller and the fetus delicate, and so the sampling should be limited to 1–2 mL of fluid and should only be done by a very well-trained team, under detailed ultrasound guidance. Pregnancy loss may be increased, but there are too few cases to be conclusive.

Hormone measurements and studies of enzyme deficiencies have been made possible by this technique: propionic acidaemia, methylmalonic aciduria, argininosuccinicaciduria, and citrullinaemia. Diagnosis of sickle cell anaemia and thalassaemia is possible by DNA analysis, and others may be possible using the polymerase chain reaction. Acetylcholinesterase electrophoresis on amniotic fluid is possible only from 12 weeks of gestation (see p. 54).

Finally, fetal karyotyping has been done from successful cultures of samples obtained at very early amniocentesis. However, the reservations regarding the risks of such early sampling mean that for testing indicated by maternal age, a minimum gestational age of 13 weeks seems appropriate.

Third trimester amniocentesis   Amniocentesis can be performed at a late stage in pregnancy, even close to term for detection of fetal distress, assessment of fetal lung maturity, amniotic bilirubin titre in cases of rhesus incompatibility, or detection of amniotic infection in threatened premature delivery or premature rupture of membranes.

Ultrasound guidance is required in these cases as well, as it allows rapid identification of a 'pocket' of fluid which can be sampled without risk of harm to the fetus or risk of sampling failure in cases where there is a lack of amniotic fluid.

Oligohydramnios or absence of fluid The absence of amniotic fluid or its presence in reduced quantity (oligohydramnios) is a common cause of amniocentesis failure. Ultrasound has considerably reduced this failure by allowing sampling in even the smallest pocket of fluid.

In order to facilitate ultrasound examination of the fetus and sampling, the amniotic cavity can be filled with some 10 mL of physiological saline at 37°C. Paradoxically, in these cases karyotyping from a fetal blood sample by cordocentesis may be simpler and more reliable than amniocentesis.

Polyhydramnios An excess of amniotic fluid does not complicate amniocentesis, and may even facilitate it. In cases of maternal discomfort due to uterine distension one can extract fluid and so relieve the mother. The excess fluid will quickly be made up, however, so this procedure is merely palliative.

Setbacks at amniocentesis

Failure With ultrasound guidance this is rare — (97.5 per cent successful at first sampling). Repeated failures at multiple samplings during the same session statistically increases the risk of pregnancy loss. It is recommended instead that the patient be seen again 8–10 days later, as a second attempt at a later date does not increase the rate of pregnancy loss.

Thanks to ultrasound guidance, the rate of repeated sampling (more than two attempts) has decreased from 8.2 per cent to 2 per cent.

Bloody fluid samples The presence of blood in the fluid is very often associated with transplacental sampling where there is an anterior placenta, but may also be a result of a needle inserted too far and damaging the placenta, the cord, or the fetus. In the first case, the first few millilitres of fluid are blood-tinged; collection of this fluid in a 2 mL syringe will permit the further suction of clear fluid. In other instances the whole fluid sample is contaminated with blood. With the introduction of ultrasound the frequency of bloody samples has decreased considerably (5.2 per cent when ultrasound is performed only before the procedure, and 1.2 per cent with continuous ultrasound monitoring). Whereas this is without consequence for some, it appears to be a cause of increased loss and fetal death for others: it depends on the type of vessel which is punctured (6.6 per cent pregnancy loss when a maternal vessel is punctured and 14.3 per cent when a fetal vessel is punctured). The risk of pregnancy loss can be predicted by observing a raise in maternal serum alphafetoprotein taken after sampling (sign of a maternal–fetal haemorrhage).

The presence of red blood cells in amniotic fluid may be responsible for a greater number of culture failures in the laboratory, as it is impossible to separate red blood cells from amniocytes.

Brown fluid If at the 17th week the fluid is of a brownish-greenish colour this is associated not with meconium but rather with a previous haemorrhage, as proved by the presence of haemoglobin and a history of metrorrhagia in early pregnancy. This does not appear to indicate an increased risk of fetal malformation, but might indicate an increased risk of pregnancy loss.

At the end of pregnancy, the tinted fluid may indicate the presence of meconium which is associated with fetal distress and requires special measures to be taken at the baby's birth. Meconium in amniotic fluid at the end of pregnancy may not be macroscopically visible, and should be confirmed by digestive enzyme assay.

Complications at amniocentesis

Spontaneous abortion or death *in utero*   A number of studies, randomized or non-randomized, have given risk figures which vary according to the population studied, the techniques used, and the particular operators.

For all pregnancies developing normally until after the 16th week, the risk of pregnancy loss or fetal death varies from 0.7 to 1.5 per cent. Several years ago amniocentesis raised this risk by 2.5–3 per cent, but with the introduction of ultrasound guidance this risk has been reduced to 0.5–0.7 per cent. Factors increasing the risk of pregnancy loss after amniocentesis are: multiple pregnancy (two- to sixfold), the presence of blood in fluid, and brown fluid. The most important factors are the operator and the techniques used.

Today, the tendency is to attribute to amniocentesis incidents occurring 3–6 weeks after sampling. Clinical signs are: uterine contractions, metrorrhagia, amniotic fluid leakage, fever. Sometimes the absence of a heartbeat on routine ultrasound examination is also attributed to amniocentesis.

A threatened abortion requires hospitalization and ultrasound evaluation of fetal viability, and appropriate treatment to permit safeguarding the pregnancy. Infection of the amniotic cavity or the loss of amniotic fluid also requires hospitalization and treatment; unfortunately, however, it most often results in pregnancy loss within 48 hours.

Fetal injury by needle   In earlier reports, the frequency was 1–3 per cent. The injuries are mostly skin lesions, visible at birth as linear scars or pits. More severe injuries have rarely been described. Today, they are extremely rare because sampling by trained operators with ultrasound guidance has minimized this risk.

Neonatal problems   Contradictory studies mention the presence of neonatal orthopaedic complications (hip dislocation, clubfoot, and foot malposition) and pulmonary problems (respiratory distress) that occur after amniocentesis. It has never been clearly demonstrated that the amniocentesis might cause such anomalies in the newborn, because the limb deformations are already present at the time of amniocentesis and the fluid taken is replaced within a few hours. It is perhaps by chronic fluid leakage due to tearing of membranes, leading to oligohydramnios, that one can observe limb compression and deformation and pulmonary hypoplasia.

Prematurity and perinatal mortality are not increased after amniocentesis.

Maternal complications

Maternal injuries   Exceptionally, injuries to the maternal epigastric artery resulting in abdominal wall haematomas have been described. Similarly, uterine wall hematomas and gut injuries (small intestine and bladder) have been described.

Rhesus isoimmunization   The risk of fetal–maternal iso-immunization in a rhesus-negative mother carrying a rhesus-positive fetus exists (3–12 per cent). This risk is often associated with a transplacental tap, and requires a search for fetal red blood cells when the aspirated fluid is bloody.

In France, this is considered to justify systematic treatment of these mothers by anti-immunoglobulin.

We can extend this risk for iso-immunizations, c, e, Kell, Kidd, and Duffy for which no prevention exists.

Conclusion

Advantages of amniocentesis

- It is a relatively simple and painless procedure, which can be performed rapidly and does not require hospitalization.
- It is a well-established procedure, implying little inherent risk to the pregnancy and therefore well suited for cases where the risk of fetal anomaly is small.

Inconveniences of amniocentesis

- It is performed at 17 weeks for most indications, with results being available from 10 days to 3 weeks later. In cases of fetal anomaly, this leads to a late termination of pregnancy (19–20 weeks after the last menstrual period), which is more difficult to achieve medically, and psychologically difficult for the patient. Recent studies have shown that amniocentesis can be done between 14 and 15 weeks with the same results and without increasing the fetal risk assuming proper use of ultrasound guidance.
- Amniocenteses performed after 32 weeks are associated with a considerable risk of culture failure.

Chorionic villus sampling

Villous branches form a trunk of conjunctive and vascular tissue surrounded by a double layer of trophoblastic cells. Inside is the cytotrophoblast with mitotic cells, and outside is the non-mitotic and hormone-producing syncytiotrophoblast.

The development of chorionic villus sampling arose from the need to establish an earlier procedure than amniocentesis. As mentioned above, amniocentesis permits only a second-trimester abortion, where the physical and psychological burden is higher.

The cytogenetic and genetic information found in the cells of the villi and fetus, originating from the fertilized egg, are identical.

Early sampling techniques

Blind transcervical aspiration   This was the first method used in China to examine sex chromatin for fetal sexing. The technique, which was soon abandoned, served to bring attention to the possibility of and increase interest in first-trimester prenatal diagnosis.

Endoscopic transcervical aspiration   In 1968, this was one of the first methods described by Scandinavian authors (Mohr 1968), using large-diameter hysteroscopes and more recently using small-diameter optics. Its drawback was a high rate of fetal loss, and it has been replaced by ultrasound-guided methods.

Ultrasound-guided methods

Counselling by the geneticist involved in prenatal diagnosis is indispensable and should, if possible, precede pregnancy because this sampling technique can be carried out so early. Certain preliminary tests may be required to assess the possibility of diagnosis, particularly, for some single-gene disorders.

The couple must be informed of the limitations of the diagnosis, appropriate timing of sampling, time required to obtain results, methods of abortion if indicated, and fetal risks of sampling.

Whatever the route and instruments used, sampling should be performed under strictly sterile conditions, using sterile gloves, and with thorough sterilization of the work area. Ultrasound before sampling is essential to determine multiple pregnancy, gestational age by crown–rump length, viability by fetal movement and heartbeat, presence of any anomalies (malformations and fibroids), uterine position, and finally, the point of insertion and accessibility of the trophoblast, where sampling should be done.

At 9–12 weeks, at the time when sampling is usually performed, the pregnancy is visible on ultrasound with the non-echogenic gestational sac in which one can see an embryo with a cephalic pole, the body with a heartbeat, and the limbs. The trophoblast, which at this time surrounds the whole gestational sac, appears as an echogenic zone at the periphery of this sac. Easily seen on ultrasound is a thicker and denser area of the trophoblast which corresponds to the placenta. On the fetal side of the placenta is the cord insertion. The yolk sac is mobile and does not provide a reliable reference point .

Longitudinal and transverse scans of the gestational sac will show the insertion of the trophoblast (anterior, posterior, fundal, low-lying), the sampling site, and the means of access, in general at the thickest area of the placenta (but at a distance from the cord insertion).

During sampling, it is essential to use ultrasound continuously to visualize the sampling instrument as it is directed to the chosen site.

Optimally, sampling is done between 9 and 12 weeks (and preferably in the 11th week). Before this, sampling is difficult and risky because the trophoblast is poorly developed and the risk of spontaneous abortion is high.

Transcervical aspiration This method is most commonly used, with the aid of a variety of instruments. The patient is positioned on an operating table as for pelvic examination, the vulva is throughly disinfected, and sterile drapes are laid down to delineate the work area. A speculum is introduced into the vagina to expose the cervix, and these areas are thoroughly disinfected. A tenaculum is placed on the anterior or posterior part of the cervix in order to align the cervical and uterine cavities during sampling.

The ultrasound, operated by an experienced colleague, is placed on the suprapubic area in order to give a longitudinal view of the genital organs, the uterus containing the gestational sac, the sampling site identified in the thickest area of the trophoblast, and the cervix and its canal.

The catheter with a flexible stylet can then be oriented in the right direction (anterior, posterior, and lateral) and introduced slowly into the cervical canal. Once on the interior side of the cervix the catheter can be directed to the sampling site. Ultrasound allows continual guidance of the entire catheter, containing an echogenic metallic stylet. Ideally, the top of the catheter is inserted into the trophoblast midway between the chorion frondosum and the decidua basilis, ensuring some distance from the cord insertion.

The stylet is slowly removed, while the top of the catheter is kept in place in the placenta (for catheters which do not retain their form). The sampling is performed by a 5–7 mL aspiration into a 20 mL syringe, attached to the free end of the catheter and containing 3 mL of heparinized culture medium. A gentle back-and-forth movement of the catheter loosens the villi.

Aspiration is maintained while the catheter is removed; the contents of the catheter and syringe are deposited in a sterile Petri dish and examined under a dissecting microscope. This ensures the presence of chorionic villi, allows evaluation of the quantity, and permits removal of maternal decidua and cervical mucus.

Initially, a 21 cm long Portex polyethylene catheter with an external diameter of 1.45 mm and an internal diameter of 1.13 mm containing an aluminium stylet was used (Old *et al.* 1982). Since then, a number of plastic catheters with diameters varying from 1.3 mm to 2 mm and with metal (steel or aluminium) stylets have been proposed. These new catheters and stylets have been introduced because both are echogenic, and once the stylet is removed the catheter retains its form. Other teams prefer flexible metal catheters with diameters of 2.3–2.7 mm and lengths of 21–23 cm.

Depending on the expertise of the team, the sampling success rate is 80–85 per cent for the first attempt and 90–95 per cent for the second. To avoid the higher risk of abortion, making more than two attempts at the same sitting is not recommended.

Transcervical microbiopsy   This technique is widely used in France and throughout Europe. Instruments include 20 cm steel (very echogenic) biopsy microforceps with a rounded tip, often used in pediatric laryngoscopy. The rounded tip is made of two mandible-like curettes, of which only the upper mandible opens in a vertical plane. The diameter of the forceps is 2 mm closed and 6 mm open.

The sampling method is identical to that described for transcervical aspiration. The forceps is introduced into the cervical canal and directed by ultrasound guidance to the trophoblast insertion.

Once the instrument is in place close to the chorionic frondosum the forceps are opened, then closed with light pressure and pulled away. These steps are easily followed by ultrasound because of the echogenicity of the forceps. When the forceps are opened at the site of sampling the chorion is pushed away; a slight distortion of the gestational sac as the forceps are withdrawn is a sign of a successful sampling.

One limiting factor is the rigidity of the forceps. However, in our experience, taking advantage of the filling of the bladder as well as manipulation of the forceps, only some laterally inserted placentas have presented any problems. The success rate is close to 100 per cent for obtaining a more than 20 mg sample of chorionic villi. Above all, the sample is perfectly pure in 95 per cent of cases.

It is advisable not to have more than three insertions at one sitting.

Transabdominal aspiration technique

Following the methodology used for amniocentesis under ultrasound guidance, Scandinavian operators use a needle guide attached to the transducer head to predetermine a needle pathway (Smidt-Jensen *et al.* 1986). After thorough cleansing of the abdominal area and application of a sterile gel to the skin, the transducer is placed in a sterile plastic bag and then attached to the sterile guidance apparatus.

A local anaesthetic is often used. The sampling site is localized on the screen, along with the pathway of the needle. It is advisable to tap in a plane parallel to the chorial frondosum, to avoid rupture of the gestational sac. First, a 15 cm 18-gauge needle is introduced through the needle guide in the desired direction through the uterus up to the edge of the trophoblast. Its role is to hold the uterus and the apparatus in a fixed position such that once the stylet is removed it is possible to introduce a 21-gauge 20 cm needle. The tip of this second needle will go in 1 cm deeper than the first needle. Using a 20 mL syringe attached to the second needle and rinsed with heparinized culture medium, the chorionic villi are slowly aspirated using a back-and-forth and rotational movement.

The villi (in a Petri dish) must be examined under a dissecting microscope because the fragments are small and maternal cell contamination is common; multiple samplings may be necessary and are possible because the needle guide is kept in place and no repeat tap is required. This technique, initially used for first-trimester sampling, has also been used for second- and third-trimester sampling for direct cytogenetic analysis. An absence of trophoblastic tissue requires repeat taps. The amount of tissue sampled is directly related to the diameter of the needle used. The success rate is 94 per cent at the first attempt, and 100 per cent at the second attempt, with 52 per cent of samples being less than 10 mg.

This technique has certainly advantages: it is the only one used after 14 weeks, or when there is a contraindication to other sampling methods (cervical or vaginal infection).

Some operators simply use a 20-gauge needle and modify the aspiration syringe to favour fluid extraction (adding a trigger which can be depressed, or a pump). Repeat taps are therefore more often necessary.

Dumez (1985) described a technique whereby microbiopsy is performed using forceps through a trocard 1.8 mm in diameter. This technique has provided quality samples, with risks similar to those for techniques used by other teams.

After sampling Ultrasound examination ensures viability, the absence of placental abruptions, and absence of hematomas at the site of sampling. Should a tenaculum be used, examination of the cervix after sampling may reveal some bleeding (often requiring swabbing).

It has been the practice to prescribe an antispasmodic for use immediately after the procedure, along with 10 days of progesterone and antibiotic vaginal suppositories, 5 days off work, and reduced activity (little walking, and sexual abstinence). The patient or her partner immediately transports the sample to the laboratory and is advised to watch for substantial bleeding (minimal bleeding may follow testing and subsides in 24 hr), fluid leakage, uterine cramps, or fever, symptoms for which the patient should immediately seek consultation.

Ten days after testing and at 20 weeks' gestation, ultrasound examination is carried out. Rhesus negative patients receive an injection of 100 μg of anti-D immunoglobulin.

Comparison of different techniques for chorionic villus sampling

Failure rates Regardless of the technique used, failure rates are low, demonstrating the simplicity of these techniques (Table 2.1).

None the less, transcervical sampling techniques are associated with a slightly larger sampling failure rate than techniques using transabdominal aspiration or biopsy with forceps. This may be due to the flexibility of plastic catheters, such that displacement occurs when the echogenic metallic stylet is removed. Techniques using metallic materials (aspirating cannula, microforceps, needles) are more precise. The failure rate of transabdominal aspiration may have been somewhat underestimated. Moreover, comparing large testing centres to centres

Table 2.1 Failure of chorionic villus sampling.
Figures in brackets are percentages. From Jackson (1988)

Method	Type of centre	Total number of cases	Sampling failure	Total failure
Transcervical aspiration	> 100 cases	19 788	403 (2.03)	(2.16)
(Portex catheter)	< 100 cases	606	38 (6.27)	
Transcervical aspiration	> 100 cases	9 548	217 (2.27)	(2.54)
(other plastic catheters)	< 100 cases	621	42 (6.76)	
Transcervical aspiration	> 100 cases	1 072	22 (2.05)	(2.09)
(metal catheter)	< 100 cases	316	7 (2.21)	
Microbiopsy	> 100 cases	2 348	24 (1.02)	(1.35)
(forceps)	< 100 cases	308	12 (3.90)	
Transabdominal aspiration	> 100 cases	3 446	20 (0.58)	(0.60)
	< 100 cases	206	2 (0.97)	

doing fewer samplings, it is clear that experience is the main factor in the success rate of these techniques, with transabdominal being the easiest technique for those centres just beginning this kind of sampling. This is perhaps because it is based on ultrasound-guided amniocentesis, a method which most teams are well versed in.

Quantity of villi   It is important to consider this since, for cytogenetic analysis indicated maternal age alone, only a small sample is required; if other analyses, such as DNA, are required, a larger sample is needed. Chorionic villi are quantified by visual assessment and comparison to photographic references or pre-weighed samples. Operators and laboratory staff are often in disagreement as to the quantity of villi actually sampled, with operators often overestimating the amount.

Transabdominal sampling provides less than 10 mg of villi in 50 per cent of cases and less than 20 mg in 70 per cent of cases. Thus, this technique may be well suited for karyotyping but not for other types of analyses.

Transcervical aspiration has a more variable success rate. At the first attempt with the Portex catheter more than 10 mg is obtained in only 12 per cent of cases, but in general at least 20 mg with the second attempt. With metallic cannulas, more than 10 mg is obtained at the first attempt in 27–35 per cent of cases. The microforceps, on the other hand, allow for more than 10 mg at the first attempt in 90 per cent of cases. Therefore, although transabdominal aspiration seems appropriate for cytogenetic analysis, for other kinds of analyses, requiring more tissue, transcervical aspiration using metallic cannula or microforceps is more successful.

Sample quality All transabdominal and transcervical samplings must be examined under the dissecting microscope at the moment of sampling to discriminate between chorionic villi, decidua, blood from passage through the cervix, and cervical mucus.

Samplings using these techniques, are more problematic and contaminated with various tissues, a concern not encountered with microforceps when the villi are stripped at the root. This last sampling method is therefore particularly satisfactory in terms of purity of sample.

Conclusion Present-day methods are almost equally useful, although the diagnostic indication may favour one method over another. The low rate of sampling failure indicates that the essential factors for success are the experience and dexterity of the operators, as well as the coordination between the ultrasonographer and the operator.

Skill in two or three different techniques is useful, making it possible to choose a method in accordance with the indication and the particulars of the pregnancy in question.

Maternal cell contamination and problems of cytogenetic abnormalities will be discussed in the section on laboratory results, but they are also a consideration in sampling quality.

Complications

Maternal complications

Metrorrhagias Bleeding immediately after testing is not uncommon, and may be due to the tenaculum injuring the cervix; a simple swabbing usually controls this. It may also come from within the cervix, and in this case it is usually moderate. Wapner (1989) calculated that bleeding occurred in 4/2700 cases, and in only one case did an abortion follow.

In the days following the test, bleeding is observed in 15–40 per cent of cases; it can vary from intermittent spotting to bleeding equivalent to menstruation. This may be associated with lower abdominal cramping which subsides with rest and use of an antispasmodic. Bleeding may last for 3–4 days or as long as 10–14 days. It is sometimes a result of a haematoma (4 per cent at the sampling site or on the pathway to the site) which in itself does not have a bad prognosis for the pregnancy, as it often disappears prior to 20 weeks. The risk is that infection occurs where the blood has accumulated, and this in turn puts the pregnancy at risk.

Intraperitoneal haemorrhage This has been observed during or after transabdominal sampling and on occasion has been reported as requiring emergency intervention because of excessive bleeding of the uterine wall.

Infection Uterine infection can occur in transcervical sampling, but it may also occur after transabdominal sampling if preventive measures have not been applied.

Uterine and embryonic infection usually occurs 2–5 days after chorionic villus sampling and is usually associated with hyperthermia, metrorrhagia, and pelvic pain comparable to uterine contraction. Spontaneous abortion then occurs rapidly. Such clinical signs require immediate hospitalization to establish intravenous antibiotic therapy and to ensure emptying of the uterus. A few exceptional cases of severe uterine infection followed by septic shock requiring radical intervention have been reported.

Prospective microbiological studies of the vaginal flora confirm the presence of a variable number of micro-organisms, without demonstrating a particular predominance of one type nor any correlation to any clinical complications which would have permitted more local or general preventive measures. Other microbiological studies of the catheter, after sampling, did not demonstrate any correlation with infection.

In conclusion, it appears that most of the complications related to infection occurred when the techniques were being pioneered. Though risk of infection with transcervical sampling seems obvious, transabdominal sampling is not devoid of risk, since rare cases of infection have been reported with amniocentesis. All authors agree:

● on the uselessness of preventive treatment;
● on the existence of contraindications to transcervical sampling or on postponement of sampling in cases of vaginal or cervical infection, IUD pregnancies, or uterine malformation making sampling risky;
● on thorough disinfection with antiseptic before sampling;
● on the use of new sampling tools for any repeated transcervical sampling (catheter, microforceps).

It is clear that sampling where there are contraindications, or in a difficult case requiring multiple insertions, increases the risk of infection and diminishes the prognosis for the pregnancy.

Rhesus isoimmunization   Maternal serum alphafoetoprotein levels measured before and after chorionic villus sampling have shown, in about 50 per cent of cases, a significant rise in its concentration suggesting a fetal–maternal haemorrhage. The passage of 60 μmL of fetal blood into the intervillous space has been evaluated in 14 per cent of cases, and presents a risk of isoimmunization. The extent of increase in alphafoetoprotein may be related to the amount sampled, the number of attempts, and the risk of miscarriage.

Cases of isoimmunization, or cases of rapid increase in levels of agluttinin in women previously immunized, confirm:

● the risk of isoimmunization in rhesus negative women justifying therapy with anti-D immunoglobulin;
● the contraindication of testing women already sensitized, in view of increasing this sensitization; the exception being those women for whom

fetal blood typing has been done and for whom only a rhesus-negative fetus can be tolerated.

Fetal complications

Perinatal complications These occur between 28 weeks of gestation and 30 days after delivery. The numbers for intrauterine fetal death, intrauterine growth retardation, neonatal death, and prematurity are equal to those observed in the general population. No specific congenital malformation seems to be associated with sampling.

A malformation sequence associating microglossia and abnormalities of limb extremities has recently been described and has been associated with transabdominal chorionic villus sampling done 56–63 days after the last menstrual period (Firth *et al.* 1991). There is no conclusive evidence to link these abnormalities with chorionic villus sampling, and most teams performing chorionic villus sampling agree that sampling should be done after 10–11 weeks, or even after 13 weeks for maternal age indication.

Abortions Table 2.2 shows how, in the largest series, the frequency of spontaneous abortion after chorionic villus sampling of pregnancies analysed as normal has evolved since 1984. The rate, which varies from 2 to 5.5 per cent, is stable for each operator and does not appear to be different with respect to sampling technique used. It is difficult to assess the real risk to the pregnancy. Indeed, if one considers studies of pregnancies not undergoing prenatal testing, but for which viability at 10 weeks has been established by ultrasound (at the time of sampling),

Table 2.2 Abortions of normal embryos after chorionic villus sampling.
Figures in brackets are percentages

Authors	December 1984	February 1986	February 1988
Brambati (Milan)	434 (3.2)	1 020 (2.7)	1 453 (3.1)
Golbus (San Francisco)	418 (5.9)	1 486 (6.1)	2 850 (4.63)
Jahoda (Rotterdam)	160 (3.5)	515 (4.2)	1 519 (4.86)
Ginsburg (Chicago)	326 (3.0)	960 (2.6)	2 633 (2.12)
Wapner (Philadelphia)	519 (1.5)	1 476 (2.0)	4 105 (1.05)

Table 2.3 Risk of spontaneous abortion after normal ultrasound and viable embryo in pregnancies not undergoing chorionic villus or amniotic fluid sampling

Authors	Number of patients	Time of normal ultrasound with viable fetus (weeks of amenorrhea)	Subsequent spontaneous abortions (per cent)	
Christiaens (1984)	274	< 10	3.28	
Gilmore (1984)	1 960	< 10	2.1	
MacFadyen (1985)	1 855	< 12	1.29	
MacKenzie (1988)	157	< 10	3.8	(total 2.0)
	343	10–12	1.2	
Wilson (1984)	920	< 10	2.13	
Cashner	489	12	2.0	

the rate of spontaneous abortion is about 2–3 per cent (Table 2.3). This risk is still 1–1.5 per cent once viability has been assessed at 12 weeks. A certain number of these spontaneous abortions are associated with chromosomal abnormalities, but some are of 'normal' embryos. With respect to chromosome abnormalities, chorionic villus sampling detects 4.5–6 per cent while amniocentesis detects 3 per cent. Also, the risk of spontaneous abortion increases significantly with a history of miscarriage.

Jahoda (1985) showed that the risk of spontaneous abortion after chorionic villus sampling increases significantly after the age of 36 (2.6–7.2 per cent) and seems to be related to the number of insertions required to obtain an adequate sample (3 per cent after one insertion, 12 per cent after three insertions) whereas before age 36 the number of insertions does not seem to modify the risk. The risk of abortion varies with the gestational age at which sampling takes place. When sampling is done prior to 9 weeks or after 12 weeks the risk increases from 2–5.5 per cent to 12.9 per cent and 17.1 per cent respectively, therefore the safest transcervical sampling time is between 10 and 12 weeks. Maternal age alone constitutes a risk of spontaneous abortion, whether a transcervical or transabdominal technique is used. The risk is four times greater before 12 weeks in patients more than 36 years of age than for younger women: at later gestational ages the risk is the same regardless of age. Thus patient's age must be taken into consideration when counselling regarding sampling risks. Taking all of this into consideration, chorionic villus sampling appears to be relatively innocuous and does not seem to increase the rate of spontaneous abortion significantly. The fact that a certain proportion of spontaneous abortions have been associated with infection definitely resulting from transcervical sampling may be an important factor to consider in attempting to improve the quality of testing.

Other abortion risk factors   The reason for testing is important, as it dictates the amount of tissue required. Biochemical or DNA studies require larger samples than cytogenetic analysis and impose a higher risk on the pregnancy. Indeed, in those cases where a larger sample is required, multiple insertions may be needed, increasing the risk of haematoma, abruptia, and infection. The consensus, then, is to limit the number of insertions to three, to change the catheter or sterilize forceps after each insertion, and to strictly observe contraindications. The obstetric team's experience is also an important consideration since it is known that though expertise in a particular technique is a measure of success, experience in a range of transcervical and transabdominal techniques allows a choice in accordance with the particular features of the case.

Conclusion
Advantages of chorionic villus sampling

- Early sampling, allowing early and quick intervention and requiring a shorter hospitalization. The result is a safer procedure (less risk of scarred uterus or late termination) with less psychological trauma for the patient.
- Direct cytogenetic analysis is possible.
- Good-quality samples for biochemical and DNA studies are possible.

Disadvantages

- An evolving technique with unresolved problems.
- Uncertainty of risk with great variation in figures available from experienced centres. In practice, one should rely on local statistics as opposed to figures from foreign or those for, average risk.
- Problems of laboratory interpretation (see Chapter 4).

Fetal blood sampling
Since the introduction of fetal blood sampling in the early 1970s there has been considerable evolution of this sampling technique and indications for such sampling have expanded.

Placentocentesis
This was the first method of fetal blood sampling, developed in Sardinia for the diagnosis of β-thalassaemia. Ultrasound localized the placenta and, under local or general anaesthetic, blind transplacental puncture with a 19–20-gauge needle was carried out in an attempt to access a vessel in the chorionic frondosum and to aspirate fetal blood, often diluted with amniotic fluid. Maternal contamination of fetal blood occurred in more than 75 per cent of cases. A high rate of fetal complications (8–12 per cent) was reported.

Fetoscopy
This allows for fetal blood sampling under visual guidance.

The ideal time for sampling is 18–20 weeks' gestation: volume of fluid is sufficient and is clear to allow good visibility, and the fetus is still small enough not to interfere with sampling.

An ultrasound precedes sampling to ensure fetal viability. This also determines the presence of twins, appropriate gestational age by fetal measurement, and possible presence of fetal malformations or uterine anomalies, and establishes the site of sampling taking into account the placental and cord insertions. It is essential to avoid the placenta as bleeding into the amniotic fluid renders it turbid, diminishes visibility, and makes for a difficult sampling procedure. An anterior placenta has long been a contraindication to fetal blood sampling. Today, ultrasound often reveals a window where sampling can take place. Under general anaesthetic, or more often after sedation and using a local anaesthetic, the skin on the abdomen is thoroughly disinfected, the sampling area is defined, and the transducer, in a sterile sac, allows continual guidance during the procedure.

Equipment includes:

- an optic 1.7 mm–2 mm in diameter and 15–17 cm long connected to a cold light;
- a 2.1 mm–2.4 mm cannula holding a trocar or an optic and having a fine passageway where a needle can be inserted;
- a trocar.

With continual ultrasound guidance the cannula with trocar is introduced through a 2 mm incision made in the maternal abdominal wall. It then crosses the uterine wall, the chorion and amnion, away from the placenta towards a pocket of amniotic fluid away from or posterior to the fetus. With the cannula in place, the trocar is replaced by the optic and, guided by ultrasound, is directed to the chorionic frondosum, where the cord insertion or vessel to be punctured is located. A 26–27-gauge needle is introduced appropriately into the cannula, rinsed with normal saline or citrate, and connected to a hypodermic syringe. Once the tip is in the visual field, it must be carefully and dexterously manipulated. In the past, samplings were made from large vessels of the chorionic frondosum but were often contaminated with amniotic fluid or maternal blood (for example from puncture of intervillous space if needle was introduced too far). Today, a less mobile large vessel is chosen, usually the vein at the base of the cord, and 1.0–1.5 mL of fetal blood is drawn under visual guidance. This allows for purity of sample with no amniotic fluid contamination. The blood is immediately analysed by electronic measurement of mean corpuscle volume (Coulter counter) or by a Kleihauer test. Once the needle is removed from the vessel, bleeding continues for a few seconds (1 mL, or less than 4 per cent of fetal blood volume) and then the cannula and optic are withdrawn and the ultrasound ensures that there are no fetal complications. Technical problems are related to visibility through the optic. The field of vision is narrow and shallow, therefore continual ultrasound guidance is essential for orientation in the amniotic cavity. Clarity of the fluid is essential. Any turbidity renders fetoscopy impossible; even slight injury to the placenta during testing, or a failed puncture followed by bleeding, does not allow for a repeated attempt.

An experienced operator is indispensable. Introduction of the cannula should be gentle so as not to damage the fetus or a posterior placenta, and at the same time firm in order not to dislodge the amnion without actually penetrating the cavity, which then would not be accessible. The puncture pressure should be well judged, because the shallow field of vision does not allow for control of a needle entered too far in the direction of the placenta or intervillous space. Also, the needles are too fine to visualize on ultrasound. Fetal movement may interfere with sampling, but sedation of the mother avoids this problem in most cases. Gestational age is a limiting factor, as the sampling can only be performed from the second trimester to 26 weeks. After this, the space taken up by the fetus may render sampling impossible.

After sampling, anti-D immunoglobulin is administered to rhesus negative mothers. A 24 hr hospitalization is advisable to monitor uterine contractions, bleeding, or amniotic fluid leakage, and on the following day good viability as well as the appropriate amount of amniotic fluid should be ensured.

Complications

1. *Immediate.* In skilled hands perforation, hematomas, or fetal injury are infrequent. Amnionitis is more common and often leads to abortion:

2. *Late.* Risks seem to be directly related to the duration of sampling and most certainly to the team's experience. Premature rupture of membranes has been described in 4–5 per cent of cases and premature delivery in about 8–12 per cent, a figure significantly higher than that observed in the general population.

The reported risks of spontaneous abortion or intrauterine fetal death varies from 2 to 5 per cent, though the apparent risk in skilled hands is estimated at 1.5 per cent and is generally related to an amniotic infection or premature rupture of the membranes. With the advent of fetal blood sampling, use of fetoscopy as practised in the early 1980s is now limited. A few teams continue to use it, but primarily for other indications (fetal visualization, etc.)

Ultrasound-guided fetal blood sampling with needle

Introduced by Daffos (1983), this technique has rapidly replaced fetoscopy. It is less invasive and relatively simple for those trained in other ultrasound-guided sampling techniques. It permits a number of fetal analyses, as well as fetal therapy through the umbilical cord. It can be performed at any time from 17 weeks to term, and even during labour, to measure fetal pH.

The procedure is done on an out-patient basis, without any premedication or local anaesthetic, but with sterile precautions; the patient lies on an operating room table. A careful ultrasound examination verifies fetal viability, allows for fetal measurements confirming expected date of delivery, and determines the presence of any physical malformations. The placenta is localized, particularly the cord insertion and a sampling site on the fixed part of the cord, an area which cannot move away from the needle, is chosen. The operator and the ultra-sonographer are gowned and gloved. The abdomen is given a sterile wipe and draped around the sampling site.

The ultrasound transducer assembly may have a single transducer angling back and forth, or a group of transducers rotating to produce a sector scan. The sampling procedure is the same in either case; the transducer is put into a sterile bag, the cord insertion is located (this can take time), and once it is found the transducer is kept in place while the operator introduces through the abdominal wall a 20–22-gauge needle whose length (9, 12, 17 cm) depends on the depth of the cord. It is important to keep the needle (and its echogenic image on the screen) within the ultrasound range which encircles the cord insertion, facilitating a gentle but firm puncture of the cord.

With needle in place, the needle's trocar is removed and a 2 mL syringe is attached. At the first appearance of blood in the syringe, it is quickly replaced by another non-heparinized or non-citrated one, depending on the tests required, and 1–2.5 mL of blood is drawn. The needle is then slowly withdrawn from the umbilical cord and the gestational sac, and the sample is examined for quality (dilution) and purity (Coulter counter and Kleihauer test). Ultrasound is repeated to observe any effects on the fetus (bradycardia, for example) and to ensure there is no haemorrhaging at the puncture site. If all is well, the patient may go home with no treatment other than an anti-D gammaglobulin injection, should she be rhesus negative.

Sampling difficulties

Timing   Sampling early in pregnancy is more difficult, because the cord is finer than it is later on; fluid volume in proportion to fetal size is greater and the needle is more likely to move around. Close to term, the larger fetus may mask a posterior, funnicular, insertion and may necessitate puncture of a free-floating cord, which is possible but much more difficult because of its mobility.

Amniotic fluid volume   In pregnancies complicated by oligohydramnios, lack of fluid makes ultrasound examination of the fetus and placenta difficult and may prevent localization of the cord insertion. None the less an area of free cord is always identifiable, and it can be punctured because absence of fluid renders it less mobile.

Placental cord insertion   When the placenta is anterior, one can guide the needle directly to the end of the cord by going through the placenta without penetrating the gestational sac. When the cord insertion is fundal or posterior, one must go through the gestational sac and guide the needle to the cord at approximately 1 cm from its insertion.

Should the cord insertion not be attainable (oligohydramnios or interference of fetus) one is then forced to puncture a free-floating cord: the tip of the needle is placed on the same ultrasound plane as the cord, and then firmly punctures it, as confirmed by ultrasound.

Patient-related complications   Sampling may be made difficult by the patient's obesity. Obesity increases the depth of sampling, and makes ultrasound guidance more difficult. Movement of nervous patients results in loss of ultrasound localization and straying of the needle, and so interferes considerably with sampling.

Failures   Should a first sampling fail, it is reasonable to make up to two more attempts at the same session. After this it is best to reschedule for sampling 8 days later. Daffos (1985) gives a total sampling failure of 0.3 per cent, with 3 per cent repeat sampling after 8 days.

Sampling quality   By implementing certain precautions (such as changing syringes once blood appears in the first syringe), dilution of the samples is rare (2.5 per cent).

A posterior placenta, or sampling too close or too far from the cord insertion, can lead the tip of the needle to the intervillous space of the placenta and thus result in maternal contamination.

In general, these problems disappear with increasing experience of the operator.

Risks and complications   No maternal complication has of yet been encountered or reported. On the other hand, a number of fetal complications can present themselves:

Immediate problems at time of sampling

- fetal injury, though this is rare in expert hands;
- haemorrhaging at the puncture site: this occurs, and can be seen on ultrasound, in 40 per cent of cases. Usually lasting less than a minute, it can occasionally last longer than 2 minutes and in cases of bleeding disorders has been the cause of fetal death;
- fetal bradycardia occurs after sampling in 9–15 per cent of cases and appears to be more frequent in the presence of fetal disease in conjunction with oligohydramnios and intrauterine growth retardation, so prudence is recommended, as well as slow and minimal sampling in these high-risk cases;

- cord haematoma, which does not seem to have any repercussions on the fetus;

Problems occurring later in pregnancy.

One must differentiate between two types of cases with respect to the type of diagnosis:

- pregnancies where there has been chronic fetal distress in general associated with growth retardation, and abnormality of fluid volume and a fetal anomaly (oedemas associated with rhesus incompatibility or other mal-formations) for which the sampling is done with a view to karyotype study and/or fetal physiological well-being;
- pregnancies where we are searching for the presence of a genetic or infec-tious disease, and which in general are not associated with immediate fetal repercussions.

In fact, those risks related to sampling and those related to the pregnancy itself are not at all the same, and these two categories of patients must be dis-tinguished if one wants to study the sampling risk itself. In pregnancies where there is no chronic fetal distress:

- the risk of premature delivery is estimated at 4–6 per cent;
- the risk of intrauterine fetal death or of spontaneous abortion is less than 1 per cent.

When sampling is carried out on a threatened pregnancy:

- the percentage of intrauterine fetal death is higher, at around 10 per cent, essentially related to fetal disease;
- the risk of premature labour doubles, but this prematurity is also related to fetal disease.

Other fetal blood sampling techniques

Intrahepatic umbilical vein sampling Following the same principal of ultrasound-guided sampling, certain authors prefer puncturing the intra-hepatic umbilical vein by crossing the anterior wall of the fetal abdomen. This area of the vein is stable enough, but this kind of sampling is only possible if the fetal abdomen is anterior and still. Thus, premedication of mother and fetus is often necessary. For certain indications, such as *in utero* transfusion in cases of rhesus incompatibility, this technique appears most suitable and greatly simplifies therapy because, once the needle is in place, it is less likely to move than when it is placed in the cord.

Intracardiac puncture Ultrasound-guided puncture of the cardiac ventricle with an 18–20-gauge needle has been described by Bang (1983). There is a theoretical risk of injuring the chordae tendinae, of rhythmic problems due to injury to the septum, of bleeding in the pericardium, and of intrauterine death due to cardiac arrest. However, according to the authors, the risk of any of this is low and the outcome identical to that experienced with umbilical cord puncture. Since the number of cases is small, evaluation after longer experience is necessary.

Conclusion

Advantages of fetal blood sampling   Fetal blood sampling permits:

- those diagnoses which can be made on blood only: immune deficiencies, certain cases of haemoglobinopathy, haemophilia, viral or parasitic infection, a rapid karyotype at the end of the pregnancy;
- confirmation of diagnosis in cases of mosaicism or unusual findings on chorionic villi or amniotic fluid;
- fetal assessment in cases of chronic fetal distress, or distress observed during delivery;
- fetal therapy (blood transfusions, platelet injection, or injection of medication).

Risks to the fetus seem minimal but require further evaluation.

Disadvantages   At present, sampling is only possible at the beginning of the 17th to 18th week, which is rather late.

References and further reading

Bang, J. (1983). Ultrasound-guided fetal blood sampling. In *Progress in perinatal medicine* (ed. A. Alberhini and P. F. Crosignani), p. 223. Excerpta Medica, Amsterdam.

Christiaens, G. C. M. L., Stoutenbeek, P. H. (1984). Spontaneous abortion in proven intact pregnancies. *Lancet*, **ii**, 571.

Daffos, F. Capella-Pavlovsky, M., Forestier, F. (1983). A new procedure for fetal blood sampling in utero: preliminary results of 53 cases. *Am. J. Obstet. Gynecol.*, **146**, 985.

Daffos, F. Capella-Pavlovsky, M., Forestier, F. (1985). Fetal blood sampling during pregnancy with use of a needle guided by ultrasound: a study of 606 consecutive cases. *Am. J. Obstet. Gynecol.*, **153**, 655.

Dumez, Y., Goossens, M., Boué, J., Poenarn, L., Dommergues, M., Henrion, R. (1985). Chorionic villi sampling using rigid forceps under ultrasound control. In *First trimester fetal diagnosis,* pp. 38–45. Springer-Verlag, Berlin.

Firth, H. V., Boyd, P. A., Chamberlain, P., *et al.* (1991). Severe limb abnormalities after chorion villus sampling at 56–66 days' gestation. *Lancet*, **337**, 762.

Gilmore, D. H., McNay, M. B. (1986). Spontaneous fetal loss rate in early pregnancy. *Lancet*, **i**, 107.

Gerbie, A. B. and Elias, S. (1980). Technique for mid trimester amniocentesis for prenatal diagnosis. *Semin. Perinatol.*, **4**, 159.

Henrion, R. and Papa, F. (1981). Risques de l'amniocentèse. *Concours med.*, **103**, 525–30.

Kappel, B., Nielsen, J., Brogaard Hausen, K., *et al.* (1987). Spontaneous abortion following mid trimester amniocentesis: clinical significance of placental perforation and blood stained amniotic fluid. *Br. J. Obstet. Gynecol.*, **94**, 50–4.

Leschot, N. J., Verjaal, H., and Treffers, R. E. (1985). Risks of mid trimester amniocentesis assessment in 3000 pregnancies. *Br. J. Obstet. Gynecol.*, **92**, 807.

Medical Research Council Working Party on Amniocentesis (1978). *Br. J. Obstet. Gynecol.*, **85**, Suppl. 2: 1.

NICHD (1976). National registry for amniocentesis study group of mid trimester amniocentesis, for prenatal diagnosis safety and accuracy. *J. Amer. Med. Assoc.*, **236**, 1471–6.

Old, J. M., Ward, R. H. T., Karagozlu, F., *et al.* (1982). First-trimester fetal diagnosis for haemoglobinopathies: three cases. *Lancet*, **ii**, 1414.

Romero, R., Jeanty, P., and Reece, E. A. (1985). Sonographically monitored amniocentesis to decrease intraoperative complications. *Obstet. Gynecol.* **65**, 426.

Smidt-Jensen, S., Hahnemann, N., Hariri, J., *et al.* (1986). Transabdominal chorionic villi sampling for first trimester fetal diagnosis: first 26 pregnancies followed to term. *Prenat. Diagn.*, **6**, 125.

Tabor, A., Madsen, M., and Obel, E.B. (1986). Randomised controlled trial of genetic amniocentesis in low-risk women. *Lancet*, **i**, 1287–1292.

Tahoda, M. G. J., Vosters, R. P. L., Sachs, E. S., Galjaard, H. (1985). Safety of chorionic villus sampling. *Lancet*, **ii**, 941–2.

Wapner, R. J. (1989). Transcervical CVS. In *Fetal physiology and pathology*, Advances in gynecology and obstetrics. Proceedings of the 12th World Congress of Gynecology and Obstetrics, Vol. 2 (ed. P. Belfort, J. A. Pinotti, and T. K. A. B. Eskes), p. 39. Parthenon, London.

Weiss, R. R., Ebert, R., and Dichter, J. (1986). Risks of amniocentesis. *Lancet*, **i**, 577–8.

Williamson, R. A., Varner, M. W., and Grant, S. S. (1985). Reduction in amniocentesis risks using a real time needle guide procedure. *Obstet. Gynecol.* **65**, 751–755.

Wilson, R. D., Kendrick, V., Wittman, B. K., McGillivray, B. C. (1984). Risk of spontaneous abortion in ultrasonically normal pregnancies. *Lancet*, **ii**, 920.

3 Laboratory techniques

Cell culture

Despite progress in the refinement of laboratory techniques it is not always possible to obtain a diagnosis directly from a fetal sample, either because there are
too few cells in the sample (amniotic fluid in a pellet, for example), or because
of a particular quality required to apply the techniques; some require live, dividing cells (cytogenetic analysis) or metabolically active cells (biochemical assay
with labelled precursors).

Cell culture is a basic requirement for a large number of diagnoses, and diagnostic success is often dependent on the quality of cell cultures and sometimes
on the quantity of cells obtained *in vitro*.

Other than for prenatal diagnosis, cell cultures are required in the following
instances:

- to demonstrate that enzyme activity in various cell types (fibroblast, epithelial cells, etc.) is expressed at a measurable level in normal cells in
  culture, so that any lack of enzyme activity can be observed;
- to serve as control in confirming a final diagnosis on fetal cells after
  pregnancy termination;
- increasingly to store cells essential to confirm an enzyme deficit, or for DNA
  analysis of informative markers in the family of an affected child whose
  chances of survival are limited.

A good genetics laboratory should have all cell culture techniques available.

Cell biology
Some knowledge of the basics of cell biology is required.

Cell division The cell cycle in humans lasts about 18 hours, which in practical
terms represents a daily doubling of the cell population (this is very little when
one starts out with the few cells in amniotic fluid). This sets the culturing time
needed to obtain the number of cells required for a particular technique.

Cell division consists of four phases: G1, approximately 6 hours; S (synthesis
and duplication of DNA), 7 hours; G2, 4 hours, and M (mitosis) less than
1 hour. Chromosomes are observed only in this M phase.

In vitro *cell proliferation* All normal cells have a limited potential for division
in vitro, and thus a finite life, in contrast to transformed cells which have unlimited potential, and thus theoretically an infinite lifespan. A cell's ability to

45

divide varies with its type, and within one cell type it is a function of the donor's age. Fibroblasts from an embryo divide many times over *in vitro* and provide a large number of cells; on the other hand differentiated cells and particularly epithelial cells cannot be made to divide for long. Despite a fibroblastic appearance, the longevity of chorionic villus cells is reduced in *in vitro* culture: one can only suppose that the tissue from which they originate was not programmed to live long.

Blood lymphocytes do not last long *in vitro*, and one must rely on short cultures after stimulation with lectin (for blood karyotypes); or, using the Epstein–Barr virus, one can transform them to lymphoblastic lines, which have an unlimited ability to divide and are a good source of DNA.

Quality of medium for tissue culture   Much has been done to improve the basic medium, particularly by replacing animal sera with serum substitutes. These serum substitutes combine growth factors and promote adherence of cells to substrate, thus increasing the number of cells which will produce colonies, as well as improving the quality of growth: These products also provide consistent quality, which is difficult to control with commercial animal sera.

Amniotic fluid cell cultures

Conditions required in amniotic fluid sampling have been described in the preceding chapter. The laboratory should receive clear yellow (lemon-coloured) fluid in a sterile container, non-toxic to cells. When the fluid arrives at the laboratory, its state should be assessed and proper labelling ensured. If it is from a twin pregnancy, the laboratory staff should confirm with the mother the particulars of the amniocentesis in relation to each sample of fluid.

The fluid is centrifuged, the cell pellet is then resuspended in growth medium, and the supernatant is put into small tubes and kept at –20°C for possible biochemical assay. It is by retrospective studies of these frozen samples that much progress has been made in prenatal diagnosis (for example the study of digestive enzymes to diagnose cystic fibrosis).

What cells are present in amniotic fluid?
Quantitative characteristics   At the usual time for amniocentesis, between 16 and 20 weeks, there are 10 000 cells per millilitre of which 10 or more per millilitre remain viable and adhere to produce colonies. Later in the pregnancy, the fluid is encumbered by many more dead cells, and therefore very few remain to produce colonies.

It is possible to obtain fluid by ultrasound-guided early amniocentesis. The number of viable cells is small until the 15th week, but with medium made up with serum substitutes there is a high success rate of cultures from fluids drawn at 14–15 weeks.

Qualitative characteristics Initially there is a large variety of cells, but the vast majority (cells originating from fetal epidermis) do not attach and grow.

Despite research on the characterization of those cells giving rise to colonies *in vitro*, our knowledge is still limited. These cells are classified as large epithelial cells, which resemble amniotic membrane, small epithelial cells (from the amniotic fluid) which are more numerous, and fibroblast cells. The proportion of each of these different types of cells is different from one amniotic fluid sample to the other: the significance of this is not known.

Knowledge of the different types of cells could be important in diagnoses based on a measure of enzyme activity; it would then be essential to select as controls cells with the same morphology as those being analysed.

Primary culture of amniotic cells Techniques for primary cultures are determined by the principal indication: the establishment of a fetal karyotype. Two techniques are commonly used:

1. *In situ* chromosome analysis. Pyrex Petri dishes 30 mm in diameter, with a slide at the bottom, are used. Into these 1.5 mL of amniotic fluid are pipetted, and an equal amount of medium is added. The centrifuged cell pellet is resuspended in medium in another set of Petri dishes.

The Petri dishes (8–10) are incubated at 37°C in an incubator containing air and carbon dioxide, maintaining the pH of the medium at 7.3. During the first 4–5 days the Petri dishes must remain undisturbed, in order to allow attachment of cells to the cover slip. From then on the medium is changed every 2–3 days. The dishes are examined under an inverted microscope to assess the presence of colonies. When a sufficiently large number of colonies has been established, chromosome preparations can be made directly on the slide at the bottom of the Petri dish.

2. Chromosome analysis after trypsinization. The primary culture is identical, but plastic flasks are used instead of Petri dishes. Once cell colonies are well grown, chromosome preparations can be made.

Media used for cell culture A minimum essential medium contains a mixture of mineral salts, amino acids, vitamins, antibiotics, and bicarbonate to stabilize pH. The medium also contains animal sera, mostly newborn bovine or fetal bovine serum (10–20 per cent), or serum substitutes alone or supplemented with a small quantity of animal sera (a commonly used substitute is Ultroser G). One medium for the culture of amniotic fluid cells is HAM F10. Ready-made media such as Chang Medium are available.

Result of culturing Failure of culture is minimal (in our experience of the order of 1/1000 with clear fluid) if the sample is suitable and elementary precautions in culturing are used (a sufficient number of Petri dishes or flasks, and use of two different culture media to minimize risk of contamination).

Bloody samples, old samples containing a large number of dead cells, and samples cultured after many hours in transport may present some problems.

Secondary cell cultures   When a considerable number of cells is required (i.e. for enzymatic assay) the primary cultures are trypsinized to detach cells from the medium in order to transfer to plastic flasks. Normal cells display contact inhibition: in other words, on any surface where one monocellular layer touches another, cell division stops. To increase the culture surface, transfer into several flasks is required to initiate new cellular proliferation.

Chorionic villus cell cultures   Chorionic villi are covered by a trophoblastic epithelium made up of two cell layers, externally the multinucleated cell of the syncytiotrophoblast and internally the cytotrophoblast. It is the latter cells that undergo numerous mitoses, permitting direct analysis. The mesenchymal axis of the villi contains a small number of dispersed fibroblasts, which can be cultured *in vitro*.

For the primary culture, the explant technique with scissors or scalpels is simplest. The villi are minced to liberate the fibroblasts from the trophoblastic layer. After a few days in culture the explants are surrounded by a crown of fibroblastic cells. As for other primary cultures involving trypsinization, transfer into several flasks is required to obtain a layer of cells. The proliferation of cells is abundant, but the number of possible transfers is limited. Medium containing the serum substitute Ultroser seems to be beneficial for these types of cultures.

Fibroblast cell cultures   One can obtain fibroblastic cell lines either from skin biopsies, or from fetal tissues (skin and lung) after interruption of the pregnancy.

Once again it is the culture of primary cell explants which is easiest. The explants are placed in small drops of medium on the inner surface of the flask, where they attach after 24–48 hours. Medium can be added to allow the culture to grow. The cells are transferred from one flask to another after trypsinization. A larger number of cells can be obtained, particularly from fetal cells.

Lymphoblast cultures   This technique has come to replace that used for fibroblasts derived from skin biopsies. The ability of the Epstein–Barr virus to transform the B lymphocytes *in vitro* is used to establish lymphoblastoid cell lines. This technique has many advantages. A sample of a few millilitres of blood is sufficient, the culture technique is simple, the cells are grown in suspension, and a large number of them can be obtained. Control studies have demonstrated that during numerous transfers the karyotype as well as biochemical properties of the cells remain stable, and above all they are a good source of DNA.

Freezing of cells   Cell storage in liquid nitrogen, with the advantage of being able to thaw and re-culture cells, is an indispensable component of a cell-culturing laboratory. All cell-lines can be stored frozen. Cells are suspended in their medium with a supplement of dimethyl sulfoxide (DMSO) which prevents crystal formation in the cytoplasm, particularly in the range from 0°C to –15°C, and is critical for maintaining the vitality of the cells. These are then stored in liquid nitrogen. Thawed to 37°C the cells will instantly proliferate, because they keep their mitotic potential.

Techniques of chromosomal analysis

In prenatal diagnosis, it is important to choose techniques which can maximize quality and success in a minimal amount of time.

Fetal karyotyping

In order to establish the fetal karyotype it is necessary to obtain metaphases in sufficient quantity and quality and to apply various chromosome staining techniques, permitting the classification of chromosomes and any possible rearrangements. Finally, and most important, a microscopic analysis by someone with long experience is required.

Obtaining metaphases Mitosis accounts for only a fraction of the cell cycle, and the metaphase stage is the most appropriate for a chromosome analysis. To obtain a sufficient number of cells in metaphase, one can take advantage of a tissue in an active proliferative state, as the number of mitoses available at the time of preparation is sufficient for analysis. This is the case in direct analysis of chorionic villi, when the trophoblastic cells provide numerous mitoses. To maximize the number of mitoses, the delay between sampling of the villous and its processing must be brief (2–3 hours at most), as a longer delay, often in transport at low temperature (20°C or lower), leads to a decrease in spontaneous cell proliferation and an absence of mitoses.

Also, one can take advantage of spontaneously dividing cells when one prepares amniotic fluid cells cultured *in situ*. Around the 10th day of culture, after the medium has been changed the day before, there are many mitoses at the periphery of the cell colonies. A widely used method of obtaining metaphase cells is the blocking of mitosis at the prophase–metaphase transition using colchecine, a mitotic agent. The advantage is that one obtains a great number of metaphases, but the quality of the chromosomes is inferior to that found when using a direct technique, where the chromosomes are more extended. This is the technique used for amniotic fluid cells, particularly for those cells cultured in flasks, and for chorionic villi when preparations are made after, say, 24 hours of incubation. In chromosomal analysis of blood cells the proliferation of lymphocytes is first stimulated by a lectin, phytohaemagluttinin.

Fixation of metaphases

It is mostly due to a fortuitous observation made by T. C. Hsu that one can obtain well-extended metaphases. The cells are dipped into hypotonic solution, which induces a swelling of the nuclei, the chromosomes disperse, and rapid fixation of the cells provides well-separated chromosomes with minimal overlap. The two essential steps in preparation are made either directly on the monolayer on a slide (*in situ*) or on cells in suspension dropped onto slides. This cell suspension is obtained either after dissociation of chorionic villi with acetic acid or from amniotic fluid cells cultured in flasks and dissociated with trypsin, or again, directly from blood.

Staining of chromosomes

Solid stain   The more common DNA stains have been used since the early days of cytogenetics, in particular Giemsa. This remains the basic staining technique because it stains the chromosome uniformly, allowing classification by length and morphology with a well-delineated centromere, distinguishing between submetacentric, metacentric, or acrocentric. With this technique alone all changes in chromosome number and gross structural changes can be detected. Greater resolution for detecting chromosomal anomalies can be obtained by using various banding techniques.

Banding techniques   These techniques permit a linear differentiation of the structure of each chromosome by producing bands of different staining intensity which allow perfect identification of each chromosome pair, identification of breakpoints in various chromosomal anomalities, delineation of heterochromatic regions, etc. The most commonly used techniques are G bands induced by trypsin, Q bands obtained with fluorescent quinacrine derivatives, R bands obtained by heating, and C bands staining the centromere and the heterochromatin.

Delineation of some structural anomalies   Certain disorders are associated with very subtle structural abnormalities, usually visible in only a small percentage of metaphases. In order to establish these diagnoses one must follow good working protocols ensuring the expression of these chromosomal subtleties. For example, in mental retardation associated with a fragile X chromosome, the structural abnormality (p. 107) is expressed only in folate-deficient media or in media containing folate antagonists. This explains why they have been overlooked, as the trend was to use rich medium to maximize the number of metaphases.

In certain diseases resulting from a DNA-repair defect one can observe chromosome lesions such as breaks and re-arrangements (Fanconi anaemia, see p. 183). These lesions can be expressed more readily by the addition of clastogenic drugs to the culture medium.

Microscopic analysis

Fetal karyotyping depends on the analysis of sufficient number of metaphases. This analysis is first made under the microscope, and requires well-trained staff. It involves a selection of good-quality metaphases where the chromosomes are well spread out with minimum overlap, but not so widely spread that the rupture of the nuclear membrane leads to chromosome loss. The count and identification of chromosome pairs in itself permits a quite precise diagnosis.

This fetal karyotype is then confirmed by the analysis of metaphases derived from various colonies, if an *in situ* technique is used, or from different flasks if Petri dishes or flasks are being used. Microphotographs of well-selected metaphases, after magnification, printing, and cutting, are used to provide a fetal karyotype.

When a change in the chromosome structure or number is identified, the change will be elucidated by making use of banding techniques selected in accordance with the suspected anomaly.

Staining of sex chromosomes on interphase nuclei

Barr body   The heterochromatic body observed by Barr in 1949 in female interphasic cells corresponds to an inactivation of the X chromosome. If there are *n* X chromosomes there are *n*-1 Barr bodies. In terms of diagnosis, the search for the Barr body is useful only in confirming a numerical anomaly of the X chromosome, for example 47,XXX or 47,XXY.

Y body   Quinacrine staining of the heterochromatic part of the long arm of the Y chromosome may be used on an interphase nucleus where the Y chromosome appears as a fluorescent body. This technique is seldom used, because it has too high a rate of error. Analysis is subjective, and because the fluorescent part of the Y chromosome may be of variable length, it may remain undetected if it is very short.

Automated chromosomal analysis

In the last 25 years efforts have been made to develop automatic chromosomal analysis by computerized image analysis. In cytogenetics, this method of image analysis has been plagued with problems which have as yet not permitted fully automated equipment. One of the first objectives was to accomplish automatic screening of metaphases on slides. Although this did not prove difficult, an automated measure of the quality of metaphases has remained unsatisfactory.

Automated screening may be used for tissue preparations poor in mitoses, such as chorionic villi, but it does not significantly speed up the search for metaphases of amniotic fluid cells, particularly when these are grown *in situ*, as colonies are already easily localized and the metaphases are found at the periphery of the colonies.

The automation of chromosomal analysis faces great difficulties due to the variable morphology of the chromosomes and, in particular, to fragments overlapping each other, or even in juxtaposition. This problem, already significant with Giemsa staining, is even more exacerbated with banding.

The use of totally automatic systems has been abandoned, and semi-automatic equipment, which provides only partial assistance, is the system of choice. The technician identifies each chromosome on the screen and classifies it; the system reconstitutes the karyotype, and decreases the time required for printing and cutting. It is not yet possible to estimate the time saved by this recently developed semi-automated equipment.

Digital recording of the banding pattern of different chromosomes and their computerized handling do not yet allow for easy identification of structural changes of the chromosome.

Despite the recent impact of semi-automatic equipment in establishing the karyotype, chromosome analysis is still an art and depends, above all, on the experience of the technician.

Other developments in chromosome analysis

The use of flow cytometry has been considered for karyotyping, because of its speed. It requires cells in metaphase, and therefore a culture time of 2–5 weeks. In addition to its prohibitive cost, this technology does not allow one to distinguish one chromosome from another, does not allow for the detection of breakpoints, and is plagued with a significant number of false positives (false diagnosis of trisomy when the karyotype is normal).

Chromosome analysis of fetal cells in maternal circulation

Fetal cells are present in the maternal circulation during pregnancy and for a few months after delivery. A measure of the number of fetal cells has been made possible by fluorescence of the Y body. The proportion of fetal cells increases steadily from 1/5000 maternal nucleated cells to 5/5000 at delivery. These are trophoblastic cells, as well as lymphocytic B cells responding poorly to mitogens. Recent developments in automated cell sorting have lead some to believe that prenatal diagnosis using these cells might be possible if they could be separated from maternal cells by flow cytometry. Results have been disappointing, and for the present there must be some reservations about this possibility. A measurable number of fetal cells is present only from the third month of pregnancy. Stimulating division of these cells to make them useful for cytogenetic analysis is not yet possible, enzymatic or molecular techniques will require a cell sorter, and finally it must be kept in mind that these cells will be maintained in the maternal circulation after the pregnancy (interrupted or not) and may therefore lead to erroneous results in a subsequent pregnancy. Sex determination on fetal cells present in maternal circulation by gene amplification (PCR) of specific DNA regions of the Y chromosome has recently been proposed, but this approach has already been severely criticized and could lead to frequent errors.

Cytogenetic diagnosis using molecular technology

The recent development of a large number of molecular probes specific to a particular chromosome region makes the diagnosis of a chromosomal anomaly possible. Several methods are applicable.

Diagnosis on DNA extracted from fetal samples   This is largely performed on chorionic villi, where DNA extraction is often done for the diagnosis of single-gene disorders.

Diagnosis of sex   Probes specific for the Y chromosome are now available, and with relatively simple techniques (dot hybridization, see p. 66), one can affirm or exclude the presence of this chromosome, in this way determining fetal sex. This technique has recently been developed for its application in the diagnosis of sex-linked disease, because cytogenetic analysis done on amniotic fluid cells in culture provides a late diagnosis. Direct cytogenetic analysis on chorionic villi allows a diagnosis in a matter of hours, eliminating the need of DNA for these diagnoses.

It must be emphasized that the diagnosis of sex by karyotyping also permits the detection of chromosome anomalies. In high-risk cases such as those involving sex-linked disease, a diagnosis of sex, overlooking a possible chromosomal anomaly, would be unsatisfactory.

Diagnosis of trisomy   With DNA probes specific to a particular autosome (chromosome 21, for example) one can perform a quantitative analysis of that probe. At present, quantitative analysis of DNA is not reliable enough to allow us to measure the difference between $\frac{2}{3}$ and 1.

Diagnosis of structural abnormalities   Molecular technology may be useful in those structural anomalies where a molecular probe can be localized close to the breakpoints.

Diagnosis by in situ *hybridization on interphase nuclei*

Recent techniques of *in situ* hybridization on chromosomes using cold probes may provide new possibilities in cytogenetic diagnosis. With molecular probes coupled to a fluorescent marker, one can visualize on interphase nuclei the chromosome(s) corresponding to the probe. One can for example, in this way, detect a trisomy 21 by observing three fluorescent dots obtained using a probe for chromosome 21. Similarly, one can demonstrate the presence of a deletion, for example, in some cases of Prader–Willi syndrome or Angelman syndrome using a molecular probe specific for the 15q site. Though fast and elegant, this technique can only determine anomalies of the chromosome in question and is therefore subject to the same limitations as diagnoses depending on Y-fluorescence.

Unless there is development of a yet unforeseeable technology, cytogenetic analysis will remain a craft based on the quality and experience of the technical staff and management. The relative absence of sophisticated equipment in comparison to other disciplines, which today tend to occupy and monopolize the limelight, must not let us forget that 95 per cent of all prenatal diagnoses still rely on cytogenetic analysis.

Biochemical analysis of fetal samples

Biochemical tests on amniotic fluid

The technique of amniocentesis has already been described (p. 31) but some practical details must be reiterated here. The presence of blood in the sample is always of concern, as it may interfere with the assays or with their interpretation. Should blood appear in the syringe at the time of sampling, one must immediately cease aspiration and change the syringe. This may happen several times, depending on the amount of fluid withdrawn. Most biochemical assays require only 1–2 mL of fluid, so it is preferable to have a small clear sample than 200 mL of bloody fluid. Should a fetal karyotype be done parallel to the biochemical assay, two tubes should be sampled.

One can distinguish between qualitative and quantitative techniques: the technical approach and interpretation of results is quite different for each of them. All these techniques are tricky in their application and their interpretation. For reliability, these assays should not be improvised or done only infrequently. It is often best to send samples to an experienced laboratory. Methods of sampling and transport should be discussed for each type of analysis.

Qualitative technique

Cholinesterase electrophoresis for the diagnosis of neural tube defects   This qualitative technique involves electrophoresis of amniotic fluid in a non-denaturing polyacrylamide gel on a horizontal support. Horizontal electrophoresis is preferred, as in vertical electrophoresis the borders may hinder interpretation in some cases.

After migration, cholinesterase activity is demonstrated using Karnovsky's dye (Karnovsky and Roots 1964): acetylthiocholine is hydrolysed by the cholinesterases, and freed thiocholine forms a brown-coloured complex with the ferricyanide and copper ions.

In order to reveal cholinesterase in this way, the enzymatic activity of the protein must be intact. Great care must be taken: in choosing reagents, particularly polyacrylamide (of all of those tested only Kodak has proved satisfactory), in the making of the gel in order to get rid of all inhibitors of enzyme activity, and in cleaning the equipment because detergents are cholinesterase inhibitors.

Normal amniotic fluid contains butyrylcholinesterase which migrates as a 'slow' band, whereas amniotic fluid associated with an open neural tube defect contains not only butyrylcholinesterase but acetylcholinesterase of neuronal origin, which migrates in two bands, one overlapping that of butyrylcholinesterase and one migrating faster. The presence of a fast band indicates a neural tube defect (Fig. 3.1).

The quantitative analysis resting on the ratio of acetyl versus butyryl activity in the presence of inhibitors should not be used, because specific inhibitors for each enzyme do not exist. Furthermore, as for any quantitative technique stand-

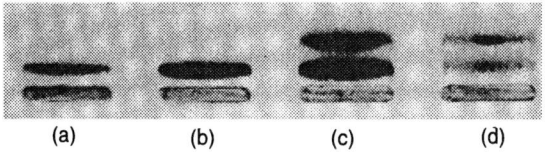

(a)   (b)   (c)   (d)

Fig. 3.1 Polyacrylamide gel electrophoresis of amniotic fluid. Cholinesterases are detected by the Karnowsky stain. *a*, normal amniotic fluid; *b*, blood-tinged amniotic fluid; *c*, amniotic fluid from a spina bifida pregnancy; *d*, cerebrospinal fluid.

ard curves must be established. In our experience this gives rise to false positives and false negatives which are not a problem with the electrophoretic technique. Also, some spina bifidas or anencephalies are associated with serum transudate or even some bleeding which increases the butyrylcholinesterase. In these circumstances the acetylcholinesterase activity appears decreased, and this may lead to a false negative. In case of blood contamination of the amniotic fluid, electrophoretic study demonstrates five bands of the serum cholinesterase in addition to the one associated with cerebral acetylcholinesterase which in most cases is perfectly clear.

The qualitative technique takes longer and is more expensive, but is more reliable and is not associated with any false positives and/or false negatives. The presence of false negatives in the quantitative technique limits its use as a screening method.

The acetyl- and butyrylcholinesterase band positions associated with omphalocoeles are so characteristic that with technical experience they can be recognized. The supernumerary bands of cholinesterase, sometimes observed in amniotic fluids sampled late, are a result of the poor quality of the reagent. The absence of bands corresponding to butyrylcholinesterase may be observed in two instances: either the sample is of maternal urine, not amniotic fluid (a simple measure of protein, sodium, and potassium eliminates this occurrence, which has been observed in 1/2000 amniotic fluids in 1987), or it is amniotic fluid, but the mother has a deficiency of butyrylcholinesterase, a rare genetic trait associated with a hypersensitivity to curare during anaesthesia. A maternal blood sample sent to a specialized laboratory can confirm this abnormality.

How is amniotic fluid sent for acetylcholinesterase studies? The electrophoresis technique requires very little fluid (20 μL); a 1 mL sample is enough. Cells do not interfere with the electrophoresis method, but it is preferable to work on the supernatant.

The red cell membrane is rich in acetylcholinesterase (called insoluble acetylcholinesterase). A bloody amniotic fluid sample can at times make interpretation of electrophoresis difficult. In practice when the amniotic fluid is bloody it should be processed as quickly as possible, and centrifuged at 1000 rev/min. The supernatant can then be frozen before analysis.

Cholinesterases are stable, and after centrifugation the amniotic fluid can be sent unfrozen by regular mail even if the sample takes several days in transit. Despite the need for a small amount of fluid, it is wise to keep a larger volume of supernatant as back-up.

Quantitative techniques

Alphafetoprotein measurements   Alphafetoprotein is fetal in origin, and its presence in fluid is determined by the physiology of fetal maturation. It is synthesized in fetal liver, and it is through the immature renal glomeruli that this protein (molecular weight 60 000) filters into the amniotic fluid. The concentration of alphafetoprotein in amniotic fluid reaches its peak at 12–13 weeks, then kidney maturation slowly limits its filtration and thus the alphafetoprotein level declines. At 17 weeks it is 15 mg/L, and at term 0.1 mg/L.

The method chosen to measure alphafetoprotein must be sensitive enough to detect these levels. Whereas an immunoenzymatic or radioimmunological method is required for the assay of alphafetoprotein in the serum, an immuno-electrophoretic technique according to Laurell (1966), or a radioimmuno-diffusion technique, is more suitable for amniotic fluid.

Whatever the technique, there are two major drawbacks to measuring alphafetoprotein in amniotic fluid. Firstly, as for any quantitative technique, each laboratory must establish a standard curve. As levels in amniotic fluid vary at each gestational age, these standards should be based on at least 100 normal amniotic fluids measured for each gestational week. While standard values are well established (95–99th percentile) for 15–20 weeks, they are not applicable beyond 20 weeks because amniocenteses done after this term are often recommended because of abnormal ultrasound findings and no longer represent normal pregnancies. Normal alphafetoprotein values, as measured using Laurell's method, are plotted in Fig. 3.2. Secondly, difficulties are related to the risk of fetal blood contamination of the amniotic fluid. The concentration of alphafetoprotein in fetal serum is 100 times that found in amniotic fluid, and although virtually impossible to measure, will none the less raise the alphafetoprotein level in amniotic fluid.

These drawbacks, added to the non-specific nature of alphafetoprotein, makes interpretation of a high value difficult. Today, cholinesterase electorphoresis to detect neural tube defects and the study of digestive enzymes for digestive tract abnormalities are techniques better adapted for each of these diagnoses. There is little indication for measuring alphafetoprotein in amniotic fluid.

Assay of digestive enzyme activity   The presence of digestive enzymes in amniotic fluid is determined by fetal physiology (see p. 12). These enzymes seep from the anal canal as soon as the cloacal membrane opens, around the 12th week of gestation, until the 20th week when the anal sphincter becomes innervated.

The study of fetal tissue has allowed us to localize and assay certain digestive enzymes. Around 18 weeks of gestation, bile contains a high level of

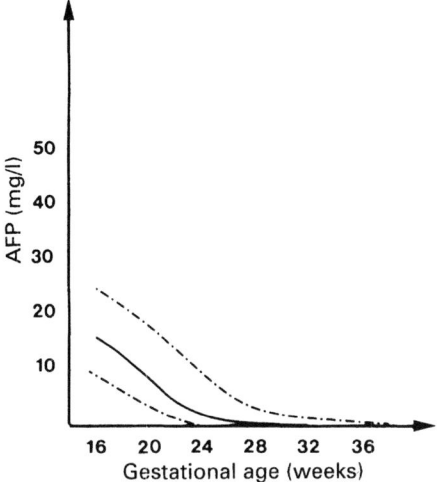

Fig. 3.2 Normal values of alphafetoprotein in amniotic fluid as a function of gestational age. Alphafetoprotein is measured by immunoelectrophoresis using Laurell's method (L. Cédard), personal communication.

activity of gammaglutamyl transpepsidase and 5' nucleotidase. Alkaline phosphatase is of hepatic origin. The intestinal villi contain gammaglutamyl transpepsidase, leucine-aminopeptidase, an intestinal form of alkaline phosphatase, and disaccharidases. These intestinal and biliary enzymes accumulate in the digestive tract to form the meconium. The activity of certain enzymes of the bile, intestinal villi, and meconium of fetuses at 18–19 weeks' gestation are given in Table 3.1. All intestinal transport abnormalities can influence the enzymatic profile of the amniotic fluid. The measurement of these amniotic fluid markers played an important role in the diagnosis of cystic fibrosis, which during fetal life is primarily reflected by a disorder of the digestive tract. The measurement of these enzyme activities is also useful in the diagnosis of intestinal anomalies found on ultrasound examination or suspected in a polymalformative complex, as for imperforate anus.

For all enzymes, assay of activity rests on colorimetric interpretation of the enzyme activity curve. Automated assay, as has been used in serum, can be used in amniotic fluid so long as it is adjusted for values to be expected in the samples. For example, the normal level of gammaglutamyl transpepsidase in serum is less than 40 IU/L, whereas in amniotic fluid at 16 weeks it is 600 IU/L. Contrary to this alkaline phosphatase has a lower value in amniotic fluid than in serum, 2 IU/L. The study of isoenzymes of alkaline phosphatase rests on the action of enzyme inhibitors, and the concentration and duration must be adapted to the equipment as well as to the experimental temperature: 25°C, 30°C, 37°C. In our centre we use phenylalanine, 5 mM, to inhibit the action of the intestinal

Table 3.1 Median values (extreme values) for the activity of digestive enzymes in fetal tissues at around 18 weeks. GGT, gammaglutamyl transpepsidase; LAP leucine aminopeptidase; PAL, alkaline phosphatase. (F. Muller, personal communication)

Activity (IU/L)	GGT	LAP	PAL	Type of PAL
Amniotic fluid	300	6	22	80% intestinal
(n = 255)	(75–818)	(10–73)	(4–73)	
Gastric fluid	700	67	48	80% intestinal
(n = 10)	(600–1400)	(54–74)	(20–74)	
Bile	7000	500	20	100% hepatic
(n = 12)	(850–54 000)	(270–670)	(5–100)	
Meconium	12 500	6500	14 500	100% intestinal
(n = 27)	(1700–136 000)	(1800–36 000)	(6000–77 000)	
Ileum	1700	850	4300	100% intestinal
(n = 23)	(80–4200)	(200–3300)	(800–11 400)	
Colon	1150	750	1000	50% intestinal,
(n = 14)	(100–6500)	(400–1800)	(10–1700)	50% kidney–liver–bone
Urine	< 2	< 1	< 1	
(n = 10)				

alkaline phosphatase; bromotetramisole, 0.1 mM, to inhibit kidney–liver–bone alkaline phosphatase; and phenylalanylglycylglycine, 1 mM, to inhibit placental alkaline phosphatase.

This quantitative approach requires establishment of standard values. Percentiles should be determined for each week of gestation for hundreds of samples, because the activities of gammaglutamyl transpepsidase and leucine aminopeptidase diminish during gestation, particularly between 16 and 20 weeks. The total activity of alkyline phosphatase is stable throughout gestation, but the level of placental isoenzyme itself increases with gestation. The data for these enzymes are plotted in Fig. 3.3.

The activity of 5′ nucleotidase can be measured in amniotic fluid, and confirms an abnormal value of gammaglutamyl transpepsidase as it is also of biliary origin. However, this enzyme has a strong affinity to plastic and is adsorbed by the tubes at the time of sampling or during storage; this prevents any interpretation of measurements.

The disaccharidase activity (lactase, sucrase, maltase) can also be measured, but the low activity of trehalase, maltase, lactase, and at 16–20 weeks' gestation makes measurement of a decreased activity very tricky. This does not reliably diagnose cystic fibrosis.

Sucrase activity is higher at this point in pregnancy, but its measurement requires amniotic fluid dialysis because the glucose in amniotic fluid interferes with its measurement. This cumbersome procedure, when applied to a great number of samples, also introduces large variability in normal values. For this

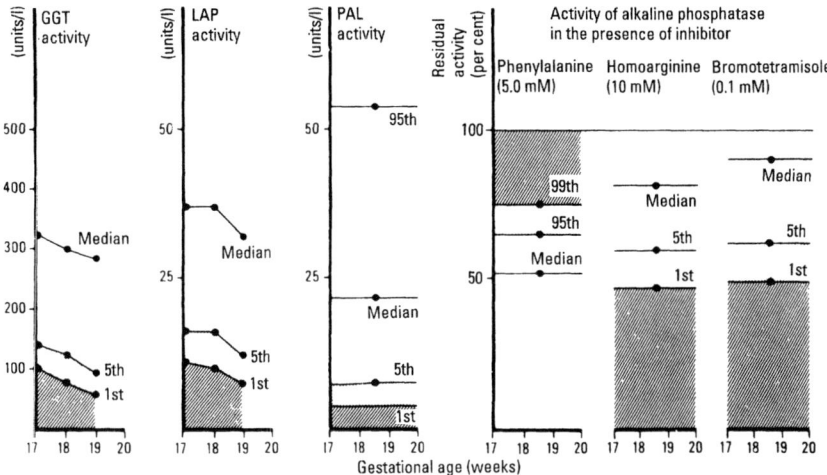

Fig. 3.3 Normal values of gammaglutamyl transpeptidase (GGT), leucine amino-peptidase (LAP), and alkaline phosphatase (PAL) and its isoenzymes in normal amniotic fluid at 16–20 weeks. From F. Muller, personal communication.

reason, we do not use disaccharidase measurement, as it would not provide supplementary information for the diagnosis of intestinal fetal anomalies.

How should a sample be prepared? Today's automated systems require very small samples. In practice, 2 mL of amniotic fluid allows for proper analysis. Fluid should be centrifuged before measurement, and blood contamination must be avoided because its level of enzyme activity is different from that of normal amniotic fluid. Alkaline phosphatase in amniotic fluid is the intestinal type, while in serum it is of the liver–kidney–bone type and is also 10 times more concentrated. A dark brownish-coloured fluid associated with earlier bleeding can hinder any interpretation of enzyme activity because of colorimetric inter-ference. In this case, it is possible to use monoclonal antibodies against the isoenzymes of alkaline phosphatase.

These digestive enzymes are stable, and the fluid, once centrifuged, can be sent to the laboratory by regular mail.

Quantitative measurement of protein   Amniotic fluid contains 4–5 g/L of total protein. A sensitive Biuret method can be used to measure these con-centrations. The more common proteins are albumin IgG, α-1-antitrypsin, trans-ferrin, α-1-glycoprotein and alphafetoproteins. They are measured by immunonephelometric methods.

Normal values must be established by each laboratory for each week of preg-nancy. Maternal blood contamination will interfere with the measurement: blood contamination makes amniotic fluid diagnoses impossible. The normal values of the most common proteins are listed in Table 3.2. Measurement of specific proteins may help in the diagnosis of the Finnish nephrotic syndrome.

Table 3.2 Protein levels (mg/L) in normal amniotic fluid at 18 weeks' gestation. Median values. (F. Muller, personal communication)

IgM	0	
IgG	320	(± 140)
IgA	16	(± 11)
C$_3$	16	(± 8)
α-1 Glycoprotein	43	(± 15)
Haptoglobin	0	
Transferrin	222	(± 108)
Albumin	2825	(± 870)
α-1 Antitrypsin	200	(± 54)
α-2 Macroglobulin	0	

Biochemical assays on fetal blood

The late timing of fetal blood sampling (after 18 weeks' gestation considerably limits the value of biochemical assays on fetal blood for numerous genetic diseases which can be diagnosed on chorionic villus sampling. For most of these disorders, there is no experience of the reliability of the diagnosis on fetal blood.

Sampling carried out for diagnosis of infectious disease of the fetus has made it possible to evaluate the constitution and biochemical components of fetal blood (Table 3.3). Normal values have been established for different stages of pregnancy. These biochemical assays of fetal blood are seldom used diagnostically, except in those cases of fetal infection where IgM titres are measured (the titre is usually less than 100 mg at 22 weeks of gestation, and a steep increase represents fetal response to an antigenic stimulation) and in those cases where the level of gammaglutamyl transpeptidase represents liver damage.

The consequences of fetal damage by toxoplasmosis or herpes virus have been evaluated. An increased level of gammaglutamyl transpeptidase may be the only sign of fetal infection. An immunological assay for specific IgM will be discussed on p. 226.

Biochemical assays of fetal urine

Only in obstructive urinary tract disorders can one sample fetal urine. In fact, where the bladder, the ureter, and the pelvis of the kidney are not dilated, urine sampling is impossible because the fetus urinates in response to the abdominal puncture. Understanding renal function through the study of fetal urine is only possible by examining cases of obstructive uropathy.

At first glance, it may seem odd that a single sample of fetal urine can accurately reflect fetal renal function. But the fetus is special in that it is in a sort of maternal dialysis, and its kidney has no role in homeostasis. Glomerular filtration and the secretion/reabsorption function in the fetus are gradually established independent of any functional role. This is why the study of fetal blood

Table 3.3 Normal levels of fetal blood components sampled between 20 and 26 weeks of amenorrhea compared to maternal serum levels (mean ± standard deviation). Data from Daffos *et al.* (1984)

Component	Units	Fetus	Mother
Glucose	mmol/L	2.8 ± 0.2	4.4 ± 0.1
Triglycerides	mmol/L	0.89 ± 0.03	1.4 ± 0.07
Cholesterol	mmol/L	1.5 ± 0.05	6.6 ± 0.2
Protein (total)	g/L	30.4 ± 0.6	69.6 ± 0.9
Albumin	g/L	21.4 ± 0.4	34.9 ± 0.5
Calcium	mmol/L	2.25 ± 0.2	2.27 ± 0.1
Phosphorus	mmol/L	2.65 ± 0.1	1.45 ± 0.06
Urea	mmol/L	2.5 ± 0.16	4.4 ± 0.2
Creatinine	μmol/L	64 ± 2	67 ± 1.5
Uric acid	μmol/L	167 ± 10	215 ± 9.5
Bilirubin (total)	μmol/L	26.8 ± 1	8.6 ± 0.4
Bilirubin (direct)	μmol/L	16.1 ± 0.6	0.9 ± 0.4
Creatine kinase	IU/L	62 ± 6	48 ± 2
Lactic dehydrogenase	IU/L	261 ± 14	132 ± 5
Aspartate aminotransferase	IU/L	21.1 ± 2	12.9 ± 1
Alkaline phosphatase	IU/L	197 ± 11	60 ± 3
Gammaglutamyltranspeptidase	IU/L	24.4 ± 9.6	19 ± 10

does not allow measure of kidney function, and why it is useless to measure the clearance and glomerular filtration rate. None the less, differentiation of the kidney plays an important role, and a urine analysis at 25 weeks is not equivalent to one performed at 35 weeks (Fig. 3.4).

The sampling site of fetal urine (bladder, ureter, renal pelvis) depends on the site of obstruction and fetal position. It is important to ensure that the urine is not contaminated with blood or amniotic fluid. A red blood cell count allows one to measure the extent of blood contamination; a measure of digestive enzyme activity allows one to exclude amniotic fluid contamination.

Biochemical assay to measure kidney function can then be carried out. The ionic and metabolic concentrations resemble those of the serum rather than those of newborn urine, so the methods used should take this into account. Table 3.4 illustrates this.

As for all quantitative assays, interpretation of fetal urine parameters rests on establishing normal values. We have observed previously that it is impossible to sample *in utero* either a bladder or pelvis if undilated, and postabortum urine cannot be used because of cell lysis. Establishment of normal values therefore rests on the values observed in those samples from cases of obstructive uropathy for which the renal function was normal at 1 month of age. Our criteria for normal function is a creatinine clearance greater than 50 mL/minute/1.73 m^2. The means and standard deviations for parameters measuring fetal renal function are listed in Table 3.4.

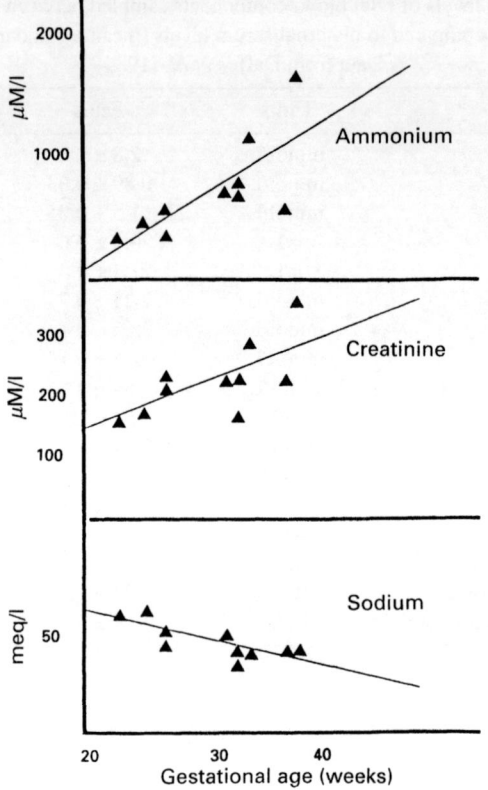

Fig. 3.4 Changing values of sodium, ammonium, and creatinine measured in fetal urine during development. From F. Muller, personal communication.

DNA analysis

Discovered and isolated as early as 1869, characterized as the material carrying genetic information in 1944, the DNA molecule was until 1970 the cell component most difficult to analyse. This difficulty, which is related to the length of the DNA molecules and to their characteristic non-random configuration of four bases in repeated sequence constituting the coded hereditary message, was overcome by the introduction of recombinant DNA technology. The length of the human genome contained in the 22 pairs of autosomes and the X/Y pair is 3×10^9 base pairs (bp), 10 per cent of which correspond to the structural genes. These genes are not only made up of coding sequences (1/10), which by cell mechanisms will be translated into proteins, but are also made up of the non-coding sequences (9/10), which play a role in gene expression. The number of genes varies between 2×10^4 and 5×10^4 and they are dispersed or clustered in gene families.

Table 3.4 Biochemical parameters in fetal and newborn urine (mean ± standard deviation). (F. Muller, personal communication)

	Units	Fetal urine	Newborn urine
Urea	mmol/L	10.5 ± 2.45	300
Creatinine	μmol/L	245 ± 66	7000
Protein	g/L	0.02 ± 0.05	< 0.10
Sodium	meq/L	51 ± 10	Variable
Chloride	meq/L	52 ± 10	Variable
Osmolarity	mOsm/L	110 ± 19	Variable
Glucose	mmol/L	0.13 ± 0.16	0
Calcium	mmol/L	0.69 ± 0.45	2.2
Phosphorus	mmol/L	0.18 ± 0.16	11
Ammonia	μmol/L	719 ± 403	20 000
β-2 Microglobulin	mg/L	0.86 ± 1.1	0.1

These figures demonstrate the difficulty or even impossibility of isolating one gene or a particular chromosomal region for all individuals to be studied, if it were not for molecular genetic technology. Indeed, it was the cloning of the first gene (globin) in 1977 which set the stage for the great technological advancements realized using Southern techniques. This leap forward rests on the unique property of DNA: it is made up of two complementary chains linked by weak chemical bonds between guanine (G) and cytosine (C) or between thymine (T) and adenine (A). It is possible, simply by heating or in the presence of salt, to dissociate the two complementary chains. These two chains can re-adhere to each other, at the same time retaining their complementarity, but they can also adhere to an identical sequence found in the 3×10^6 bp of an individual's genome.

Gene analysis by Southern technique relies both on 'chemical scissors', restriction enzymes which cut DNA into fragments, and on specific molecular probes. These probes are made up of precise copies of nucleotide sequences forming part or all of the whole gene under study. These copies, obtained by methods of DNA technology (cloning), can be formed of either deoxyribonucleic acid (DNA) or ribonucleic acid (RNA). Currently on the market today there are a number of restriction enzymes (bacterial enzymes) which cut the DNA at recognition sites comprised of nucleotide sequences specific to each of them (Fig. 3.5). DNA from different individuals can therefore be fragmented at predictable and identical sites by each enzyme. This cutting of DNA constitutes the basis for most of the diagnoses of mutation.

These studies have shown that the non-coding genetic DNA (introns and regulating sequences) and the DNA between genes (90 per cent) as well as the coding sequences (exons), could be altered by mutation. These modifications in the DNA sequence are not associated with any recognized phenotypic con-

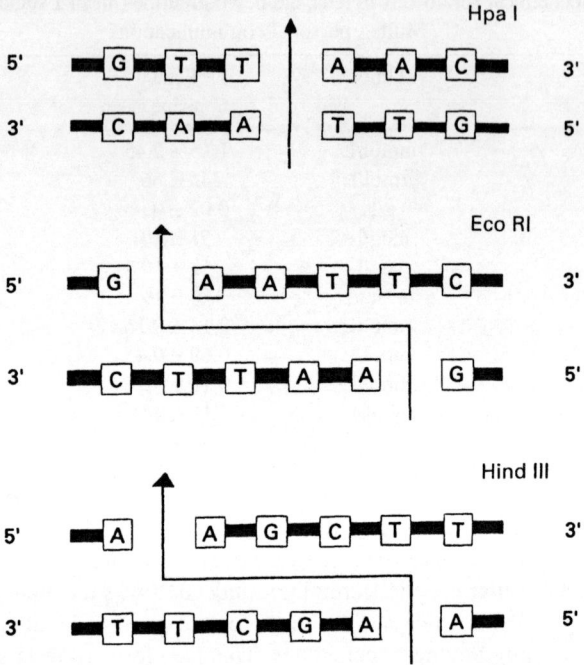

Fig. 3.5 DNA digestion by restriction enzymes. The specific DNA sequences recognized here by three frequently used restriction enzymes, Hpa I, Eco RI, and Hind III, are called restriction sites. They are made up of a variable number of base pairs (four, six, or more) and are palindromes because the nucleotide sequence on each strand is the same when it is read in the same direction, from the 5′ end to the 3′ end. The way in which the enzyme cuts the double-stranded DNA varies from one enzyme to another (represented by the arrow).

sequences but could affect the recognition of this sequence by a restriction enzyme. These modifications may be encountered by a restriction enzyme. These modifications may be encountered once in every 100 bp. This implies that for any two unrelated individuals and for a given sequence, 99 per cent of the restriction sites will be identical. None the less, these small differences have been the basis for the greatest discoveries in human genetics in the last few years. These variations which are genetic polymorphisms are transmitted, following Mendelian rules, as a dominant trait for which the transmission can be followed in a given family. Thanks to these minor modifications, of which the great majority have no phenotypic effect, it is possible to follow the transmission of a small chromosomal region carrying precisely the mutant gene in question.

This chapter is not written in an attempt to describe at length all the methods of molecular biology, rather to illustrate by means of a limited number of techniques, all derived from the Southern method and circumventing laborious cloning of genes, how one can explore different cases.

Techniques

Obtaining DNA   DNA can be extracted from any nucleated cells. In practice it is today extracted from leucocytes in whole blood (10–30 mL) using EDTA or heparin as anticoagulant. One cell contains on average 5 ng of DNA, and the Southern technique requires 10 μg for each experiment. All cell lines can be used, because they provide a continual source of material. Fibroblasts are inconvenient because they necessitate a skin biopsy, and lymphoblastoid cell lines transformed by Epstein–Barr virus require only 10 mL of heparinized blood sterilely sampled. On the other hand, the DNA obtained from chorionic villi or amniocytes cultured or not, is limited: 10–100 μg.

This limit to the quantity of material available for analysis sometimes makes a complete study impossible. However, development of the technique of amplification of specific sequences by the polymerase chain reaction (PCR) should overcome this difficulty.

DNA transports well. Total blood can be sent at room temperature within 48 hours. It stores well, either as whole blood or purified DNA at –20°C. Freezing does not require the preliminary extraction of DNA, which itself takes up to 2 days. Only lymphoblastoid cell lines pose any restrictions. When whole blood is transported at room temperature, leucocyte extraction must be done within 48 hours; in practice this limits transportation of the specimen to the beginning or middle of the working week.

Hybridization of probes to genomic DNA

cDNA probes   These deoxyribonucleic acid probes are exact replicates of a part of the messenger RNA, and therefore correspond to coding sequences.

Genomic DNA   The properties of these probes are related to their sequence: gene fragments (coding and/or non-coding segments), or an anonymous, unique, or repetitive sequence.

Synthetic oligonucleotides   It is possible to synthesize any sequence, for example: a sequence of 20 bp surrounding a mutation in a specific gene, or short sequences which flank that to be amplified and serve as primers to synthesize that DNA fragment several times over, then to analyse it by classic or more simplified methods, or again, minisatellite sequences, which allow detection of highly polymorphic sequences in the genome.

cRNA probes   These probes may be the complementary copy of RNA or, after cloning in an appropriate vector, may be the copy of a DNA or cDNA sequence. cDNA and genomic DNA probes are double-stranded oligonucleotides, and RNA probes are single-stranded. Depending on their structure, these sequences can be identified by incorporation of ^{32}P-labelled nucleotides, using various enzyme techniques such as labelling with a polymerase (nick translation or primer extension) or labelling with a polynucleotide kinase. These radiolabelled single-stranded or rendered single-stranded sequences can then hybridize with the complementary sequence in the genome of the individual under study. The unique properties of these radiolabelled probes allow the recognition of a complementary sequence to the probe from among several million sequences.

Studying DNA

Dot blot   Total DNA is mechanically reduced to smaller fragments and laid on a membrane. The radioactive probe is then applied. Either a complementary sequence will be found in this DNA and hybridization will occur, which will be revealed by autoradiography as a black dot; or the sequence is mutated or absent and therefore hybridization will not occur.

This technique is applicable in only a few cases but is much faster than the one described next.

Southern blot   This technique, perfected by E. Southern in 1975, consists of a number of steps and requires 5–10 days, depending on the number of samples to be run and the intensity of the observed radioactive signal. As well exemplified by the variation in different laboratory protocols, the many parameters of this technique have still not been completely mastered, because they rely on the quality of commercial products available: stability and purity of enzymes, chemical reagents and probes, and the heterogeneity and reliability of membranes used. Laboratories go through 'dark' periods where results are not always interpretable. These difficulties, for which it is often impossible to identify a source because of the multiplicity of parameters involved, slow down the obtaining of results even further (Fig. 3.6).

1. DNA is first cut by a specific restriction enzyme in appropriate conditions.
2. The millions of DNA fragments obtained are separated according to their size by electrophoretic migration in an agarose gel.
3. Prior to transfer, DNA is denatured, in other words rendered single-stranded by the immersion of gel in an alkaline solution.
4. In order to facilitate hybridization of the DNA contained in the gel with the probe, the DNA is blotted onto a nylon membrane which is stronger and easier to handle than the gel. There are a number of ways of anchoring the DNA, depending on the type of membrane, and thus allow repeated de-hybridization and hybridization, facilitating the study of the same membrane using numerous probes.
5. The filter is pre-hybridized with a solution containing substances that can attach to the filter in such a way that they prevent non-specific binding of the probes to the filters.
6. The radioactive probe is bound to the filter overnight and the unbound material is washed away with an appropriate saline solution.
7. The filter is exposed to a radio-sensitive film for a certain amount of time: a few hours to several days may be necessary for this autoradiography.

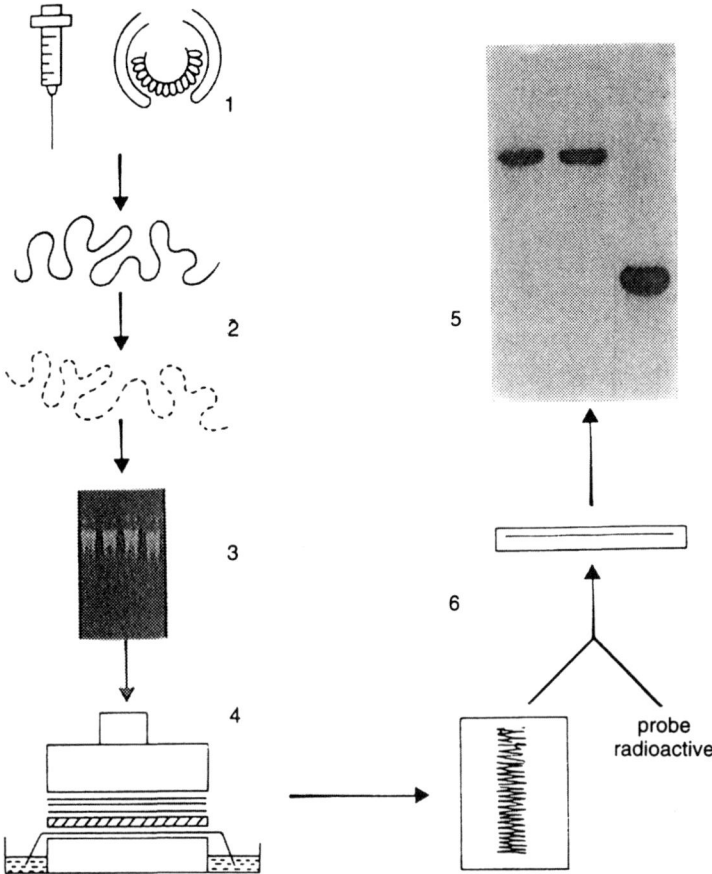

Fig. 3.6 Southern blot method. 1. DNA is prepared from a blood or villus sample. 2. High-molecular-weight DNA is cut by an appropriate restriction enzyme. 3. The fragments obtained are separated according to size by agarose gel electrophoresis. 4. The gel DNA is transferred to a nylon membrane. 5. The membrane DNA is hybridized with a radioactive probe. 6. DNA sequences which the probe hybridizes to are revealed by autoradiography.

8. The film is processed using fixing and developing agents which reveal in black the DNA fragment(s) which have attached to the probe.

Though a number of controls are done in conjunction with each test sample, none escapes the possibility of failure: this can be the result of degradation, contamination, incomplete digestion of DNA, or a weak signal due to a small quantity or poor quality poorly-labelled probe.

Pulsed-field gel electrophoresis   The principle behind this method is not very different from the Southern method just described. Instead of using restriction enzymes which cut the DNA into fragments smaller than 25–30 kb (the limit of the separation ability of the Southern method), the enzymes used cut DNA much less frequently, generating much larger fragments.

Despite the difficulty of migration of these large fragments in the agarose gel, one can nevertheless, with use of appropriate electrical fields, separate fragments of up to 5000 kb. The numerous methods published testify to the inherent difficulties of this technique, which none the less has the advantage of being able to examine larger areas of DNA using a single probe.

Studying mRNA

Unlike DNA which is present in all nucleated cells of the organism, mRNA is present only in those cells where a gene is expressed. Because of the omnipresence of ribonuclease, sterile precautions are necessary in order to prevent degradation; the biopsy sample should be immersed in liquid nitrogen as soon as possible.

Dot blot   The principle is the same as that used for DNA.

Northern blot   The term 'Northern blot' is a play on words. After Southern described hybridization of DNA on to filters, the term 'Northern blot' was given to the procedure of transfer of RNAs, separated by electrophoresis, on to filters and visualization by molecular hybridization. With this method, one can measure the size of RNA (the size of the fragment being inversely proportional to its electrophoretic mobility) and its concentration. The concentration can be estimated by the intensity of hybridization of a radiolabelled probe with an RNA sample on filter, without prior separation of the fragments (dot blot method). Electrophoresis takes place in conditions of denaturation. The quality of results depends on the quality and quantity of RNA obtained. Although the principle is identical to that of Southern blotting, there are nevertheless differences due to the fact that the nucleic acids are those of RNA not DNA.

Nuclease SI or RNase A mapping   These techniques allow the detection of sequence differences between a radioactive probe and the RNA under study. SI nuclease will cut a DNA probe if mismatching is greater than 3 bp, whereas RNase A will be able to cut the RNA probe even with a mismatch of 1 bp. This enzyme is particularly useful in studying a point mutation, whether hereditary or acquired (by activation of an oncogene). Measuring the intensity of the band in a nuclease SI protection assay is also an extremely sensitive method of detection and quantification of minority classes of RNAs.

These methods allow for detection of abnormal messenger RNA and elucidation of the mechanism of a hereditary disease.

Applications A disease caused by a congenital or acquired genetic mutation can be analysed at the level of the mutant gene product and its RNA when they are present, or directly at the gene level. However, this latter study is only possible when a probe recognizing the sequence of the gene is available; that is, when the gene is cloned. If the gene is not cloned, characterization or identification of the mutation is impossible. In that case an indirect approach is required, using marker genes relatively close on the chromosome to the unknown site of the mutant gene. This indirect approach is only useful when there is no doubt as to which chromosome the gene under study is localized.

Direct studies

Deletions and insertions

1. Small (several hundred to several thousand base pairs): When the mutation involves a sufficient number of base pairs it can easily be detected on a Southern blot. These mutations are associated with the loss or change in size of the fragment, revealed through molecular hybridization of radioactive probes specific to the normal gene (Fig. 3.7a, b).

2. Large (several thousand to a sub-chromosomal region): The loss of a large region will translate itself not through a quantitative change, but rather through a difference in intensity (Fig. 3.7c). This intensity difference in the fragment recognized by the probe can be measured. However, appreciation of the number of gene copies is not easy; it requires a statistical analysis relying on several measurements, and this is not therefore a method of choice for prenatal diagnosis.

Point mutations, microdeletions, or microinsertions

The identification of these requires much more sophisticated techniques.

1. *Building a DNA genomic library, screening for detection of a mutant clone, determination of base-pair sequences.* The method is cumbersome for large genes (close to 200 kb for the factor VIII gene and 2000 kb for the DMD gene). By using probes which recognize exons exclusively (for example, a DNA segment complementary to messenger RNA) it is possible to focus analysis on those, ignoring an intronic mutation which may lead to a splicing error.

2. *Digestion of DNA by various restriction enzymes*, each recognizing different sequences, and hybridization to Southern blot with specific probes (Fig. 3.8a). Although over 100 restriction enzymes are presently known, this method does not recognize all possible sequences! In addition, it is cumbersome and expensive. Finally, when an abnormal cleavage site is recognized (or loss of a normal cleavage site recognized) it is not possible to predict whether the change observed is due to the disease or simply to a coincidental polymorphism.

3. *Protection assay against RNase A digestion of a genomic DNA/RNA hybrid* (Fig. 3.8b). This method uses RNA probes made available in recent years by the construction of plasmids containing a transcription initiating site, the transcription being carried out with a very specific RNA polymerase. Once this RNA

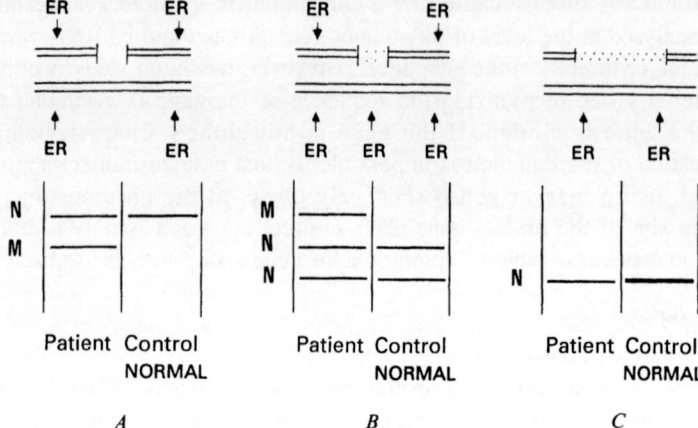

Fig. 3.7 Detection of deletions. Depending on the position and size of the deletion or insertion (M), the DNA fragment resulting from restriction enzyme digestion (ER) will be either smaller than the normal fragment (N) [situation *(A)*] or larger [situation *(B)*], or will not be qualitatively detectable by the probe [situation *(C)*].

is rendered radioactive and hybridized to a complementary DNA strand, it becomes insensitive to RNase A digestion. However, the mismatch of only 1 bp results at this level in a cleavage site that is easily recognized because of modification of the size of the RNA. This relatively new method undoubtedly holds great promise. It should permit the analysis of any uncloned genomic DNA fragment, when complementary probes are available. However, even though this method may indicate the site of the mutation it does not reveal its nature; elucidation of this requires the sequencing of the cloned mutated fragment.

4. *Search for a mutation at a known site by synthetic oligonucleotides* (Fig. 3.8c). Certain mutations are frequent (for example, thalassemias, mutations of codons 12 and 61 of the *c-ras* oncogene in cancers) and therefore the problem is to determine the existence of such mutations and not to screen the whole gene. Oligonucleotides of 17–18 bp are used. Their hybridization to a totally homologous sequence is significantly more stable than that with a sequence having even one modified base pair, and this allows one to rapidly explore the existence of a sequence mutation, as well as identifying its nature.

5. *Amplification of the mutated region* (Fig. 3.8d) This method, (polymerase chain reaction, PCR) consists of amplifying the mutant region several thousand times over by recopying it, using nucleotide primers. This technique facilitates all earlier methods for fine characterization of mutant regions. As in the previous technique described, one is looking for particular mutations previously characterized in other cases. This technique, which requires being able to synthesize the oligonucleotides serving as primers, can only be applied once the precise

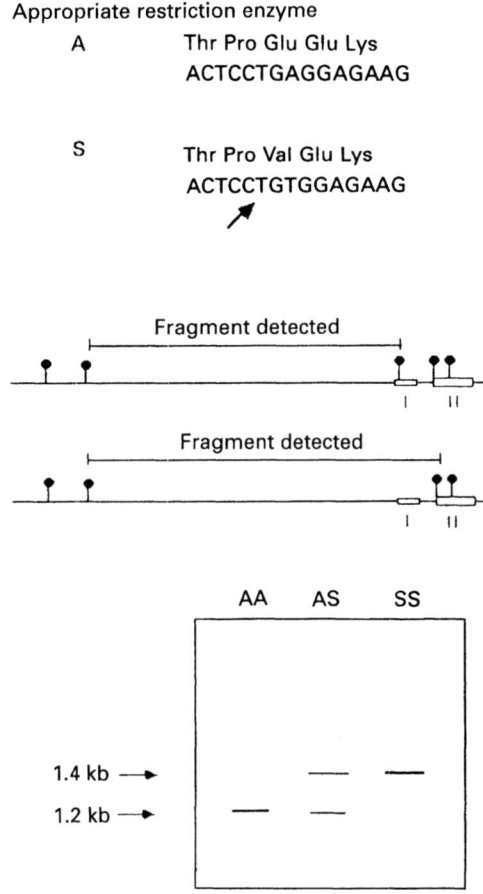

Appropriate restriction enzyme

A   Thr Pro Glu Glu Lys
         ACTCCTGAGGAGAAG

S   Thr Pro Val Glu Lys
         ACTCCTGTGGAGAAG

Fragment detected

Fragment detected

AA   AS   SS

1.4 kb →

1.2 kb →

Fig. 3.8a Detection of point mutations using a restriction enzyme whose restriction site has been modified by the mutation. Here, the MstII enzyme no longer recognizes the characteristic sequence of haemoglobin β^S and the restriction fragment is longer (1.4 kb) than the fragment obtained with normal haemoglobin β^A (1.2 kb).

region of the gene to be amplified is identified, around which the appropriate nucleotides can be placed.

In summary, it must be remembered that precise identification of a known gene mutation is now always possible. Some techniques are relatively simple and can be applied to a large number of samples (identifying a deletion or a 'known' mutation using synthetic oligonucleotides), others remain very cumbersome and are the exclusive domain of experienced laboratories. This must be borne in mind each time a point mutation in an unknown gene site is being looked for.

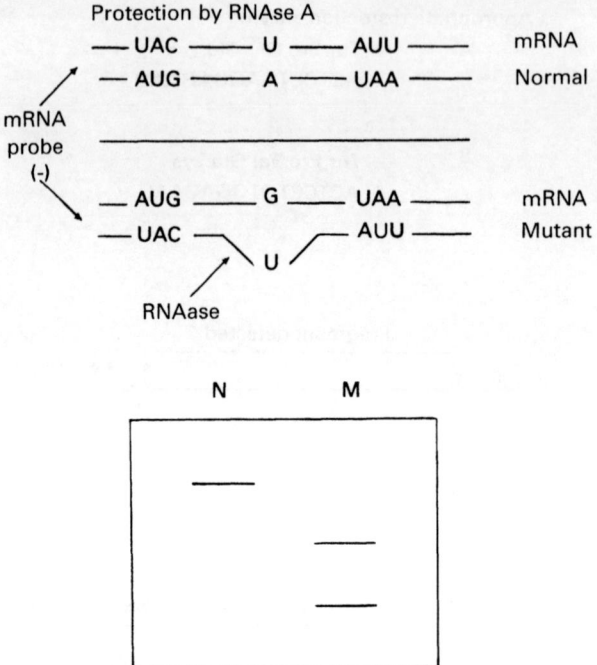

Fig. 3.8b Detection of point mutations by digestion with RNAase. If the message is normal, the cRNA probe binds perfectly and the message is protected from digestion by RNAase A (specific to single-stranded RNA). When the RNA message is mutant, binding at the mutation is not possible and the probe is cleaved by RNAase A. Fragments are submitted to electrophoresis (Northern), and demonstrate cleavage when there is a mutation.

Indirect analysis

Restriction fragment length polymorphisms (RFLPs)   One of the more spectacular breakthroughs in terms of genetic diagnosis was the use of restriction fragment length polymorphisms as genetic markers of a disease.

DNA differs from one individual to another, at the level of the gene which forms the basis of their individuality, as well as in their intergenic sequences. Variability is even more striking in the non-coding, non-regulatory sequences (where mutations can accumulate without consequence) than in the gene exons (coding regions) and control regions of gene expression.

Between two individuals, this variability in DNA at a same locus may change the recognition site of different enzymes and therefore their cleavage sites. In this first kind of polymorphism there are two different alleles, A_1 or A_2, (Fig. 3.9a) with individuals being homozygote A_1A_1, A_2A_2 or heterozygote A_1A_2. The frequency of heterozygotes, A_1A_2, in the population, may reach a maximum of 50 per cent. In practice, in order to use an informative marker the frequency of heterozygotes must be higher than 10 per cent.

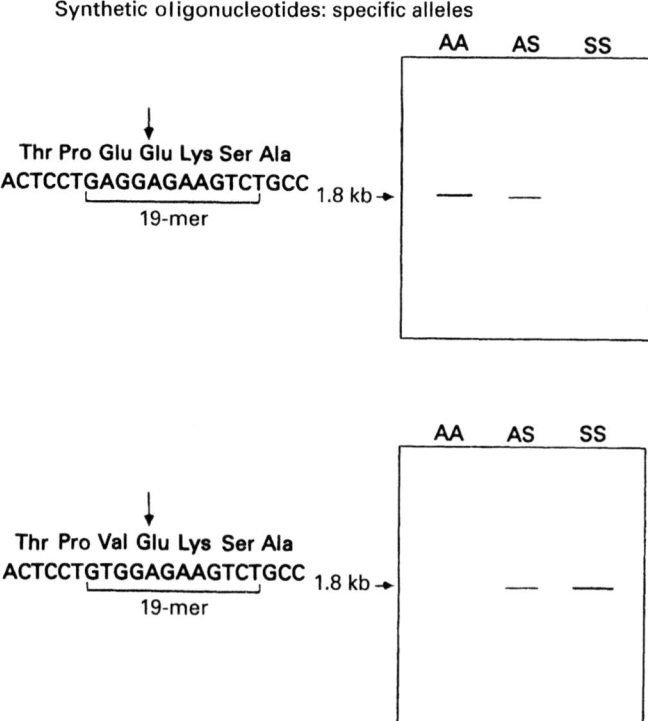

Fig. 3.8c Detection of a particular point mutation by Southern blot hybridization using synthetic oligonucleotides. Nineteen-residue oligonucleotides complementary to the region under study are synthesized and are constructed in such a way that the altered base is found in the middle of the oligonucleotide. These oligonucleotides specific to the normal gene will hybridize with a normal fragment but not with the fragment corresponding to the mutant area. An oligonucleotide complementary to the mutant gene will hybridize with the mutant gene but not with the normal gene.

Another type of polymorphism in the non-coding regions is the existence of variable-number tandem repeats. Here it is the size of the fragment between two restriction sites which varies depending on the insertion or deletion of a variable number of tandem repeats between individuals (Fig. 3.9b). In this second type of polymorphism there may be a large number of different alleles. As each individual has two alleles, one of maternal and one of paternal origin, the proportion of heterozygotes may be larger and in some instances may be as high as 90 per cent. This type of marker may be much more informative.

Phenotype–genotype relationship It is important to point out that the nature of these markers has nothing to do with the gene mutation causing the disease. The only relationship between this random change at the DNA level and the gene

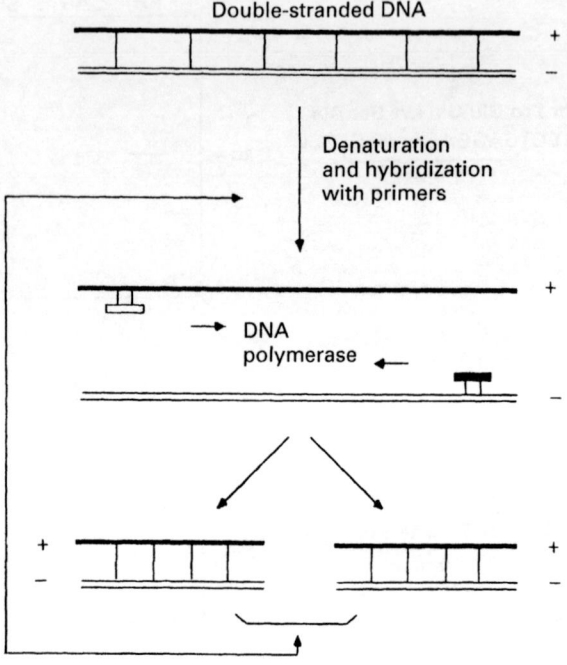

Fig. 3.8d Detection of point mutations by amplification of a particular region of genomic DNA. The two strands of these regions are separated by denaturation, and then combined with oligonucleotides which are perfectly complementary to one end of each strand. These oligonucleotides serve as primers for DNA polymerase, which will re-copy each of the strands. Therefore after the first cycle, there are two exact double-stranded copies of the DNA region. By denaturing these two copies and re-copying in the presence of primers and radioactively labelled oligonucleotide, one can obtain four, eight, ... copies.

itself is their close proximity on the chromosome. When it is impossible directly to identify the gene or its mutated state, one takes advantage of the marker to distinguish the chromosomal segment adjacent to the normal gene from that region surrounding the mutated gene. There remains a risk that a similar genetic defect could be due to a so far undetected or undetectable gene mutation. Figure 3.10 illustrates the different possibilities.

I An alteration in a structural gene leads to a particular phenotype, for example HbS and sickle cell anaemia.

II Different mutations in the same structural gene leads to phenotype A, B, or C, all different from one another. For example, point mutations of the β-globin gene which may lead to unstable haemoglobin, sickle cell anaemia, or methemoglobinaemia.

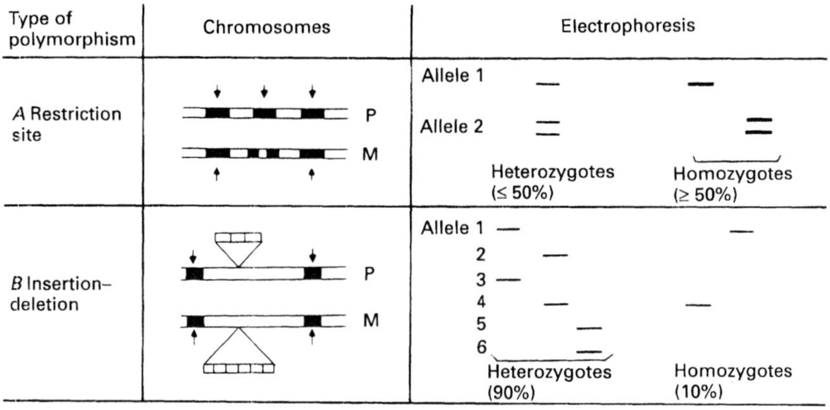

Type of polymorphism	Chromosomes	Electrophoresis		
A Restriction site	[P chromosome with arrows] P [M chromosome with arrows] M	Allele 1 — Allele 2 ═	— ═ Heterozygotes (≤ 50%)	Homozygotes (≥ 50%)
B Insertion–deletion	[P chromosome with insertion] P [M chromosome with deletion] M	Allele 1 — 2 — 3 — 4 — 5 — 6 ═	Heterozygotes (90%)	— — Homozygotes (10%)

Fig. 3.9 Two kinds of polymorphisms. *(a)*, restriction site polymorphisms; *(b)*, insertion–deletion polymorphisms; P and M represent chromosomes of paternal or maternal origin respectively.

III An alteration in two different structural genes may lead to a similar phenotype, for example haemolytic anaemia due to a defect in one of the enzymes of the glycolysis pathway.

IV The product of a structural gene (A) may be altered by post-transcriptional or post-translational modifications. These modifications may be controlled by the product of other structural genes, B or C, which may themselves be modified by mutation. The phenotype, being the net result of the alteration in the gene product, will be the same. Examples are the diseases due to collagen abnormalities.

These examples emphasize the danger of over-reliance on DNA markers when the culprit gene cannot be identified with certainty.

Obviously, because of the crossing-over phenomenon, resulting in exchange

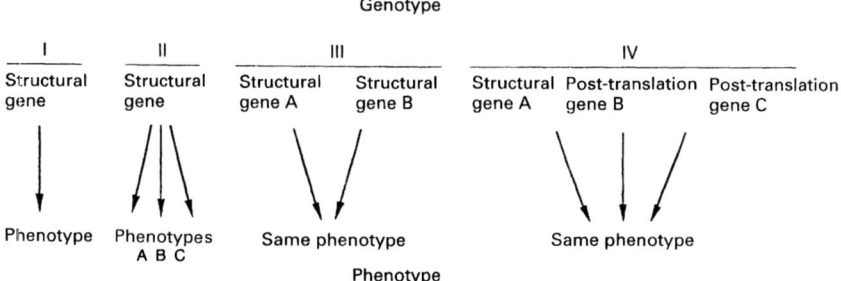

Fig. 3.10 Phenotype–genotype relationships.

of maternal and paternal homologues during meiosis, the DNA marker must be as close as possible to the gene itself.

Here we will examine two different situations:

1. The marker being used is either intragenic or so close to the gene that the probability of crossing-over is almost nil.
2. The gene itself is not known, but it has been mapped on the chromosome. One can then consider the use of DNA markers located on the same chromosome region.

Cloned gene   The use of RFLPs provides another genetic approach when the mutation is different from one family to the other and the use of synthetic oligonucleotides is therefore impossible, or when the mutation site cannot be recognized by the restriction enzyme, but after analysis of the protein product the mutation is shown to be in the gene itself. Two approaches may be considered.

Family studies   Figure 3.11 illustrates the use of RFLPs to study the segregation of the mutated gene. A comparison of polymorphic alleles (A_1 and A_2) in normal and affected individuals shows that the disease gene co-segregates with the A_1 allele. It then becomes possible, after study of fetal DNA, to assess whether it has inherited from its affected mother the chromosome carrying the A_1 allele (mutated gene) or the chromosome carrying the A_2 allele (normal gene). From this analysis one can determine whether the fetus is affected (A_1) or unaffected (A_2). As this DNA marker has no relationship whatsoever to the disease, it is obvious that, in another family, the disease may travel with the A_2 form of the allele. This approach therefore requires a family study to assess which marker allele segregates with the disease allele.

Linkage disequilibrium   For certain diseases, it has been possible to demonstrate (in a particular geographical area or ethnic group) that the disease gene is preferentially associated (always or most often) to a particular marker allele or to several neighbouring alleles on the same chromosome forming a specific haplotype (e.g. A-b-C-d-E) retrievable with a different frequency in individuals carrying the mutation. One can take advantage of this preferential association, called linkage disequilibrium, to detect heterozygous individuals, particularly in the case of recessive diseases. One can indeed provide an explanation for this preferential association: for a given geographical area the carriers all descend from the same ancestor (who may be very distant) and have all inherited the same mutation, even if they are not related. The recognition of an association between a particular haplotype and sickle cell disease allowed for identification of individuals at risk (Kan and Dozy 1978). However, once mixing of populations occurs it is important to extend the study to include several affected and normal individuals of the same ethnic origin.

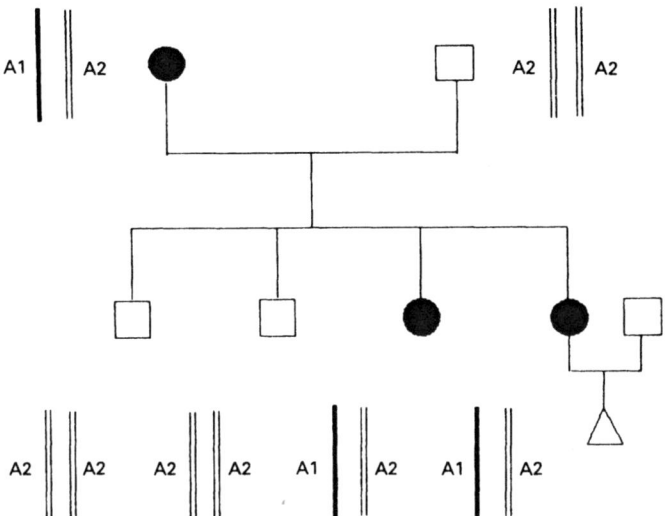

Fig. 3.11 Studying the transmission of a trait using RFLPs.

Non-cloned gene   Though rapid progress has permitted cloning and mapping of several hundred genes during the last 10 years, the identification of unknown genes for which only chromosome location is known remains difficult although it is possible.

Reverse genetics positional cloning   This method, which proceeds from the initial mapping of the disease on a chromosomal segment to the isolation of the gene and its corresponding protein, was successful for retinoblastoma, chronic granulomatosis disease, Duchenne muscular dystrophy, cystic fibrosis and myotonic dystrophy. Similarly, although the initial localization of the Huntington's disease gene on to chromosome 4 was in 1983 (Gusella *et al.*), the gene and associated mutation were not described until 1993 (Huntington's Disease Collaborative Research Group).

Gene mapping   The necessary but insufficient condition for considering the diagnosis of a disease for which the gene has not been cloned is that its chromosomal map be known. This mapping relies on the existence, in affected individuals, of a chromosomal rearrangement specific to a chromosomal region, for example deletion 13q14 and retinoblastoma. These chromosomal abnormalities are rare, and more often than not family studies are required.

Linkage studies   On the same lines as family studies undertaken until recently, using blood group markers or HLA antigens, these linkage studies are now carried out with RFLPs. Because of the 2000 anonymous DNA markers and the hundreds of mapped and cloned genes, the ability to identify a link between a marker gene and a disease gene has almost doubled. Once this link is established it is necessary to determine the position of the marker or markers relative to the disease gene; that is, whether they are centromeric or telomeric. These studies also provide an estimate of their genetic distance, which is directly proportional to the observed meiotic recombination. Generally, although the genetic distance is proportional to the physical distance, one must consider that the ratio between these two factors may vary with the sex of the individual, the chromosome, or chromosome region, and finally that variation may exist between two individuals.

Prerequisites to performing prenatal diagnosis are the following:

1. *Markers* have to be close, informative and numerous, and surrounding the gene.

2. *The family has to be informative and accessible*, and a diagnosis of heterozygosity must be possible.

3. *Establishing the phase* is the recognition of the marker allele travelling with the disease, possible through a preliminary family study only if the key individual is a double heterozygote: heterozygous for the disease mutation and heterozygous for the polymorphism recognized by the marker. One can then determine in the progeny which marker allele is present in children carrying the disease gene and/or which marker allele is present in the children carrying the normal gene. Should an individual not be heterozygous for a first tested marker, one would test that individual for further markers until an appropriate one was found. Hence the necessity to have available a sufficient number of close and informative markers (Fig. 3.12).

4. *The informativeness of a probe* depends on the frequency of the different alleles: for a two-allele polymorphism the maximum frequency of heterozygosity is 50 per cent if the frequency of each allele is almost identical. The frequency of heterozygosity is even lower when one of the alleles is rare in the population.

For multiallelic polymorphisms, since a person cannot have more than two alleles (one on the paternal chromosome and one on the maternal chromosome), the frequency of heterozygosity, which can reach more than 90 per cent, will also be dependent on the frequency of each of the alleles.

5. *The detection of heterozygotes for the disease gene* is hindered by several factors which depend most often on what the disease is and in particular on the mode of inheritance. Phase determination then relies on the family study and obviously on the accessibility of key individuals. As a rule of thumb, the affected parent(s) must be heterozygous for the marker. This, however, is not sufficient, because, depending on the disease's mode of inheritance, the spouse (healthy or not) should fulfil certain criteria. Moreover, for phase determination, grandparents must be studied and, particularly if the child is deceased, it is necessary to know which grandparent is carrier of the mutant gene. If these criteria are not fulfilled, diagnosis is more difficult.

6. *Autosomal dominant inheritance*. By definition, carriers are affected. However, because of incomplete penetrance the disease may not be expressed, or variable expressivity may make the diagnosis difficult. Certain conditions

PHASE

Distribution of alleles on both chromosomes

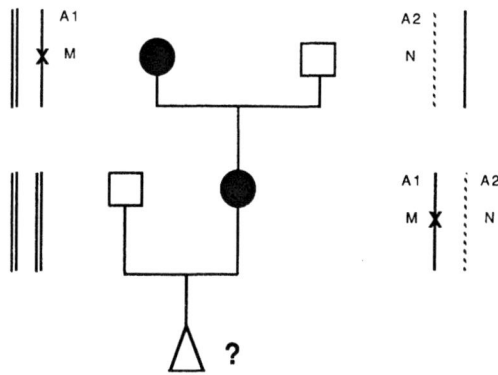

Fig. 3.12 Definition of phase. The individual must be doubly heterozygous for the marker and the disease, in order for the two chromosomes to be differentiated. The diagram shows the distribution of different alleles on the two chromosomes.

may be of late onset (Huntington's chorea) and it is not always possible to determine whether a young apparently healthy individual is affected. Here, the informativeness rests on the heterozygosity of the affected parent. The healthy parent may have any genotype except one: he/she cannot have the same alleles as the affected parent unless the affected child is homozygote (Fig. 3.13*A*, *B*). If the affected child is deceased, the grandparent's genotype must determine the phase. The grandparent's genotype must also be informative for the marker and disease alleles (Fig. 3.13*C*).

7. *Autosomal recessive inheritance.* By definition carriers are healthy and, in general, not detected clinically. Only a laboratory analysis will allow for a qualitative or quantitative measure of the gene product permitting diagnosis (example: a 50 per cent decrease in enzymatic activity or an abnormal electrophoretic migration). In order to provide a diagnosis parents must be heterozygous for different alleles or, when heterozygous for the same allele, the affected child must be homozygous for one or the other allele. Here, one must establish two types of phase: the allele associated with the mother's mutant gene and that associated with the father's mutant gene. This is why the affected child's DNA must be available for study (Fig. 3. 14). If the child is deceased, study of the grandparents may allow phase determination. In the case of consanguinity only one type of phase need be determined.

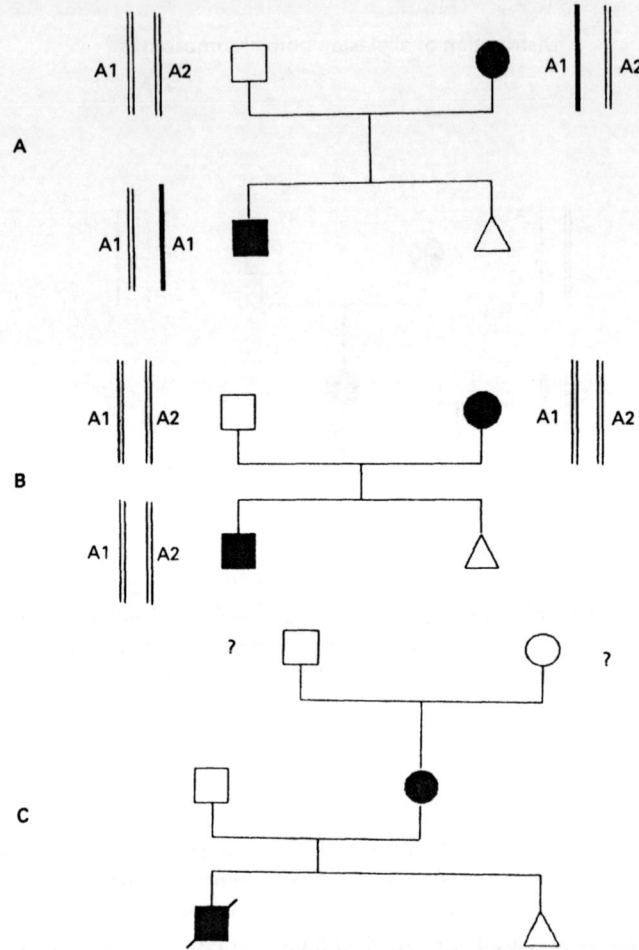

Fig. 3.13 Definition of phase: autosomal dominant. *(A)*. Diagnosis possible for the current pregnancy. *(B)*. Diagnosis not possible for the current pregnancy because it is impossible to predict the maternal or paternal origin of alleles A1 A2 present in either parent. *(C)*. Diagnosis not possible. Phase cannot be determined: (1) the affected child is deceased, (2) grandparents are apparently healthy. It may be a new mutation, or the affected grandparent may be asymptomatic because of incomplete penetrance.

8. *X-Linked recessive inheritance*. All male carriers are affected. Depending on the disease in question, and due to random X-inactivation, a certain number of female carriers do not show any signs of disease. Detection of heterozygotes rests on subtle or even absent clinical findings. For prenatal diagnosis of male fetuses, study of the father is useless as he would have transmitted his Y chromosome and not his X chromosome. Only the mother must be heterozygous

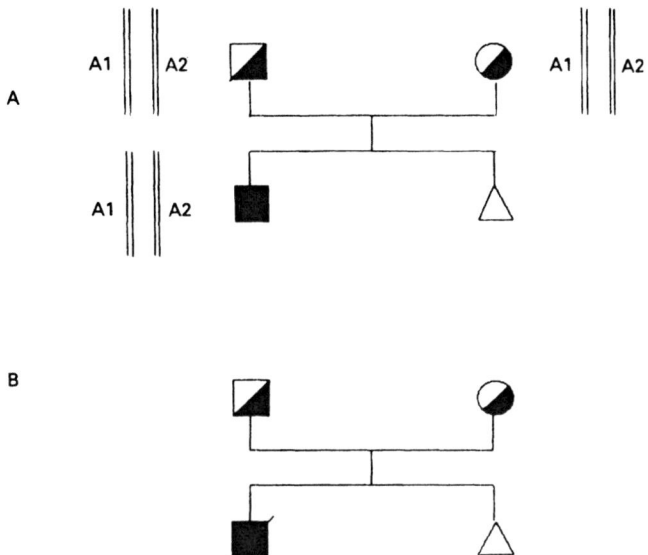

Fig. 3.14 Definition of phase: autosomal recessive. *(A).* Diagnosis impossible: neither phase can be identified. (B). Diagnosis impossible: affected child deceased.

for one marker. For phase determination one must be able to study either the grandparents, or male individuals of the family, and in their absence, women for whom the carrier status is known. If grandparents are available, the disease may be inherited from the grandfather and therefore transmitted by his X chromosome to all of his daughters, or may be inherited from the grandmother (Fig. 3.15). Though one cannot describe all possible situations here, these general rules and the few illustrated examples demonstrate the difficulties and even impossibility of establishing such a diagnosis if there is not a sufficient number of individuals to determine phase, or a sufficient number of markers to satisfy all prerequisites. It is therefore apparent that, in order to meet all requirements, time is essential: time to collect samples from all necessary individuals, time for clinical examinations permitting identification of heterozygotes or those with variable expression of the disease, time to study these subjects with different probes. The cost of such tests justifies attention to limiting time and expense by judiciously selecting the individuals initially studied in order not to conduct useless studies of individuals with uninformative probes which will not contribute any relevant information to the diagnosis.

Conclusion

The simplicity of blood sampling should not allow one to forget the difficulties mentioned here, which render this type of study completely different from the lab-

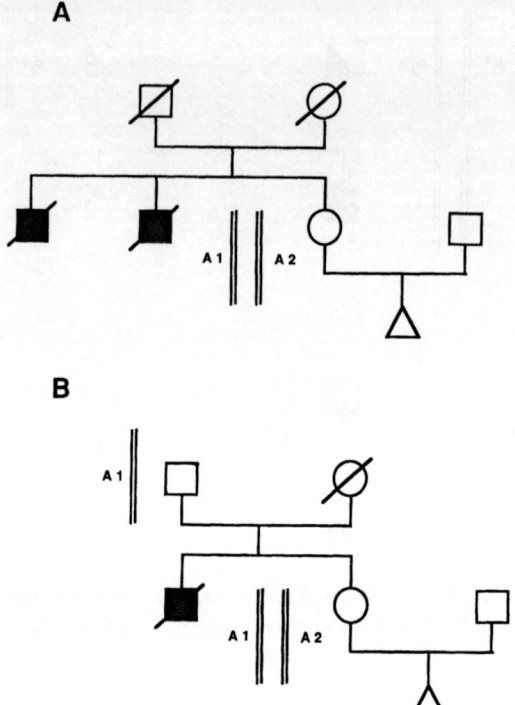

Fig. 3.15 Definition of phase: X-linked recessive. (A). Diagnosis impossible: key individuals (grandparents, parents, and affected uncles) are deceased. (B). Diagnosis possible; the chromosome carrying allele A_1 must carry the normal gene from the unaffected father.

oratory analyses previously used. The notion of a 'result' must also be revised. These studies involve different stages which are negotiated step by step and therefore do not allow for a definitive result, or at least an absolute certainty, when an indirect approach with RFLPs is used.

References and further reading

Chromosomal analysis

Boué, J., Nicolas, H., Barichard, F., *et al.* (1979). Le clonage des cellules du liquide amniotique, aide dans l'interprétation des mosaïques chromosomiques en diagnostic prénatal. *Ann. Genet.*, **22**, 3–9.

De Grouchy, J. and Turleau, C. (1982). *Atlas des maladies chromosomiques*, 2nd edn. Exp. Scient., Paris.

Gusella, J. F., Wexler, N. S., Conneally, P. M., *et al.* (1983). A polymorphic DNA marker genetically linked to Huntington's disease. *Nature*, **306**, 234–8.

Gosden, J. R., Gosden, C. M., Christie, S., *et al.* (1984). The use of cloned Y chromosome-specific DNA probes for fetal sex determination in first trimester prenatal diagnosis. *Hum. Genet.*, **66**, 347–51.

Gray, J. W., Trask, B., Vand den Engh, G., *et al.* (1988). Application of flow karyotyping in prenatal detection of chromosome aberrations. *Am. J. Hum Genet.*, **42**, 49–59.

Huntington's Disease Collar borative Research Group (1993). A novel gene containing a trinucleotide repeat that is expanded and unstable on Huntington's disease chromosomes. *Cell*, **72**, 971–83.

Junien, C., Bazin, A., Guyot, B., *et al.* (1986). Rapid prenatal diagnosis of Down's syndrome with in-situ hybridization of fluorescent DNA probes. *Lancet*, **ii**, 863–4.

Kan, Y. W. and Dozy, A. M. (1978). Polymorphisms of DNA sequence adjacent to human beta globin structural gene: relationship to sickle cell mutations. *Proc. Natl. Acad. Sci.*, USA, **75**, 5631–5.

Biochemical analysis of fetal samples

Boué A., Muller, F., Nezelof, C., *et al.* (1986). Prenatal diagnosis in 200 pregnancies with a 1-in-4 risk of cystic fibrosis. *Hum. Genet.*, **74**, 288–97.

Daffos, F., Forestier, F., Capella-Pavlovsky, M., *et al.* (1984). Diagnostic prénatal. In *EMC Obstétrique*, Paris, 6.

Karnovsky, M. J. and Roots, L. A. (1964). 'Direct coloring' thiocholine method for cholinesterases. *J. Histochem. Cytochem.*, **12**, 219–21.

Laurell, C. B. (1966). Quantitative estimation of protein by electrophoresis in agarose gel containing antibodies. *Ann. Biochem.*, **15**, 45–52.

Muller, F., Dumez, Y., and Massoulie, J. (1985). Molecular forms and solubility of acetyl-cholinesterase during the embryonic development of rat and human brain. *Brain Res.*, **331**, 295–301.

Muller, F., Cedard, L., Boué, J., *et al.* (1986). Diagnostic prénatal de fermeture du tube neural. Intérêt de l'éctrophorese des cholinestérases. *Presse Med.*, **15**, 783–6.

Muller, F., Oury, J. F., Dumez, Y., *et al.* (1988). Microvillar enzyme assays in amniotic fluid and fetal tissues at different stages of development. *Prenat. Diagn.*, **8**, 189–98.

PART II PREDICTABLE RISK OF ANOMALY

Introduction

It is important to consider prenatal diagnosis within the framework of birth defects.

Frequency of congenital malformations and genetic disorders

Data from the European Surveillance Program based on 770 000 births from 1980–1983 in 17 European centres (Dewals and Lechat, 1986), provides an assessment of different types of malformations observed at birth (Table I).

Other major childhood diseases are not always observable at birth, for example genetic diseases such as inborn errors of metabolism and myopathies. Table II gives some figures for the more common ones.

Table I Frequency of congenital anomalies in 17 European registries from 1980 to 1983. (Dewals and Lechat 1986)

Anomalies	Number per 10 000 births	
Nervous system malformations	31.4	
Anencephaly		8.2
Spina bifida		10.9
Encephalocoele		1.8
Hydrocephaly		5.1
Microcephaly		3.3
Cardiovascular malformations	52.1	
Digestive system malformations	19.0	
Malformations of external genitalia	17.6	
Hypospadias		10.5
Genitourinary malformations	12.4	
Renal agenesis		3.4
Cleft lip and palate	15.1	
Limb malformations	59.1	
Musculoskeletal malformations	32.1	
Duodenal wall (pyloric)		6.1
Diaphragm		2.7
Eye malformations	5.8	
Ear malformations	8.1	
Total proportion of births with malformations	226	

Table II Diseases with Mendelian inheritance

Disease	Incidence
Autosomal recessive inheritance	
Cystic fibrosis	1/2000
Phenylketonuria	1/15 000
21-Hydroxylase deficiency	1/7000
Mucopolysaccharidosis (all types)	1/2500
Galactosemia	
Branched-chain ketoaciduria	< 1/100 000
Methylmalonic acidemia	
X-linked recessive inheritance	
Duchenne muscular dystrophy	1/7000
Haemophilia	1/10 000
Autosomal dominant inheritance	
Huntington's chorea	1/5000
Polycystic kidney disease	1/3500
Steinert's myotonic dystrophy	1/5000

Mode of inheritance of congenital anomalies

It is estimated that about 3 per cent of live births have a major birth defect. Knowledge of their mode of inheritance is essential to establish risks for future pregnancies and to anticipate management of these pregnancies. Chromosomal anomalies account for 15–20 per cent of the total number of congenital anomalies: different types of anomaly are shown in Table 4.1. The great majority (90 per cent) of chromosomal anomalies with clinical consequences are changes in the *number* of chromosomes in offspring of parents with normal karyotypes. Only some unbalanced chromosome rearrangements, about 5 per cent, result from mal-segregation of a balanced chromosomal rearrangement carried by one of the parents. Mendelian disorders represent approximately 15 per cent of birth defects. Those genetic disorders that may lead to prenatal diagnosis are transmitted mainly in two ways: by autosomal recessive inheritance, or by X-linked recessive inheritance. In fact, for the vast majority of birth defects the mode of inheritance or cause remains unknown. For some, genetic factors are suspected even though the nature of the condition is not clear (neural tube defects, certain cardiac malformations). For other malformations the cause remains unknown and recurrence risks have not been established.

In practice, it is only for a certain number of birth defects with known recurrence risks, that a prenatal diagnosis can be offered to couples early in pregnancy. This is well illustrated by a survey of the French prenatal diagnosis centres (Table III).

Between 1981 and 1987, cytogenetic analyses represented, a total of 60 000 diagnoses, 50 000 for maternal age (14 000 diagnoses in 1987 alone), 7000 in which the indication was a previous child with a numerical chromosomal

Table III Diagnoses carried out between 1972 and 1988
by the Laboratoire Unité 73, INSERM

Inborn errors of metabolism	Amniotic fluid sampling	Chorionic villus sampling	Total
Lysosomal disorders			
Sphingolipidoses			
Tay–Sachs	10	7	17
Sandhoff	4	5	9
Landing	9	5	14
Gaucher	8	8	16
Niemann–Pick	10	3	13
Krabbe	19	5	24
Fabry	2	3	5
Metachromatic leucodystrophy	15	12	27
Wolman	2	0	2
Mucopolysaccharidoses			
Type I(Hurler)	18	4	32
Type II(Hunter)	21	18	39
Type III(San Filippo)	3	2	5
Type IV(Morquio)	2	0	2
Type VI(Maroteaux–Lamy)	2	0	2
Type VII(β-Glucuronidase deficiency)	1	0	1
Glycoproteinoses			
Fucosidosis	2	0	2
Mannosidosis	2	2	4
Mucolipidosis type II	5	4	9
Sialidosis	2	0	2
Glycogenoses			
Type II(Pompe)	17	8	25
Pyruvate carboxylase deficiency	2	0	2
Galactosemia	6	0	6
Peroxysomal diseases			
Zellweger	0	6	6
Adrenoleucodystrophy (autosomal recessive)	0	1	1
Adrenoleucodystrophy (X-linked)	0	6	6
Refsum	0	2	2
Aminoacidopathies			
Methylmalonic acidemia	11	2	13
Propionic acidemia	4	4	8
Glutaric acidemia	5	0	5
Orotic aciduria	0	1	1
Argininosuccinic aciduria	5	1	6
Citrullinemia	7	2	9
Branched-chain ketoaciduria	12	4	16
Tyrosinaemia	4	2	6

Table III *cont'd.*

Homocystinuria	0	1	1
Xanthene oxidase deficiency	3	2	5
Nucleic acid disorders			
Lesch–Nyhan	20	10	30
Xeroderma pigmentosa	7	4	11
Disorders of mineral metabolism			
Menkes	5	7	12
Porphyria			
Günther	2	0	2
Methemoglobinaemia	7	0	7
21-Hydroxylase deficiency	75	32	107
Total	328	173	512
Cystic fibrosis	400	20	430
Muscular dystrophy (Duchenne, Becker)	118	150	268
(sex determination followed by DNA studies)			
Haemophilia	79	10	89
(sex determination followed by DNA studies			
Chromosomal anomalies	10 000		

anomaly, and 3000 where one parent carried a balanced chromosomal rearrangement.

For inborn errors of metabolism, the number of prenatal diagnoses in 1981–1987 was 800 (150 diagnoses in 1986 and 1987) and there were 100 diagnoses of cystic fibrosis for 1984–1987. Diagnoses relying on molecular biology (haemoglobinopathy, haemophilias, myopathies, 21-hydroxylase deficiencies, cystic fibrosis) represent approximately 200–300 analyses per year.

Other more sophisticated diagnoses — immunodeficiency, skin disorders — account for about 10 diagnoses. Table III summarizes the diagnoses performed from 1972 to 1988 by INSERM Unit 73, and carried out by that laboratory or in collaboration with other laboratories. The great variation in the frequency of the various tests requested is obvious.

References

Dewals, P. and Lechat, M. (1986). Surveillance of congenital anomalies, years 1980–1983 (Eurocat I). Department of Epidemiology, Catholic University of Louvain.

4 Chromosomal anomalies

Definitions and mechanisms

Chromosomal anomalies can be of *number* or of *structure*.

Numerical chromosomal anomalies

The cause of numerical chromosomal anomaly is a mechanical error, either at the time of gametogenesis, at conception or during first division of the zygote. The majority of parents are chromosomally normal.

Error during gametogenesis At the first or second meiotic division, segregation of one particular chromosome may go awry; rather than two gametes with 23 chromosomes each there is one with 22 and one with 24. These gametes then fuse with a normal gamete, resulting in a *monosomic* (45 chromosomes) or *trisomic* (47 chromosomes) conceptus. Of all the numerical anomalies, it is this abnormal segregation or chromosomal non-dysjunction which is most frequent. Thanks to fluorescent heteromorphisms, it is possible to determine the maternal or paternal origin of the additional chromosome and to determine whether the error occurred in the first or second meiotic division. This has been particularly studied in trisomy 21: all four possible outcomes have been observed, but errors in the maternal first meiotic division are the most frequent, accounting for about two-thirds of all observations.

During meiotic division an error involving a whole chromosome set can result in a diploid gamete (46 chromosomes), which after fusion with a normal gamete will result in a triploid zygote (69 chromosomes) by diandry or digyni depending on whether the error occurred in spermatogenesis or oogenesis.

Error at the time of conception Dispermy, resulting from the fertilization of one egg by two spermatozoa, leads to a triploid zygote.

Error in early division of the zygote A tetraploid zygote (92 chromosomes) results from a division of chromosomes in the absence of cell division (meoisis without mitosis). Segregation errors of a chromosome during the early mitotic divisions result in several different types of *mosaic*: in other words, a zygote with cell populations having different chromosomal complements, normal and abnormal.

Structural chromosomal anomalies

Structural anomalies due to chromosome breaks may involve one or several chromosomes, homologous or not, resulting in abnormal rearrangement of the chromosomes. These structural anomalies may be *de novo*, where the parents are chromosomally normal and the event has occurred during maternal or paternal gametogenesis, or inherited from one of the parents carrying a balanced rearrangement. About 50 per cent of the observed chromosomal rearrangements are inherited.

Deletions   A deletion — loss of a chromosomal fragment — results in a partial monosomy for this chromosomal region and for the genes within it.

Duplication   Duplication of a chromosomal segment results in a partial trisomy. Identification of the precise origin of this fragment is possible with molecular cytogenetics or when this aberration is transmitted (see translocation).

Inversions   Inversions mostly occur around the centromere. They are pericentric, and there is no loss of genetic material, but gene sequences are inverted.

Translocations   These involve an exchange of chromosomal material between two chromosomes.

1. *Robertsonian translocations* involve two acrocentric chromosomes which fuse at the centromere. There is therefore a 45-chromosome complement, two acrocentric chromosomes being replaced by one metacentric chromosome.

2. *Reciprocal translocations* result from the breakage of two different chromosomes and exchange of the fragments so formed. Should there be no loss of genetic material at break points, the genetic complement is complete although arranged differently; the individual still has 46 chromosomes.

Structural rearrangements such as translocations or inversions, which in a balanced state are without phenotypic consequence in the individual, might be transmitted in an unbalanced form during gametogenesis. These structural rearrangements are not rare. In the general population, a balanced translocation is observed in 1 in 550 individuals and an inversion of chromosome 9 is observed in 1 in 100 individuals.

Incidence of chromosomal anomalies

Frequency of chromosomal anomalies in the liveborn

Systematic chromosomal analysis of over 50 000 live births has permitted assessment of the incidence of chromosomal anomalies (Table 4.1). These are found in 1/175 live births. Some are without any phenotypic consequence: these

Table 4.1 Incidence of chromosomal anomalies at birth

Chromosomal anomalies	Males (per cent)	Females (per cent)	Both sexes (per cent)
Anomalies of number			
Sex chromosomes			
47XYY	0.93 ⎫		1.3 ⎫
47XXY	0.93 ⎬ 2.6		
Others	0.74 ⎭		⎬ 2.05 ⎫
45X		0.10 ⎫	
47XXX		1.04 ⎬ 1.5	
Others		0.37 ⎭	0.75 ⎭ ⎬ 3.49
Autosomes			
47,+21			1.25 ⎫
			⎬ 1.44
Others			0.19 ⎭ ⎭ ⎫
Anomalies of structure			⎬ 6.04
Balanced			
Robertsonian			0.72 ⎫
DqDq			0.19 ⎬ 1.95 ⎫
DqGq			0.84 ⎬
Reciprocal			0.20 ⎭ ⎬ 2.55
Others			
Unbalanced			
Translocations			0.19 ⎫
			⎬ 0.60 ⎭
Others			0.41 ⎭

are balanced chromosome translocations. Others have varying consequences: such as the sex chromosome anomalies, 47,XXX and 47,XYY. Finally, others are associated with major anomalies: autosomal trisomies and unbalanced chromosomal rearrangements. It is this last group that precipitated the development of prenatal diagnosis.

Chromosomal anomalies resulting in spontaneous abortion and stillbirths

Chromosomal anomalies detected in live births represent only a fraction of those conceived. Cytogenetic studies of spontaneous abortions and stillbirths have clearly illustrated the important contribution of chromosomal anomalies to these outcomes.

Spontaneous abortions   The large frequency of chromosomal anomalies in spontaneous abortions is widely recognized (Boué *et al.* 1985). Ninety per cent of clinically recognized spontaneous abortions occur in the first trimester; a chromosomal anomaly can be detected in 60 per cent of these cases. A majority of these anomalies are associated with an early arrest in development (3–7 weeks) followed by a missed abortion, the maternal hormonal system continuing to function for some time. What are some of the chromosomal anomalies observed in spontaneous abortions (Table 4.2)?

Table 4.2 Occurrence of different types of chromosomal anomalies in spontaneous abortions

Anomaly	Frequency (per cent)
Numerical anomalies	
Monosomy X	15–20
Autosomal monosomies	rare
Autosomal trisomies	50–60
Triploidy	12–20
Tetraploidy	3–7
Mosaics	0.5–4
Structural anomalies	3–6

Monosomies   Monosomy X (45,X) is one of the most common chromosomal anomalies observed in spontaneous abortions, and would result in Turner syndrome. Less than 1 per cent of 45,X conceptuses reach term. Autosomal monosomies are rarely reported, in contrast to the greater frequency of autosomal trisomies.

Autosomal trisomies   Almost all autosomes in trisomic state have been observed in spontaneous abortions, but there is a great variation in the relative frequency of the various trisomies; trisomy 16 alone represents one-third of all the trisomies. Trisomies 13, 18, and 21, the only trisomies observed at term, are also frequently observed in spontaneous abortions and stillbirths.

Triploidy   Always lethal, triploidy (69 chromosomes) is frequent in spontaneous abortion and is compatible with only a few weeks of embryonic life.

Stillbirths   Cytogenetic studies of intrauterine fetal deaths and stillbirths reveal a chromosomal anomaly in 6 per cent of cases. If one limits the cytogenetic observations to multiple malformed stillbirths, the frequency of chromosomal anomalies reaches 25 per cent; mostly trisomies for chromosomes 13, 18, and 21.

From data on spontaneous abortions and stillbirths, one can estimate the frequency of developmental arrest at different stages of development and the percentage of chromosomal anomalies associated with these arrests (Fig. 4.1). These data are critical when interpreting the results of prenatal diagnoses performed during the first and second trimester.

Cytogenetic indications

Chromosomal anomalies represent the most common cause of genetic disease in the newborn. One technique alone, fetal karyotyping, allows detection of all numerical and structural abnormalities. The issue is therefore to select the preg-

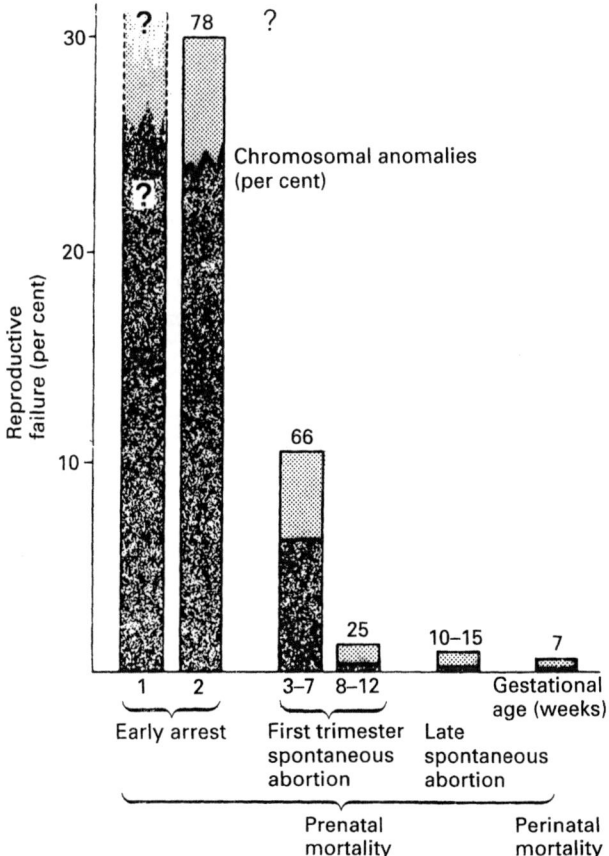

Fig. 4.1 Frequency of arrested pregnancies and percentage of chromosomal anomalies according to gestational age.

nancies at risk for these abnormalities, which can then benefit from these tests. Although there is common consensus about certain cytogenetic indications (parent carriers of balanced chromosomal rearrangement, mother over 40 years old) a policy on screening for chromosomal anomalies is limited by practical considerations of the technique and its cost on the one hand, and evaluation of the risk of the chromosomal anomaly relative to the risks inherent in the screening technology (risk to mother or fetus, risk of failure or error) on the other hand. The latter risks must remain lower than the risk of anomaly.

Maternal age

This is the most common indication for prenatal diagnosis (80 per cent in France). Prenatal diagnosis is recommended for this group because of the observation of an increased frequency of babies born with trisomy 21 to women 40 years old and over, confirmed by studies of spontaneous abortions which also extended this phenomenon to other trisomies, in particular 13 and 18. Results of cytogenetic analysis of fetal cells at amniocentesis have largely confirmed the above observations. Table 4.3 summarizes the data on diagnoses made in France between 1980 and 1985. It is clear from this table that the frequency of chromosomal anomalies increases drastically after 40 years of age. Other studies on women 35–37 years old show a sharp decrease in chromosomal anomalies below the age of 38 (Ferguson-Smith and Yates 1984).

Table 4.3 Chromosomal anomalies observed in women of 38 years old or over in France, 1980–1985. Figures in brackets are percentages.

Maternal age	Number of diagnoses	Number with anomalies	Proportion with trisomy 21
38	7 237	101 (1.40)	56 (0.77)
39	6 624	93 (1.40)	52 (0.79)
40	5 135	122 (2.38)	68 (1.32)
41	3 338	119 (3.57)	75 (2.25)
42	2 045	87 (4.25)	55 (2.69)
43	1 150	73 (6.35)	52 (4.52)
44	615	37 (6.02)	28 (4.55)
45+	560	51 (9.11)	34 (6.07)
Total	26 704	683 (2.56)	420 (1.57)

Table 4.4 illustrates the different types of chromosomal anomalies found. In comparison to the frequency of chromosomal anomalies in full-term babies born to women of the same age, one observes a higher frequency of anomalies at the time of amniocentesis (17 weeks of gestation), which can be explained by intrauterine death occurring during the second and third trimester of pregnancy. This has been demonstrated by an American study which looked at women who

Table 4.4 Chromosomal anomalies observed at the time of
amniocentesis for maternal age reasons in women of 38 years old or over.
Data from French laboratories 1980–1985

Anomalies of number	
Anomalies of number	
Trisomy 21	420
Trisomy 18	121
Trisomy 13	27
47XXY	46
47XXX	40
47XYY	9
45X	10
Anomalies of structure	
Balanced translocations	51
Unbalanced translocations	13

had an anomaly diagnosed at amniocentesis and decided to pursue the
pregnancy (Hook 1978).

From Table 4.5, one can see that these fetal deaths involve mostly monosomy
X and trisomy 18, followed by trisomy 21, but hardly ever involve sex chromosome anomalies (47,XXX, 47,XXY, 47,XYY). In the chapter on ultrasound
indications for amniocentesis, we will see that it is mainly the lethal anomalies
that are detected.

Table 4.5 Percentage of fetal deaths after the diagnosis of a chromosomal anomaly
following a 17-week amniocentesis (in women having continued the pregnancy
after diagnosis of an anomaly). Data from Hook (1978)

Type of anomaly	Percentage of fetal deaths
Trisomy 21	30
Trisomy 18	68
Monosomy X	75
47XXX	0
47XXY	8
47XYY	3
Balanced structural anomaly	3

Parent carrier of a balanced structural chromosome rearrangement

Table 4.1 gives the frequency of balanced chromosome rearrangements in the
general population, and Table 4.6 indicates how these anomalies are ascertained
within families. Without taking into consideration pericentric inversion of
chromosome 9, which is observed in 1 per cent of the population and not found

Table 4.6 Diagnosis of a carrier of a balanced chromosomal anomaly.
From Boué and Gallano (1984)

Anomaly	Mode of ascertainment of diagnosis			
	Child carrier of unbalanced anomaly	Spontaneous abortions	Others[a]	Total
Robertsonian translocation involving chromosome 21	174	12	9	195
Robertsonian translocation not involving chromosome 21	35	94	88	217
Reciprocal translocations	193	168	184	545
Inversions	6	20	96	122
Total	408	294	377	1079

[a] Mainly perinatal deaths leading to a chromosomal analysis of the parents

in an unbalanced form, in 1/100 to 1/200 couples one member is a carrier of a balanced structural rearrangement. This group of individuals has a high risk of a chromosomally unbalanced conceptus.

There is a wide difference between the theoretical genetic risk at conception and the birth incidence of children carrying an unbalanced chromosome rearrangement. Recognition of this difference is important in the management of each couple.

Factors to consider are the type of chromosomal rearrangement, type of chromosomes involved, the carrier of the rearrangement — father or mother — and the mode of ascertainment of the chromosomal rearrangement in the family. The data on the incidence of unbalanced chromosomal rearrangements detected at amniocentesis are provided by the European Collaborative Study (Boué and Galliarno 1984).

Type of chromosomal rearrangement

Robertsonian translocations   These are the most common structural chromosomal rearrangements, and Table 4.7a clearly indicates the large variation in the incidence of their unbalanced form.

When chromosome 21 is involved in the translocation (in particular t14q;t21q) and the mother is the carrier of its balanced form, the risk of the unbalanced form is high, 10–15 per cent; on the other hand it is small when the father is the carrier. When translocation 13q;14q is involved the risk is very small whether the mother or father is a carrier. Although in population studies translocation 13q;14q is four times more frequent than translocation 14q;21q, at the time of prenatal diagnosis it is present with the same frequency as translocation 14q;21q because most of the carriers of 13q;14q go undetected.

Table 4.7a Segregation of Robertsonian translocations. Figures in brackets are percentages. Data from Boué and Gallano (1984)

Type of translocation	Carrier parent	Number diagnosed	Unbalanced anomalies
13q14q	Mother	157	0
	Father	73	0
13q21q	Mother	20	2 (10)
	Father	11	0
14q21q	Mother	137	21 (15.3)
	Father	51	0
15q21q	Mother	9	1 (11)
	Father	5	0
21q22q	Mother	19	3 (15.8)
	Father	30	0

Reciprocal translocations The variety of reciprocal translocations is infinite: it is dependent on the chromosome and breakpoints involved, and therefore there are virtually never two identical reciprocal translocations. Whether transmitted by the father or the mother the incidence of unbalanced chromosomal rearrangements is the same, 11 per cent (Tables 4–7a, b).

Table 4.7b Segregation of reciprocal translocations. Figures in brackets are percentages

Carrier	Number of cases	Fetal karyotype		
		Normal	Balanced	Unbalanced
Mother	231	97	107	27 (11.7)
Father	378	168	166	44 (11.6)

The risk of detecting an unbalanced form of the translocation at prenatal diagnosis can be better assessed by considering two interdependent criteria:

1. The mode of ascertainment of the rearrangement in the family (the consulting couple or their relatives). Table 4.8 clearly shows that if the unbalanced rearrangement has been observed in a congenitally malformed livebirth the recurrence risk is much higher (20 per cent) than when a couple's karyotype reveals a balanced form of the rearrangement at the time of spontaneous abortion.

2. The length of the chromosome segment involved in the unbalanced form of the rearrangement.

Table 4.8 Frequency of unbalanced fetal karyotype with respect to the mode of ascertainment of structural anomaly in the family. The denominator of each fraction is the number of diagnoses, the numerator the number of unbalanced fetal karyotypes. Figures in brackets are percentages

Anomaly	Mode of ascertainment		
	Child with unbalanced form	Spontaneous abortion	Other
Reciprocal translocation	54/260 (20.8)	7/205 (3.4)	10/144 (6.9)
Inversion	6/8	0/25	1/85

These variations are a reflection of the degree of genetic inbalance, whose consequence for fetal development is arrest and spontaneous abortion occurring before the time of amniocentesis, leading to a decrease in the incidence of these unbalanced rearrangements found at that time.

Inversions   These are mostly pericentric inversions. In an unbalanced state, only a few inversions are compatible with the development and delivery at term of a malformed child; in these cases the recurrence risk is high (Table 4.8). On the contrary, most of the inversions lead to a greater genetic imbalance resulting in an early developmental arrest and therefore a small incidence of the unbalanced form of the rearrangement at the time of amniocentesis.

Parent carrier of a numerical chromosomal anomaly

This happens, for example, when one member of a couple carries a sex chromosome anomaly (47,XXX, 47,XYY) in complete or mosaic form. In such cases an increased risk of sex chromosome anomalies in fetal cells is not observed. Prenatal diagnosis is offered only as a form of reassurance for the parents.

A previous child born with a chromosomal anomaly

This most often concerns a couple who have had a child with a trisomy 21. One must first confirm that there is a numerical abnormality, and not a rearrangement. Overall the recurrence risk is low (1 per cent) and does not vary significantly with the mother's age or with the type of trisomy in the child (trisomy 21, 18). Recurrence can involve a different trisomy, which implies that the likelihood of undetected parental mosaicism is low.

Paternal age

A possible paternal age effect has been suggested, based on data from a German study (Stene *et al.* 1984). Analysis of data on a large series, French, British and American, has not confirmed any paternal age effect, which therefore cannot be maintained as an indication for prenatal diagnosis.

Other indications

Given the incidence of chromosomal anomalies in the liveborn there is a small risk for any pregnancy, which explains the pressing demand of many pregnant women, and their raised anxiety particularly when they are over 35 years old or when they have trisomic children in their immediate surroundings. Certain centres have been able to offer prenatal diagnosis to women who do not have any appreciable genetic risk. In this group, at diagnosis, there is a 1 per cent risk of a chromosome anomaly (a difference in figures observed at this time in comparison to those at birth represents the fetal mortality occurring during this time). In the 1 per cent detected, one-third are trisomies, one-third are sex chromosome anomalies, and one-third are structural anomalies, usually balanced. Therefore only 0.4 per cent of anomalies will have phenotypic consequences.

Chapter 9 considers strategies which could be applied to screen all pregnancies.

Problems in cytogenetic diagnosis

Interpretation of certain chromosomal anomalies

Most chromosomal anomalies do not cause any problem of interpretation, as they are found in all analysed mitoses and are either of the common type (trisomy) or expected (an unbalanced rearrangement), but the cytogeneticist can be faced with difficulties in interpretation.

Unexpected structural rearrangements

Apparently balanced translocations, reciprocal or Robertsonian translocations, inversions   These are not unusual: 3.4/1000 (Hook and Cross 1987), 3.9/1000 (Crandall 1980), 4.3/1000 (Boué *et al.* 1982).

Study of chromosomal anomalies demonstrate that two-thirds are inherited (Table 4.9). In these cases one can assume that the anomaly is without consequence to the child. One must establish whether a *de novo* translocation is

Table 4.9 Frequency of chromosomal structural anomalies per 1000 diagnoses when the indication for prenatal diagnosis is maternal age

Type of anomaly	Balanced anomalies	
	De novo	inherited
Robertsonian translocation	0.3	0.4
Reciprocal translocation	0.55	1
Inversion	0.15	1
Total	1	2.4

Table 4.10 Outcome of pregnancies where an apparently balanced *de novo* translocation has been diagnosed by amniocentesis. Data from Warburton (1987)

Type of anomaly	Number of observations	Number of malformed babies
Robertsonian translocation	32	1
Reciprocal translocation	81	3
Inversion	16	2

truly balanced and without phenotypic consequence. Table 4.10 provides results of an American study, and it is obvious that a vast majority of cases are normal (Warburton 1987).

Unbalanced rearrangements　Study of parental chromosomes indicate that one third of unbalanced rearrangements result from the malsegregation of a balanced rearrangement. In *de novo* rearrangements, where there is extra chromosomal material, it would be difficult to determine the origin of this material.

Supernumerary marker chromosome　Under this heading are included all those chromosomes which defy classification. Often these are smaller than the smallest autosomes (21 and 22), often containing heterochromatic chromosomal material, and often resembling an acrocentric or metacentric chromosome. They sometimes have satellites. It is essential to use all available techniques. The incidence of these markers at the time of prenatal diagnosis is not negligible, 1/1000 to 1/2000. In 50 per cent of cases they are inherited: in these cases the child is phenotypically normal. More difficult is the prognosis, when the marker is *de novo*. Few prospective studies are available, and they indicate that markers with satellites have a good prognosis; in markers without satellites, phenotypic consequences have been cited in 8 per cent of cases.

Mosaicism

The finding of mosaicism is problematic when observed on fetal amniotic fluid cells (Table 4.11). One must first define mosaicism in accordance with the cell culturing techniques used. With *in situ* preparations, each cell colony can be analysed separately and on different slides. It can then be established whether there is pseudomosaicism; metaphases where aberrations are limited to one colony, either entirely or partially. Mosaicism can be confirmed when the aberrant and normal karyotypes are homogeneously observed in different colonies and on different slides (Fig. 4.2). When chromosome preparations are from trypsinized cells in culture flasks, the interpretation of mosaicism may be more difficult. Mosaicism will only be confirmed when the two types of metaphases

Table 4.11 Outcome of 395 cases of mosaicism detected in amniotic fluid cells after amniocentesis (percentages). Data from Hsu (1987)

Chromosomes involved in mosaicism	Mosaicism confirmed in fetus or newborn	Phenotypically abnormal fetus or newborn
Autosomes	51.8	34.8
Sex chromosomes	86.4	8.4
Markers	85.7	13.3

are observed in two (or three) culture flasks. Trisomy 20 in mosaic is by far the most frequent type observed in amniotic fluid cells at the time of prenatal diagnosis. This high incidence is particularly striking, as in cytogenetic studies of spontaneous abortions this abnormality is rarely observed and there is no well-documented case at birth. The consensus is that trisomy 20 cells in amniotic fluid are derived from non-embryonic tissue, although in rare circumstances trisomy 20 has been observed in fetal tissue after pregnancy termination. In the 50 or so cases where the pregnancy was continued, all the children were born normal and trisomy 20 was not observed in blood or in other tissues of the child.

With available data, and even though the origin of mosaic trisomy 20 remains unexplained, one must conclude that this finding does not justify termination, fetal blood sampling is useless, and good ultrasound monitoring is sufficient.

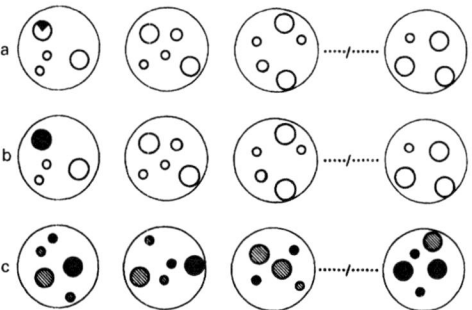

Fig. 4.2 Mosaicism: various possibilities. Each row represents the set of slides on which cell colonies from a single amniotic fluid sample have been cultured. The small open circles represent colonies with a normal karyotype. The black and shaded circles are colonies with abnormal karyotypes. *a*, a region of a cell colony with an abnormal karyotype; *b*, a single colony where all cells have an abnormal karyotype; *c*, two cell populations with different karyotypes found in different cell colonies and on different cover slips.

Discovery of a chromosomal anomaly without major phenotypic consequence

Essentially these are the sex chromosome anomalies 47,XXX, 47,XXY, and 47,XYY.

Some prospective studies of newborns with 47,XXX and 47,XXY show that these children are intellectually within the normal range, but in one-third of the cases the IQ is at the lower limit of normal. Recent studies of adult 47,XXY males followed for 20 years show an improvement in intelligence with time. From results obtained in 1985 and 1986 in French centres, of the 35 47,XXY prenatal diagnoses, 16 pregnancies continued, and of the 27 47,XXX, 18 were continued.

Direct chromosomal analysis of chorionic villus samples

Results of a collaborative study (Mikkelsen and Aymé 1987), encompassing all chromosomal anomalies, correlates well with those data available from diagnoses made on amniotic fluid. The total frequency of chromosomal anomalies detected on chorionic villus sampling — trisomy 13, 18, and 21, and unbalanced chromosomal rearrangements — is higher than that observed at amniocentesis (approximately one and a half times), which can be explained by the proportion of chromosomal anomalies which would have led to fetal loss between the 11th and 17th week of gestation.

It is important to stress those problems of interpretation of chromosomal analyses on chorionic villus samples which may lead to false positives and false negatives.

False positives

Numerical change　On the one hand there are those chromosomes which are occasionally observed in a trisomic state at birth, and on the other hand there is monosomy X. In a number of cases (trisomies 7, 9, 14, 15, 16, and 22) these anomalies have not been confirmed on fetal tissue after termination nor seen in normal babies brought to term. When such a chromosomal anomaly is diagnosed, a detailed ultrasound examination must be performed to detect either a developmental arrest or abnormalities which are associated with trisomy or lethal monosomy X.

If ultrasound examination demonstrates proper development, one must suspect that the chromosome complement does not represent the fetal genotype; for example trisomy 16 is very common in early spontaneous abortion, and is not compatible with development past the 3rd week.

In any case, an amniocentesis and possibly fetal blood sampling is recommended to confirm the fetal chromosome complement.

Mosaicism

Mosaicism can involve autosomal trisomies, numerical sex chromosome anomalies, or a marker chromosome (of 43 cases of mosaicism, 36 showed no abnormality in fetal tissue).

All mosaicism found in chorionic villi either by direct analysis or by culture analysis must be followed by a control amniocentesis.

False negatives

Although they are much less frequent, some false negatives have been reported. The chromosomal anomaly was detected either through analysis of cultured chorionic villi or at birth. The large number of discordances between fetal chromosome constitution and karyotypes obtained from direct chorionic villus analysis may be explained by the origin of the different types of cells observed in early stages of embryogenesis as described in Chapter 1, page 18. To reduce such errors, certain authors recommend backing up direct analysis of chorionic villi with culture analysis, which prolongs laboratory investigations and delays results. Based on results of various published data, one can estimate that the frequency of false positives is 1/100 and that of false negatives 1/1000 (Tomkins and Vekemans 1989). This last figure should be compared to results obtained from amniotic fluid cell analyses carried out for all prenatal diagnoses in recent years in France; the frequency of false negatives is less than 1/10 000 diagnoses.

Choice of prenatal sampling techniques for various indications

Most data available on the prenatal diagnosis of chromosomal anomalies is derived from the analysis of a large series of prenatal diagnoses performed on amniotic fluid cells sampled at 16–17 weeks of pregnancy. The introduction of chorionic villus sampling, at 10–11 weeks, for the diagnosis of chromosomal anomalies, presents a choice in sampling technique based on indication. Two criteria should be considered in this choice:

1. Sampling risk of the technique; not the theoretical risk found in the literature, but the actual risk relevant to the particular circumstances in which the woman is undergoing these tests.
2. Risk of failure and, more importantly, risk of error in diagnosis. Risk of false positives leads to termination of a normal pregnancy, and risk of false negatives leads to the birth of an affected child.

Given present-day results, it seems reasonable to limit cytogenetic analysis on chorionic villus sampling to those cases where the risk of a chromosomal anomaly is high.

Structural anomalies

The case will be managed differently depending on the type of structural anomaly (Robertsonian or reciprocal translocation), the carrier of the balanced form (father or mother), the mode of ascertainment of the family (malformed child, spontaneous abortion), and the cytogenetic techniques required to diagnose the unbalanced form with certainty. Thus, for a maternal 14;21 Robertsonian translocation, where the recurrence risk is high, the recommendation will be chorionic villus sampling at 10–11 weeks. For a reciprocal translocation, ascertained through spontaneous abortion, where the risk of the unbalanced form at birth is low, it is preferable to diagnose on amniotic fluid cells, sampled at 17 weeks, after the time when a large number of fetuses carrying an unbalanced form of the translocation have already been aborted spontaneously.

A young couple having had a baby with trisomy 21

The recurrence risk is very low (<1 per cent), and prenatal diagnosis is mainly offered as reassurance: why impose a risk on a pregnancy which has an excellent chance of a normal outcome? Amniocentesis is the best choice.

Maternal age

It must be questioned whether this is a good indication, as it is known that the associated risk of the procedure is already high and increases with maternal age (fibrotic uterus). Although early diagnosis means that termination of the pregnancy is associated with less psychological trauma, it remains to be determined whether, when the risk of abnormality and thus the chance of terminating the pregnancy is around 3 per cent, it is reasonable to run a 5–8 per cent risk for the 97 per cent of normal births which are so highly desired by the parents. This should be evaluated in the context of a group of women with a lower fertility. Table 4.12, from Tomkins and Vekemans (1989), give the predictive value of

Table 4.12 Predictive value of cytogenetic findings.
Data from Tomkins and Vekemans (1989)

Maternal age (years)	Estimated rate of all chromosomal abnormalities at CVS including lethals[a]	Positive predictive value based on false-positive rate	
		1 in 100	1 in 50
35	1/110	0.48	0.31
36	1/83	0.55	0.38
37	1/64	0.61	0.44
38	1/48	0.68	0.51
39	1/37	0.73	0.57
40	1/28	0.78	0.64
41	1/21	0.83	0.70
42	1/16	0.86	0.76
43	1/12	0.89	0.81
44	1/9	0.92	0.85
45	1/7	0.93	0.88

[a] Based on the data of Hook *et al.* (1988). Note that these data excluded all discrepant diagnoses and balanced structural rearrangements.

direct analysis in function with the risk of anomaly related to maternal age. The risk of error is not small: in the 38–39 age group, it is equal to the risk of detecting a chromosomal anomaly.

Mental handicap associated with fragile X

Mental handicap associated with fragile X is, next to trisomy 21, the most common chromosome abnormality in the liveborn: 1/1500 boys is affected. The higher frequency of mental retardation in boys has been known for a long time. Lubs (1969) observed the presence of a satellited X chromosome in mentally retarded males and transmitting females. This observation was forgotten until 1976, when several groups also noted this chromosome change in a number of families where boys presented with mental retardation and macroorchidism (Turner and Turner 1974; Giraud *et al.* 1976; Sutherland and Ashford 1979). This association permitted the delineation of a new pathological condition, and fragile X syndrome is now well defined. Affected boys have a robust stature with little dysmorphism other than a large prominent jaw giving the appearance of a long face, thick lips, the lower lip being everted, and large ears. At younger ages marcoorchidism is not always evident but is frequent at adolescence; it can be quite striking, but is inconsistent. Mental retardation is variable, ranging from moderate deficiency in 70 per cent of cases to profound deficiency in 30 per cent of cases. There is inter- and intrafamily variation. These boys always have speech and behavioural problems, and autism is sometimes noted.

In fragile X families, there is a significant proportion of carrier females, also demonstrating mental deficiency. The retardation is usually less severe than that observed in the boys.

Cytogenetic analysis

Until 1990, diagnosis relied solely on cytogenetic analysis, where a fragile site is observed in the terminal region of the long arm of the X at q27q28. This fragile site can be expressed by an actual break, a non-staining region, or a constriction sometimes giving the impression of a pseudosatellite (Fig. 4.3). This finding must be observed in more than 2 per cent of examined mitoses to be of diagnostic value.

A number of cytogenetic techniques have been described to optimize expression of the fragility of the X chromosome in lymphocyte cultures. These methods aim at creating particular culturing conditions in folate-deficient media, with or without the addition of drugs antagonistic to folic acid. Methotrexate is the agent most commonly used, and increases the percentage of fragile sites. The cytogenetic expression of the fragile X is therefore a culture-mediated artefact, and in some cases it may be difficult to observe the characteristic fragility of the X chromosome.

In affected boys the fragile site is relatively easy to express, but it is often difficult to express the fragile X in transmitting females, particularly in mothers

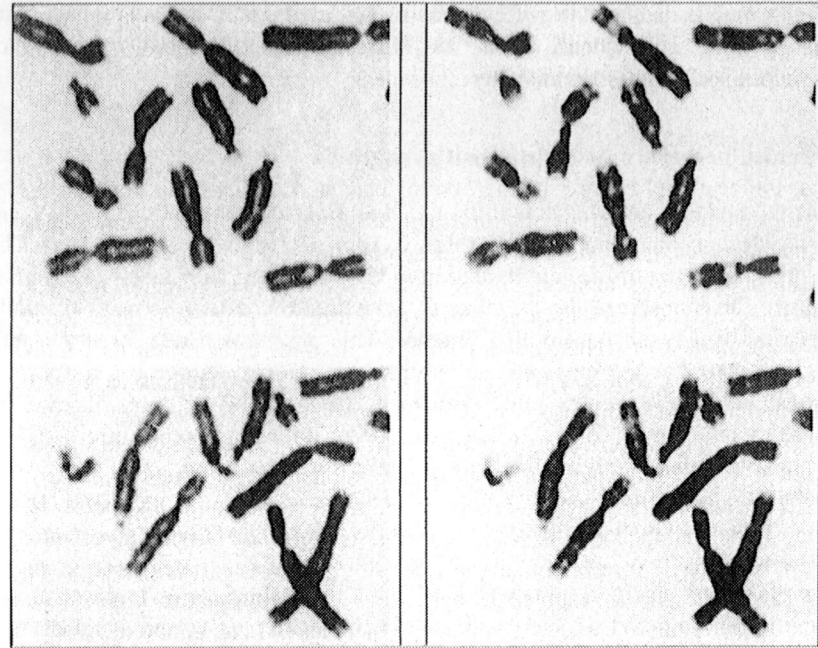

Fig. 4.3 Metaphase preparation, demonstrating the fragile X chromosome using two different stains. (*a*), solid Giemsa; (*b*), G-banding. From Boué and Deluchat.

of affected children, even though they are obligate heterozygotes. This becomes even more difficult with age, particularly over the age of 30, and it is often through the cytogenetic analysis of a young daughter expressing the fragile X site that one can determine that the mother is a carrier. The unreliability in the expression of fragile X in cultured lymphocytes is nothing compared to the unreliability of detecting it in other tissues (fibroblasts, amniotic fluid cells, chorionic villi).

Molecular biology   Early work in molecular biology allowed the localization of the gene responsible, but the distance of the markers used, as well as the high rate of recombination, did not permit practical use of this technology.

The situation at the end of 1990   Family studies done using molecular markers surrounding the fragile site have allowed the following understanding of the segregation of the chromosome transmitting the disease.

Transmission of the fragile X syndrome is not characteristic of that observed in other X-linked diseases such as Duchenne muscular dystrophy or haemophilia. Families are often found where the affected cases (boys or girls) have received from their normal mother the mutated X chromosome which she herself had received from their grandfather, also normal. Several hypotheses have been advanced suggesting the existence of a premutation transmitted from the grandfather to his daughter, as well as the existence of a mechanism of imprinting occurring during transmission of the mutation to her children (boys or girls).

The situation in early 1991 Rapid progress in the early months of 1991 completely altered our perceptions of the fragile X syndrome. This progress is the result of vigorous international competition: one must cite J. L. Mandel's team (Oberle' *et al.* 1991) in association with French cytogeneticists and the Australian (Sutherland), Dutch, and American teams (Houston and Atlanta).

To summarize what is now known, a segment of DNA containing the responsible gene has been identified (the precise gene, and the coded protein, are now being studied).

1. There is a region (GpG island) with a CGG repetitive sequence on this segment of DNA. In a normal subject, this sequence is made up of 30 CGGs (the delta is 0 base pairs). In a normal subject with a premutation, there is elongation of this sequence by 100 to 500 base pairs. In an affected subject with the mutation, there is even greater elongation to 1000 to 3000 base pairs.

2. In those cases affected with mental retardation this CGG region is abnormally methylated, which means that this DNA region is inactivated and there is therefore no gene expression (the corresponding messenger RNA is absent in the brains of the affected subjects); see Verkerk *et al.* 1991.

Based on the two premises above, for which we do not know the relationship, one can construct a model of the molecular mechanism of transmission of the fragile X (Fig. 4.4).

A healthy man carrying the premutation on his X chromosome will transmit this chromosome to all his daughters without modification. To his healthy girls the premutation may be on the active or the inactive X chromosome. During oogenesis, both Xs become reactivated in oogonia in order to segregate into the occytes.

If the premutation is on the active X, there is no need for reactivation and this premutation will be transmitted without modification to the children, boys and girls, who will be healthy transmitters of the premutation. It is thought that this is how the mutation persists over many generations, because in those family studies done to date no new mutation has been revealed and it has been possible to go back to ancestors in the seventeenth century (Sweden, Finland, and Holland).

If the premutation is on the inactive X, at the time of reactivation this segment of DNA remains inactivated because of the methylation of the repetitive sequence. There is also a lengthening of the repetitive sequence, showing heterogeneity, indicating meiotic or somatic mutations during the first cell divisions of the fertilized egg and resulting in mosaicism.

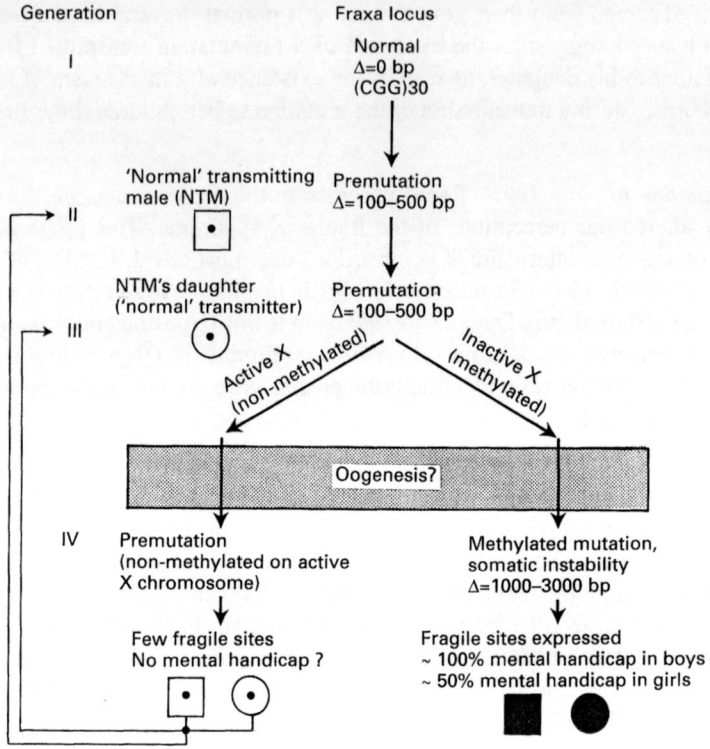

Fig. 4.4 Hypothetical example of the role of X inactivation in the change from pre-mutation to mutation. Elongation of the fragment Δ is measured in base pairs. It has not been formally demonstrated that this elongation results from amplification of the $(CGG)_n$ sequence. *A priori*, the premutation can appear in either sex, and the complete mutation of a normal allele remains possible (although it has not yet been observed). Expression of the fragile site would be due to the difficulty in replicating the very elongated methylated region. Mental retardation (MR) and the morphological anomalies may be explained by inhibition either of the initiation of transcription or of translation (amplification of the CGG sequence). The above simplified example does not take into consideration certain rare cases (males mosaic for the premutation and the mutation, possible reversal of the mutation to premutation state). NTM = normal transmitting male. From Rousseau *et al.* (1991*b*).

One in two boys in these families is affected; for girls the mental retardation depends on whether the mutation is on active or inactive X.

Family studies using J. L. Mandel's probes show that in the sibship of a pre-mutated mother there are either affected or healthy children or premutated or healthy children, and by exception in the same sibship, affected, premutated and healthy children (Rousseau *et al.* 1991*a*). This observation favours the hypo-thesis that most often an oocyte is derived from one primordial cell.

References and further reading

Definitions and mechanisms

Boué, A. and Gallano, P. (1984). A collaborative study of the segregation of inherited chromosome structural rearrangements in 1356 prenatal diagnosis. *Prenat. Diagn.*, **4**, 45–67.

Boué, J., Girard, S., Thepot, F., *et al.* (1982). Unexpected structural rearrangements in prenatal diagnosis. *Prenat. Diagn.*, **2**, 163–8.

Boué, A., Boué, J., and Gropp, A. (1985). Cytogenetics of pregnancy wastage. *Adv. Hum. Genet.*, **14**, 1–57.

Crandall, B. F., Lebherz, T. B., Rubinstein, L. D., *et al.* (1980). Chromosome findings in 2500 second trimester amniocentesis. *Am. J. Med. Genet.*, **5**, 345–56.

Ferguson-Smith, M. A. and Yates, J. R. W. (1984). Maternal age specific rates for chromosome aberrations and factors influencing them: report of a collaborative European study on 52 965 amniocentesis. *Prenat. Diagn.*, **4**, 5–44.

Hook, E. B. (1978). Spontaneous deaths of fetuses with chromosomal abnormalities diagnosed prenatally. *New Engl. J. Med.*, **299**, 1036.

Hook, E. B. and Cross, P. K. (1987). Rates of mutant and inherited structural cytogenetic abnormalities detected at amniocentesis: results on about 63 000 fetuses. *Ann. Hum. Genet.*, **51**, 27–55.

Hsu, L. Y. (1986). Prenatal diagnosis of chromosome abnormalities. In *Genetic disorders and the fetus* (ed. A. Milunsky), 115–83, Plenum, New York.

Mikkelsen, M. and Aymé, S. (1987). Chromosomal findings in chorionic villi: a collaborative study. In *Human genetics* (ed. F. Vogel and K. Sperling), 597–606, Springer-Verlag, Berlin.

Simoni, G., Fraccaro, M., and Gimelli, G. (1987). False-positive and false-negative findings on chorionic villus sampling. *Prenat. Diagn.*, **7**, 671–2.

Stene, J., Stene, E., and Mikkelsen, M. (1984). Risk for chromosome abnormality at amniocentesis following a child with a non-inherited chromosome aberration. *Prenat. Diagn.*, **4**, 81–96.

Tomkins, D. J. and Vekemans, M. J. J. (1989). False positive and false negative-cytogenetic findings on chorionic villus sampling. *Prenat. Diagn.*, **9**, 139–40.

Warburton, D. (1987). De novo structural rearrangements at amniocentesis: outcome and nonrandom position of breakpoints. *Am. J. Hum. Genet.*, **41**, A145.

Fragile X

Arveiler, B., Oberle, I., Vincent, A., *et al.* (1988). Genetic mapping of the Xq27-q28 region: new RFLP markers useful for diagnostic applications in fragile-X and hemophilia-B families. *Am. J. Hum. Genet.*, **42**, 380–9.

Giraud, F., Ayme, S., Mattei, J. F., *et al.* (1991). Constitutional chromosomal breakage. *Hum. Genet.*, **34**, 125.

Lubs, H. A. (1969). A marker X chromosome. *Am. J. Hum. Genet.*, **21**, 231.

Mattei, J. F., Mattei, M. G., Auger, M., *et al.* (1986). Le retard mental lié á la fragilité du chromosome X: connaissances actuelles. *J. Genet. Hum.*, **74**, 93–7.

Oberle', I., Rousseau, F., Heitz, D., *et al.* (1991). Instability of a 550-base pair DNA segment and abnormal methylation in fragile X syndrome. *Science*, **252**, 1097.

Rousseau, F., Heitz, D., Biancalana, V., *et al.* (1991a). Direct diagnosis by DNA analysis of the fragile X syndrome of mental retardation. *New Engl. J. Med.*, **325**, 1673.

Rousseau, F., Heitz, D., Oberle', I., *et al.* (1991b). Le syndrome du X fragile: des mutations étonnamment ciblées et instables, et un gene à la recherche d'une fonction. *Medécine/Sciences*, **7**, 637–9.

Sutherland, G. R. and Ashford, P. L. C. (1979). X-linked metal retardation with macroorchidism and the fragile site at Xq27 or 28. *Hum. Genet.*, **48**, 117–20.

Sutherland, G. R. and Mulley, J. C. (1990). Diagnostic molecular genetics of the fragile X. *Clin. Genet.*, **37**, 2–11.

Turner, G. and Turner, B. (1974). X-linked mental retardation. *J. Med. Genet.*, **11**, 109.

Verkerk, A. J. M. H., Piereti, M., Sutcliffe, J. S., *et al.* (1991). Identification of a gene (FMR–1) containing a CGG repeat coincident with a breakpoint cluster region exhibiting length variation in fragile X syndrome. *Cell*, **65**, 905.

Winter, R. M. and Pembrey, M. E. (1986). Analysis of linkage relationships between genetic markers around the fragile X locus with special reference to the daughters of normal transmitting males. *Hum. Genet.*, **74**, 93–7.

5 Prenatal diagnosis of single-gene disorders

Inborn errors of metabolism

Enzymopathies make up the majority of single-gene disorders. They are inborn errors which consist of absences, deficiencies, or alterations in the metabolic pathway of an enzyme or group of enzymes.

Their huge numbers, low incidence, and great clinical, genetical, and biological heterogeneity are factors which complicate their diagnosis and require the collaboration of many specialists and sophisticated methodologies. We will limit ourselves here to those conditions of known etiology which can be diagnosed by assay of enzyme activity (Table 5.1). In the prenatal diagnosis of inborn errors of metabolism the methods used must be adapted to each disorder, which explains the numerous techniques used and the large diversity of investigations required. Methods depend on analysing gene expression by measure of enzyme deficit, which can be the consequence of various abnormalities at many different stages of enzyme synthesis and enzyme maturation (Fig. 5.1). Successful diagnosis rests on judicious choice of tissue and techniques to demonstrate the enzyme deficiency.

Selection of tissue type

Gene expression varies from one tissue to another: thus in the prenatal diagnosis of inborn errors of metabolism there are indications and contraindications as to the type of tissue used.

Amniotic fluid   Sampled at 16–17 weeks of pregnancy, amniotic fluid may be used in the prenatal diagnosis of some inborn errors of metabolism with varying degree of precision.

Indications
   1. Amniotic fluid analysis is indicated in:

   ● certain aminoacidopathies in which the increase or decrease of a particular metabolite can be assessed using indirect methods. They can be detected by separation, identification, and quantification of amino acids;
   ● congenital adrenal hyperplasia;
   ● cystic fibrosis;
   ● Zellweger syndrome: autosomal recessive disease due to a peroxisomal disorder involved in the metabolism of very long-chain fatty acids, as well

113

Table 5.1 Diseases diagnosed by enzymatic methods

Lysosomal disease	Enzyme deficiency
Sphingolipidoses	
Tay–Sachs	Hexosaminidase A
Sandhoff	Hexosaminidase A and B
Landing	β-Galactosidase
Gaucher	β-Glucosidase
Niemann–Pick	Sphingomyelinase
Krabbe	Cerebroside β-Galactosidase
Fabry	α-Galactosidase
Metachromatic leucodystrophy	Arylsulfatase A
Mucopolysaccharidoses	
Type I (Hurler)	α-L-Iduronidase
Type I (Scheie)	α-L-Iduronidase
Type II (Hunter)	L-Iduronide sulfatase
Type III (Sanfilippo A)	Sulfamidase
Type III (Sanfilippo B)	α-Glycosaminidase
Type IV (Morquio A)	6 Sulfate-sulfatase
Type IV (Morquio B)	β-Galactosidase
Type VI (Maroteaux-Lamy)	Arylsulfatase B
Type VII	β-Glucuronidase
Glycoproteinoses	
α-Mannosidosis	α-Mannosidase
β-Mannosidosis	β-Mannosidase
Fucosidosis	α-Fucosidase
Mucolipidosis II	Acid hydrolases
Sialidosis	Neuraminidase
Glycogenoses	
Type II (Pompe)	α-Glycosidase
Peroxysomal diseases	
Zellweger	Oxidase
Adrenoleucodystrophy	Fatty acid CoA ligase
Refsum	Phytanic acid oxidase
Aminoacidopathies	
Branched-chain ketoaciduria	Branched-chain ketoacid decarboxylase
Methylmalonic acidemia	Methylmalonyl CoA mutase
Propionic acidemia	Propionyl CoA carboxylase
Glutaric acidemia I	Glutaryl CoA dehydrogenase
Orotic aciduria	Orotidyl decarboxylase
Argininosuccinic aciduria	Arginosuccinate lyase
Tyrosinosis I	Fumaryl acetoacetase

Table 5.1 *cont'd.*

Homocystinuria	Cystathionine synthetase
Citrullinemia	Arginosuccinate synthetase
Cystinosis	Cystine transport protein
Xanthinuria	Xanthine oxidase
Nucleic acid disorders	
Lesch–Nyhan	Hypoxanthine guanine phosphoribosyl transferase
Xeroderma pigmentosum	DNA ligase
Disorders of mineral metabolism	
Menkes	Copper binding P-type ATPase
Porphyrias	
Günther	Uroporphyrin III cosynthetase

as pepicolic acid, and the intermediates of biliary acids. The diagnosis rests on high-pressure liquid chromatography and the separation of free fatty acids from methyl ester.

2. Analysis of amniotic fluid for a measure of a group of substances in order to direct investigations when information available is general, for example:

- an increase in aminoglycans in mucopolysaccharidoses is an indication of that group of disorders but not of the specific disease. To assess the particular disease, one can in some cases separate the aminoglycans by bidirectional electrophoresis;
- fucosidosis is suspected when the level of α-fucosidase is decreased in amniotic fluid;
- mucolipidoses types II and III are associated with a significant increase in lysosomal enzymes in amniotic fluid.

As controls, fresh amniotic fluid taken from a pregnancy not at risk for the particular disease and of the same gestational age must be used. However, the diagnoses of these disorders should not rest on this type of analysis alone.

Contraindications The presence in amniotic fluid of specific enzymes which are not related to the enzymopathy being looked for may sometimes contraindicate this type of analysis: for example in glycogenosis type II (Pompe disease), which is due to a deficit in acid α-glycosidase. Throughout pregnancy, there is high activity of α-glycosidase in amniotic fluid because of the presence of an isoenzyme, presumably of fetal origin, but genetically independent and not involved in glycogenosis type II (Fig. 5.2). Prenatal diagnosis of this disease cannot be made on the basis of α-glycosidase activity in amniotic fluid.

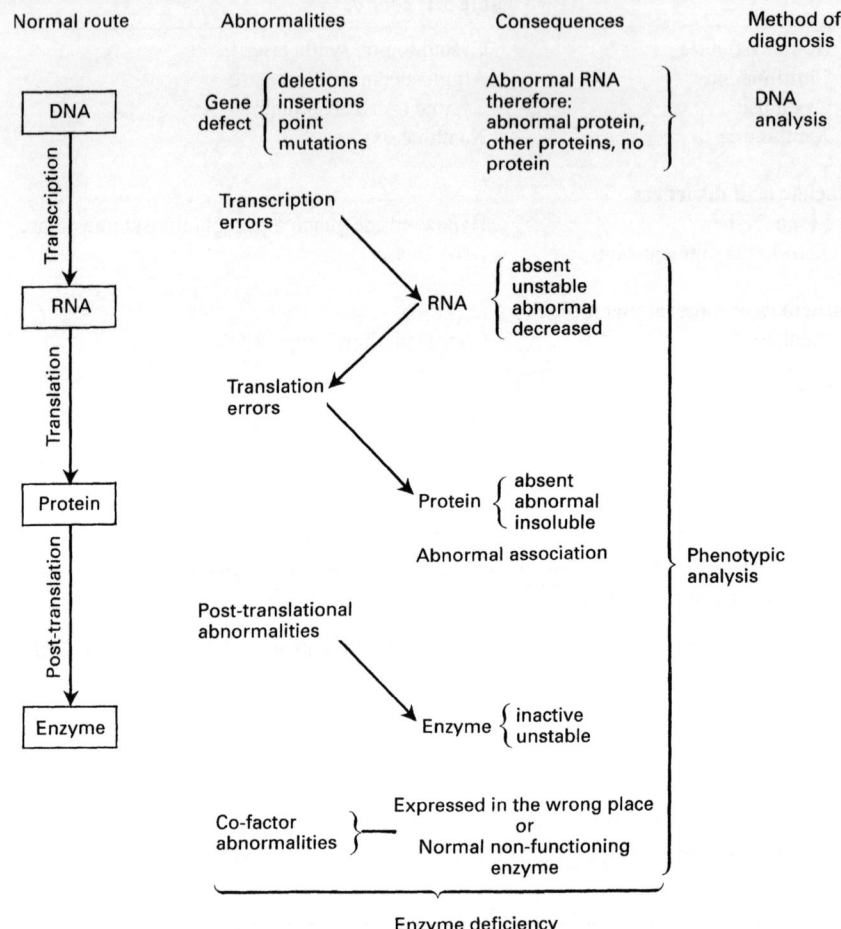

Fig. 5.1 Genetic anomalies leading to enzyme deficiency.

Non-cultured amniotic cells   The cell pellet obtained after centrifugation of amniotic fluid can provide some indication of a decrease in hexosaminidase (as in Tay–Sachs disease and Sandhoff disease) (Fig. 5.3). The ratio of the various isoenzymes is, however, different from that found in other tissues or even in cells in culture. Experience tells us that it is not appropriate to use this technique for other conditions, because the large proportion of dead cells can alter the various analyses.

Cultured amniotic cells   Cultured amniotic cells are the basis of prenatal diagnosis of enzymopathies and have been the tissue of choice in this area. These cells can be used in the study of most inborn errors of metabolism amenable to

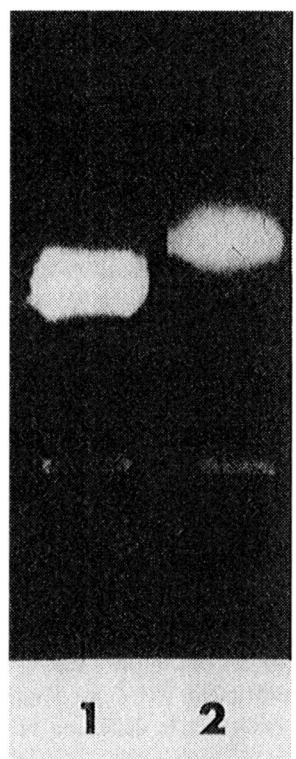

Fig. 5.2
Electrophoresis of
α-glycosidase.
1, amniotic cells;
2, amniotic fluid..

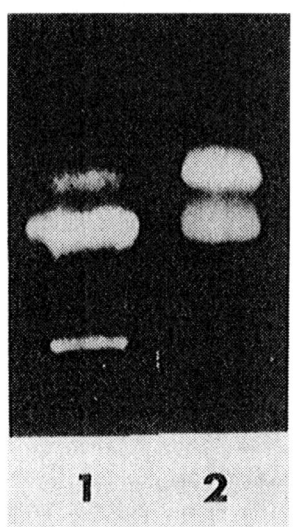

Fig. 5.3
Electrophoresis of
hexosaminidase.
1, amniotic cell
pellet; 2, cultured
amniotic cells.

prenatal diagnosis, and results are reliable. However, some guidelines must be adhered to:

- results must be compared to control amniotic cells and to the proband's fibroblasts cultured under the same conditions and in the same laboratory;
- in those disorders where enzyme measurement is difficult (as when enzyme activity is normally low, or residually high) the cells must be analysed in a primary culture and in a sub-culture because there is great variability in enzyme activity from one passage to the other (e.g. α-glycosidase);
- cells must be maintained in culture until a diagnosis is finalized in case there is a need to repeat.

The major drawback of this method, if practiced at 17 weeks of pregnancy, is the lateness of the diagnosis should a termination be required (20–22 weeks gestation). There have been promising results from cells cultured after early amniocentesis.

Fetal blood   Fetal blood sampling, at around 18–20 weeks of gestation, has been used exceptionally for those cases of lysosomal disease and amino-acidopathies. Mucolipidosis type II or III is however an indication, because this disorder can be diagnosed in serum and does not require white blood cells. Only a few microlitres of serum is required. DNA analysis can now be done on chorionic villi for these conditions.

Other fetal sampling methods   Liver biopsy has been used in the diagnosis of two enzymopathies which are not expressed in other tissues: carbamyl phosphate synthetase deficiency and ornithine transcarbamylase deficiency.

Chorionic villus sampling   Introduced as a routine sampling technique in 1984 (Poenaru *et al.* 1984), chorionic villus sampling is performed between 8 and 12 weeks of gestation. It is essential to assess the purity of the sample under the microscope in order to eliminate any deciduous maternal tissues. Villi are transported in sterile physiological saline or in culture medium. After a transition period necessary to ensure that enzymopathies are expressed in trophoblast, this tissue is now used in a large majority of these cases. In 1987, 90 per cent of prenatal diagnoses done in our laboratory were done on chorionic villus samples taken in the first trimester of pregnancy. The primary advantage is the early timing of diagnosis because in the vast majority of cases analysis is direct and a result can be obtained 24–48 hours after the biopsy. For some diagnoses culturing of chorionic villi is indispensable (Table 5.2); this postpones results to 10, 12, and 13 weeks of gestation. European experience in September 1987 showed that among 447 pregnancies at risk, of which 289 were at risk for lysosomal disorders, 42 metabolic diseases were diagnosed prenatally on chorionic villi (Poenaru 1987). For 33 diseases diagnosis can be considered precise, because affected fetuses have been recognized from villi and the defect has been

Table 5.2 Diseases for which prenatal diagnosis is possible on chorionic villi

Direct analysis of chorionic villi

Pompe	Niemann–Pick Type A
Gaucher	Lesch–Nyhan
Tay–Sachs	Menkes
Sandhoff	Citrullinaemia
Landing	Leucinosis
Mannosidosis	Tyrosinosis
Mucopolysaccharidosis type I (Hurler)	Propionic acidaemia
Mucopolysaccharidosis type II (Hunter)	Chondrodysplasia punctata
Mucopolysaccharidosis type III (San Filippo)	Wolman
Fabry	

Direct analysis and analysis of cultured cells as back-up
Adrenoleucodystrophy
Zellweger
Krabbe
Metachromatic leukodystrophy
Mucopolysaccharidosis type VI
Partial deficiencies
All atypical cases

Chorionic villus cell cultures necessary
Sialidosis
Mucolipidoses II and III
Xeroderma pigmentosum
Niemann–Pick Type C
Diseases in Table 5.3, until a deficiency is recognized in villi

confirmed on abortuses. Nine disorders where a positive diagnosis has not been made, probably due to the small number of studies in each condition, remain as diseases presumably amenable to diagnosis by chorionic villus analysis, until a diagnosis is confirmed on abortuses (Table 5.3).

Problems Our experience in the diagnosis of metabolic disorders on chorionic villi reveals two types of problems.

1. *Sampling difficulties* (Table 5.4). To circumvent these problems, it is essential that the obstetrician sample using the method in which he or she has experience, and discuss with the laboratory the tissue requirements for the particular analyses foreseen. Maternal cell contamination is a serious source of error, rendering the enzyme analysis valueless. Close microscopic examination of villi at the site of sampling or in the laboratory helps prevent this occurrence. DNA analysis has been proposed to rule out maternal contamination, but this is primarily useful where prenatal diagnosis also relies on DNA analysis.

Table 5.3 Diseases for which prenatal diagnosis on chorionic villi may be possible (deficiencies not yet diagnosed)

Glutaric aciduria
Chondrodysplasia punctata
Fucosidosis
Mucopolysaccharidosis Type VII
Orotidyldecarboxylase deficiency
Wolman

Table 5.4 Difficulties in trophoblast sampling

Sample too small
Bloody sample
Failed sampling
Maternal contamination
Inconsistent enzyme activity in several samples of the same case
Twins
Metal contamination (Menkes)

---

2. *Enzyme expression in trophoblastic tissue* (Table 5.5). A certain number of these difficulties are inherent to the trophoblastic tissue type, but because they are known in advance they can be avoided. It is important to consider:

- choice of direct analysis (Pompe, Gaucher) or analysis on cultured cells (sialidosis, Hurler) taking into consideration the optimal enzymatic expression;
- analysis of the proband's fibroblasts in atypical forms of the disease;

Table 5.5 Problems with enzyme expression

Differences in enzyme activity between chorionic villi in direct analysis, cultured villi, and cultured amniotic fluid cells

Presence of trophoblast-specific isoenzymes

Usually weak enzyme activity (e.g. neuraminidase)

Absence of expression of the defect in chorionic villi analysed directly (e.g. mucolipidosis type II)

Atypical cases (variants)

Pseudodeficit (apparent deficit)

Association with a chromosomal anomaly

- analysis of cultured villi which ensures the diagnosis of the disease where it is not expressed in trophoblast (mucolipidosis II);
- study of parents who are healthy but where there is a pseudodeficiency.

Study of the karyotype in the prenatal diagnosis of metabolic disorders reduces the likelihood of misdiagnosis. Chorionic villi is the tissue of choice for metabolic disorders because of its reliability and the early availability of results, at around the 10th week of pregnancy. There are some pregnancies which cannot benefit from this early diagnosis and for which an amniocentesis or transabdominal chorionic villus sampling is necessary:

- women who present themselves too late in pregnancy;
- late diagnosis of proband, after a new pregnancy is under way;
- same-sex twins when one cannot sample from each embryo;
- obstetrical contraindications.

Diagnostic methods

Methods used vary depending on the metabolic abnormality and the type of biological material available. The wisest choice among the numerous available techniques is determined by the expression of the disease. The method of investigating enzymopathies may address:

- the metabolites (physiological substrate);
- specific protein defect (enzyme or extraenzymatic factors);
- the mutated gene itself.

Indirect method of substrate study   Before the molecular identification of genetic anomalies, demonstration of the accumulation or of the excessive excretion of certain metabolites was the only course to follow in identifying many of the enzymopathies, and a variety of methods for this indirect analysis were established. Adapted to tissues derived from the fetus, some of these methods are still in use for primary diagnosis or to complement other methods of diagnosis:

1. Measurement of metabolites in tissue or amniotic fluid; for example measurement of aminoglycans in amniotic fluid. An increase is pathognomonic of mucopolysaccharidosis, but the specific type of disorder remains to be determined.

2. Sometimes enzymes are themselves substrates for other enzymes. This is the case in mucolipidosis types II and III where the etiology is a deficiency in phosphotransferase which acts on several lysosomal enzymes by phosphorylating unphosphorylated mannose. When these lysosomal enzymes are not phosphorylated they are not recognized by the receptor specific for the mannose-6-phosphate and they are not transported into the lysosome. Measurement of lysosomal enzymes in cultured cells (amniocytes, chorionic villi, fibroblasts)

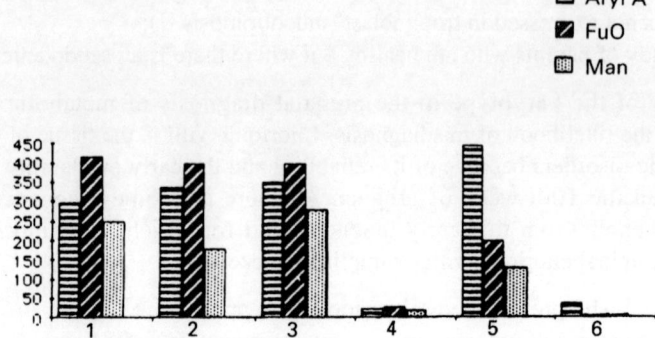

Fig. 5.4 Expression of lysosomal enzymes in mucolipidosis type II (MLII). 1, normal chorionic villi (direct analysis); 2, MLII chorionic villi (direct analysis); 3, normal chorionic villi (in culture); 4, MLII chorionic villi (in culture); 5, normal amniotic fluid cells (in culture); 6, MLII amniotic fluid cells (in culture).

permits this diagnosis by demonstrating reduced levels. This decrease is not observed in non-cultured trophoblasts studied directly (Fig. 5.4).

3. Isotopic dilution using a substrate analogue allows recognition and measurement of organic compounds present in very small amounts.

4. Mono- or bidirectional chromatography on cellulose acetate allows identification of specific spots of glycosaminoglycans with Alcian Blue stain. A larger spot corresponding to a specific glycosaminoglycan demonstrates an absence of the enzyme responsible for its degradation. Table 5.6 lists the types of glycosaminoglycans which accumulate in each type of mucopolysaccharidoses and illustrates the difficulty of interpretation in different disorders characterized by the accumulation of the same glycosaminoglycan, especially now that so many different forms of mucopolysaccharidoses have been described. A measure of the enzyme itself would give a more precise diagnosis.

5. Gas chromatography linked to mass spectrometry provides good separation and specificity for organic acids.

6. In cases of mucopolysaccharidoses, radioactively labelled sulphate is incorporated in cultured amniotic fluid cells or cultured trophoblastic cells and labelled glycosaminoglycan is measured. In normal cells, the level is low because glycosaminoglycans are rapidly metabolized in the presence of specific enzymes; in the cells of a mucopolysaccharidose-affected fetus, on the other hand, these labelled glycosaminoglycans accumulate.

7. For a large number of aminoacidopathies, the release of carbon dioxide from labelled substrates is studied. In branched-chain ketoaciduria, labelled leucine is used and in glutaric acidemia type II, the substrate is ^{14}C-butarate. Other examples of incorporation of labelled precursors used are labelled copper in Menke's disease and labelled cystine in cystinosis.

Table 5.6 Mucopolysaccharidoses

Type	Deficiency	Accumulated glyclosaminoglycans
1 (Hurler)	α-L-Iduronidase	Dermatan sulfate
I (Scheie) (formerly Type V)	α-L-Iduronidase	Heparan sulfate
II (Hunter)	α-L-Iduronidase sulfatase	Dermatan sulfate Heparan sulfate
III (Sanfilippo)	A Sulfamidase B α-Glucosaminidase C α-Glucosamine-N-acetyl-transferase	Heparan sulfate
IV (Morquio)	α-Glucosamine-6-sulfate-sulfatase β-Galactosidase	Keratan sulfate Chondroitin sulfate
VI (Maroteaux–Lamy)	Arylsulfatase B	Dermatan sulfate Chondroitin sulphate
VII (Sly)	β-Glucuronidase	Dermatan sulfate
VIII (Di Ferrante)	α-Glucosamine-6-sulfate-sulfate	Keratan sulfate Heparan sulfate

Direct measure of enzyme An increasing number of genetic disorders have been identified and recognized as being the final expression of the same enzyme defect. Hexosaminidase is a case in point. The hexosaminidase pathway from the gene starts with the transcription of two specific messages for the α and β subunits, translation, association [α,β (Hex A), β,β (Hex B)], glycosylation, and phosphorylation to mannose-6-phosphate. The latter is a recognition marker for transport to the lysosomes, which is carried out by means of specific membrane receptors. The last stage in the post-translational process takes place in the lysosomes, and consists of limited proteolysis giving rise to the functional enzyme.

A block can occur at any level of synthesis, maturation, or regulation. It results, in all cases, in a deficiency in hexosaminidase resulting in clinical heterogeneity (Table 5.7). For the α subunit alone a number of gene defects have been described and are responsible for this diversity. They range from nonsense point mutations to intron mutations and from mutations of a few base pairs to deletions of up to several thousand bases. Biochemical and clinical heterogeneity has been demonstrated for most of the enzymopathies. In these circumstances the detection technique which covers all possible variations of the defect becomes the method of choice; that is, the measure of enzyme activity with synthetic or natural substrates.

Enzyme assay is generally performed using fluorescent synthetic substrates (derived from 4-methylombelliferone), chromogenic substrates (derived from paranitrocatechol or paranitrophenol), or radioactive substrates. These synthetic substrates are commercially available, easy to use, and give a rapid response.

Table 5.7 Heterogeneity in hexosaminidase deficiency

Clinical expression	Origin	Anomaly of biological expression
Type B (Tay–Sachs disease)		
Hexosaminidase A deficiency and defective α subunit		
Classic infantile type		
	Ashkenazi	Protein (–) RNA (–)
	French Canadian	Protein (–) RNA (+)
	Italian	Insoluble protein
	Other	Labile catalytic activity
Late infantile type	French	5 per cent normal enzyme present
Adult	German	Abnormal $\alpha\beta$ subunit association
Juvenile	German	Abnormal $\alpha\beta$ subunit association
Asymptomatic	German	Abnormal maturation
Type O (Sandhoff disease)		
Deficiency in hexosaminidase A and B and defective β subunits		
Classical	US	Protein (–) RNA (–)
		Protein (–) RNA (+)
	French	Protein (+), Abnormal RNA splicing
Asymptomatic	French	Protein B (–), abnormal association of β subunit
		Protein A (+), altered catalytic activity
		β precursor of greater molecular size
Type AB		
Classical	French	Normal enzyme, absence of protein activator

However, simple measurement with an artificial substrate is not always conclusive. Therefore, in pseudodeficits (apparent enzyme deficiency with normal clinical presentation) resulting from a double genetic mutation, one classically found in the disease and the other responsible for a deficiency only observed with the artificial substrate, the diagnosis is made using the natural substrate which is not affected by the second mutation.

For certain diseases (Krabbe disease, Niemann–Pick disease) measure of the labelled natural substrate is the rule for the diagnosis. Enzymes made up of many isoenzymes, where in a disease only one is deficient, must be separated. In Tay–Sachs disease, for example, absence of hexosaminidase A is established by electrophoresis on cellulose acetate and incubation in the presence of 4-methylumbelliferyl β-glucosaminide (Fig. 5.2). Column chromatography (DEAE cellulose) or chemical inactivation may also be used for the separation of isoenzymes, but is much more laborious and is not usually used for purposes of prenatal diagnosis.

Immunological methods   Use of antibodies specific to an isoenzyme (a homogeneous protein) provides a technological advantage in complex biological cases. Their great specificity means that these methods sometimes prove to be the only way of identifying a particular enzymatic form.

The presence of many forms of arylsulfatase in chorionic villi makes the measure of a deficit of arylsulfatase A, associated with leucodystrophy, very difficult. Electrophoresis of immunoprecipitated anti-arylsulfatase A antibodies makes diagnosis of leucodystrophy possible and definite.

To obtain reliable results in prenatal diagnosis, it is sometimes necessary to combine various methods. Therefore, in the diagnosis of metachromatic leuko-dystrophy, an assay of paranitrocatechol sulfate is completed by immuno-precipation–electrophoresis and revealed by 4-methylumbelliferyl sulfate.

Strategy

The strategy in the prenatal diagnosis of inborn errors of metabolism involves co-ordination of numerous steps indispensable to obtaining a fast, reliable, precise diagnosis. The difficulty of co-ordination is a direct consequence of the subtleties in the diagnosis of these conditions, and exists when:

- the diversity of techniques which must be adapted to each disorder makes it such that one laboratory cannot do everything;
- there is an indication for prenatal diagnosis of inborn errors of metabolism only where, with a few exceptions, an index case has been recognized and assessed. This implies being careful about the phenotype specific to the family.

The process is different depending on whether one is dealing with an autosomal recessive or X-linked recessive condition. Autosomal disorders constitute the majority of defects detectable prenatally. Their large number, rarity, and diversity, and the complexity of the techniques needed to diagnose them, render any hopes of systematic screening illusory.

Recognizing families at risk

Identification of the proband (first affected family member)   Screening for index cases in the population is the hardest part. It takes place mainly in the neonatal period, sometimes in adolescence, and, for late onset disorders, in adulthood.

Co-ordinating a thorough clinical investigation encompassing all types of tests (radiological, hematological, biochemical) provides direction for more in depth assessment, which remains the specialist's privilege.

Even though in some disorders the clinical phenotype is classical, and the underlying enzyme defect is already suspected, it is impossible to consider prenatal diagnosis if the proband's diagnosis is purely a clinical presumption. The precise tissue localization of the enzyme deficit is indispensable. This is particularly so in lysosomal disorders, where in addition to the clinical similarities of a group of diseases, the causes are different (for example mucopolysaccharidosis). The existence of different forms of the same disease also requires that the precise biochemical defect be delineated in the first-affected child, thus identifying the deficiency to look for, and what method to use for prenatal diagnosis.

In the case of severe inborn errors of metabolism with a poor prognosis, where the early death of the child does not allow for detection of the biochemical defect, it is important to culture fibroblasts, and to store samples of blood, urine, leucocytes, and liver which will serve to identify the particular deficit. Prenatal diagnosis will then be possible for these families.

Another precautionary step is to study the parents to eliminate a pseudodeficit, where there is a clinically normal individual with an apparently deficient enzyme. This phenomenon has been described for several enzymes, including hexosaminidase, and arylsulfatase A. The most plausible explanation for these findings is the presence of a double genetic mutation: one mutation typical of the genetic disease, and the other controlling only the enzyme activity for the artificial substrate. This explains the absence of clinical signs and the level of enzyme activity in the heterozygote obtained with the natural substrate.

Heterozygote detection   In the absence of biochemical testing of the proband an attempt can be made to determined heterozygosity in the parents for the disease in question. With few exceptions, the main difficulty one encounters in trying to determine heterozygosity for inborn errors of metabolism is the wide range of normal values in enzyme levels.

There are two circumstances where optimal conditions for determination of heterozygosity exist:

- when clinical findings in the proband are highly suggestive, for example in galactosaemia;
- within a high-risk ethnic group, a classical example being Tay–Sachs disease in Ashkenazi Jews. Automated screening programs have been set up in the United States and Israel. Of 400 000 screened, 14 000 heterozygotes have been detected and 333 at-risk couples have been identified before the birth of an affected child.

Our evolving knowledge

Once the family's risk has been established and the phenotype delineated, prenatal diagnosis is possible. The difficulties are due to the variety of circumstances which arise. Research in this area has given a better understanding of the diseases and has in many cases elucidated their etiopathogenesis, revealing new aspects which must be taken into consideration.

1. *New diseases* have been discovered, for example β-mannosidase deficiency and α-N-acetylgalactosaminidase deficiency.

2. *New etiological entities* have been discovered among syndromes and diseases already recognized clinically: 'variant' forms. Examples are Morquio

disease (mucopolysaccharidoses type IV) types A and B, or San Filippo disease (mucopolysaccharidoses type III), where types A, B, C, and D are each caused by a different enzymatic defect.

3. *Clinical and biological heterogeneity* is due in particular to the fact that the mutation can occur at different levels: gene, transcription, post-transcription, post-translation, during molecular maturation, or at the level of genes for extra-enzymatic factors, as in the inhibitor involved in the double deficiency of β-galactosidase and neuraminidase or the protein activator of the glycolipid, GM2, present in the AB form of hexosaminidase deficiency. Table 5.7 shows the diseases now known to be due to deficiencies in hexosaminidase, demonstrating their great heterogeneity.

4. *Atypical cases* are represented by patients who have signs distinguishing them from the etiopathogenetic group to which they belong as a result of a majority of their clinical and biological signs. Examples are atypical muco-lipidosis type II and atypical Tay–Sachs disease where clinical manifestations are milder.

5. *Expression of an enzyme*, be it normal or abnormal, is at times different from one tissue to another. We have shown that some enzymes are expressed differently in the uncultured trophoblast, amniotic fluid cells, and cultured chorionic villi. A good example is mucolipidosis type II.

6. *Early diagnosis* is another new aspect. Perfection of obstetric fetal sampling techniques as well as diagnostic methods allowing for an early result (sometimes at 8–10 weeks of gestation) changes attitudes of different specialists with respect to at-risk families.

A decade ago, even when a pregnancy was begun, the detection of proband and therefore of a family at risk allowed identification of the biological defect and preparation for prenatal diagnosis only at 20 weeks (17 weeks for amniocentesis and 3 weeks of tissue culturing). Today, the earliness of chorionic villus sampling means that the nature of the defect itself and peculiarities of the disease within the family must be assessed soon after the proband is identified.

Sometimes, uncooperative families and the difficulties inherent in long-distance collaboration between specialists leads to an awkward situation where prenatal diagnosis must be done without a clearly identified risk. These complications make diagnosis uncomfortable. Therefore, considering the exponential increase in our knowledge of pathological aspects of inborn errors of metabolism, the increase in public awareness of prenatal diagnosis, and the earliness of this medical intervention, the following guidelines should be strictly observed:

- delineate the biochemical defect in the proband;
- eliminate the possibility of pseudodeficit by looking at parents;
- establish a cell line from the proband, particularly when the diagnosis was made in a laboratory other than the laboratory doing prenatal diagnosis;
- have available in the laboratory, information on the family (clinical aspects, tests done and results, address of referring physician, etc.) before testing the fetus.

In order to meet these requirements, a frank and close relationship between specialists and between physician and family is mandatory. Any undue difficulty in co-ordinating all of this can be a major obstacle, for family and physician, to obtaining an uncomplicated prenatal diagnosis.

In practice

Ideal situations

Proband identified, phenotype established prior to a subsequent pregnancy   The laboratory has made the diagnosis and transmitted the results to the referring physician, and given the family a written assessment of the biochemical tests done as well as the prenatal diagnosis to be anticipated. At the beginning of a new pregnancy, the mother informs her physician and the laboratory is alerted; the date, the form of sampling and the amount of tissue required are determined according to the disease. At that time the subject of termination of pregnancy is broached, and extensively discussed with the parents.

Once sampling and biological testing are completed, the result is transmitted immediately to the obstetrician and the family. In the case of an affected fetus, the date for termination of pregnancy is agreed upon by the physician and the laboratory which will receive the products of termination for confirmation of the diagnosis. When there is a normal fetus on direct analysis, confirmation is made on cultured chorionic villi.

Other circumstances

Proband unidentified, pregnancy already begun   Identification of the proband and the biochemical phenotype must be established with urgency.

Proband deceased prior to biochemical diagnosis   Depending on the disease suspected, samples of serum, urine, tissue samples (preferably liver) are frozen. Fibroblasts derived from skin are immediately cultured. One can attempt to identify heterozygosity in the parents, but so far this is possible only for classical Tay–Sachs disease. Prenatal diagnosis is postponed until 17 weeks of gestation in order to do an amniocentesis. One can sometimes do chorionic villus sampling transabdominally and reduce the time by 3–4 weeks. In any case, the success of prenatal diagnosis is dependent on proper communication between all specialists involved in the case.

X-linked disorders

Diagnosis of X-linked recessive conditions consists on the one hand of the diagnosis of carrier females, and on the other hand the prenatal diagnosis itself which is done in two steps: sex diagnosis and, in the case of male fetuses, diagnosis of the disease itself. These types of diagnoses have been improved, in the last few years, by two major developments: chorionic villus sampling techniques, and molecular biology. For several years, the prenatal diagnosis of several X-linked metabolic disorders has been done by enzyme assays on cultured amniotic fluid cells sampled at 17 weeks of gestation. Technically, fetal karyotyping and enzyme analysis was easy enough, but the lateness of results led to a late termination of pregnancy at 20 weeks (4 1/2 months), when an affected fetus was diagnosed; this occurred in half of the male fetuses.

Since 1984, the development of chorionic villus sampling early in pregnancy, around 10–11 weeks, has made testing conditions more acceptable (Poenaru 1984). Direct cytogenetic techniques on chorionic villus samples permit the completion of a fetal karyotype in a few hours, allowing rapid sexing. It also allows for a direct biochemical assay on fresh chorionic villi providing results in 24–48 hr (Table 5.8). As a precaution, a portion of the chorionic villi is usually put into culture: biochemical assays on these cells serve to confirm results of direct analysis or to remove any ambiguous findings.

Table 5.8 X-linked diseases

Disease	Determination of diagnosis
Adrenoleucodystrophy	Long-chain fatty acids
Fabry	α Galactosidase A
Lesch–Nyhan	HGPRT
Menkes	Copper metabolism
Mucopolysaccharidosis type I (Hunter)	Iduronate sulfatase
Ornithine transcarbamylase deficiency	OTC (liver biopsy)

This is the strategy used for the prenatal diagnosis of Hunter (mucopolysaccharidosis type II), Lesch Nyhan, Menkes, Fabry, and adrenoleucodystrophy disease. Should an affected fetus be diagnosed, a pregnancy can be terminated before the third month of pregnancy; three-and-a-half-months if diagnosis requires analyses on culture.

Diagnosis of carrier females

Obligate carriers   Women who are obligate carriers include those having two or more sons affected with a metabolic disorder, or those having an affected son as well as an affected brother, uncle, nephew or maternal cousin. In an isolated case, where a woman has only one affected son, she is usually a carrier, as new mutations are rare for most inborn errors of metabolism. Duchenne muscular dystrophy is an exception, as it has been shown that one-third of cases are new mutations.

Possible carriers   Diagnosis of women related to an affected male is an important issue for these families, as the maternal sisters, aunts, nieces, and cousins are all possible carriers. Theoretically, the diagnosis of carriers can be established at the level of the gene by means of: direct expression of the gene mutation (clotting factor for haemophilias), biochemical assays (long-chain fatty acids for adrenoleucodystrophy), enzyme levels in some metabolic disorders (exceptional), or biochemical abnormalities related to the disease (creatine kinase in myopathies). The interpretation of results however is always difficult because of lyonization of the X chromosome.

Lyonization   Inactivation of the X chromosome occurs very early on in embryonic development. The inactive X may be of maternal or paternal origin from one cell to another in the same organism, but once the decision is made, all daughter cells will inactivate the same X. Inactivation is therefore random, but fixed.

The study of X inactivation is made possible by the expression of a gene carried by the X chromosome, the gene for glucose-6-phosphate-dehydrogenase (G6PD) which has two isoenzymes, variants, A and B.

In cloning the cells from a woman heterozygous for G6PD, we obtain a clone G6PDA and a clone G6PDB. The two electrophoretic variants are expressed, and there is no hybrid band; this shows that, even when cells are *in vitro,* the X inactivation is an irreversible phenomenon. With enzyme assays, it is theoretically possible, using complex cloning techniques, to identify carriers of some X-lined disorders (for example Hunter disease and Lesch–Nyhan disease).

These techniques involve establishing a fibroblast cell culture from a skin biopsy, and from this culture a preparation of clones which will carry one or the other active X, and so enzyme assays must be done separately on each clone. Despite the accuracy of the technique and the study of a large number of clones (at least 20) this technique does not give a diagnosis with 100 per cent accuracy. Lyonization does not always, in every tissue, lead to an equal number of cells with one or the other X inactivated. There are examples where the distribution of cell-types is unequal and where the mutant allele is found in excess; this may explain why there are milder forms of the disease expressed in carrier women, for example in Duchenne muscular dystrophy. This variation in the distribution of cell types explains the limits of enzyme assays (coagulation factors and creatine phosphokinase or CPK) in diagnosing carrier females.

In other cases, there may be a somatic selection during development and cells expressing the mutation do not live as long as the normal cells. For example, in Lesch–Nyhan disease, (Hypoxanthine-guanine phosphoribosyl transferase or HGPRT deficiency), one finds the two cell populations (*HGPRT+, HGPRT–*) in fibroblasts from skin biopsies of carrier mothers, but in serum only *HGPRT+* cells are observed. A similar phenomenon is observed in carriers of X-linked severe combined immunodeficiency, where the mature T lymphocytes show a non-random distribution of cells, favouring those carrying an active normal X. Due to this observation, carrier detection relies on molecular diagnosis by DNA analysis on lymphocytes of suspected carrier females.

Molecular biology is a technology which is of increasing importance in the identification of other X-linked conditions, in addition to Duchenne muscular dystrophy and haemophilia which are already being identified using this method. A number of diseases for which the gene is cloned can already benefit from this technology, in particular when a gene deletion can be identified (ornithine transcarbomylase deficiency, chronic granulomatosis). When the gene has not been cloned, study of polymorphic markers surrounding the gene in an informative family allows for detection of the mutant X.

This method has contributed information complementary to the biochemical methodology in detecting carriers of adrenoleucodystrophy and recently for Hunter disease (Fig. 5.5a); a long costly, family study and DNA analysis of the proband were required in order to identify the informative markers for each family.

Is it worth detecting carriers where a specific and early method of prenatal diagnosis for the disease exists? Scientifically, it is worthwhile: it is satisfying and essential to perfect these techniques. Medically, it is open to discussion. DNA study should indeed allow detection of aunts, sisters, and cousins who are carriers but, considering the ever-present risk of recombination between marker and genes, the biochemical assay would still have to be done. As for the psychological impact, more than 15 years of genetic counselling has proven that it is at times disasterous; in some instances at least ignorance leaves room for hope!

At present and in some conditions, it is reasonable to provide accurate prenatal diagnosis by biochemical analysis to all women in a family, without determining beforehand whether they are carriers or not.

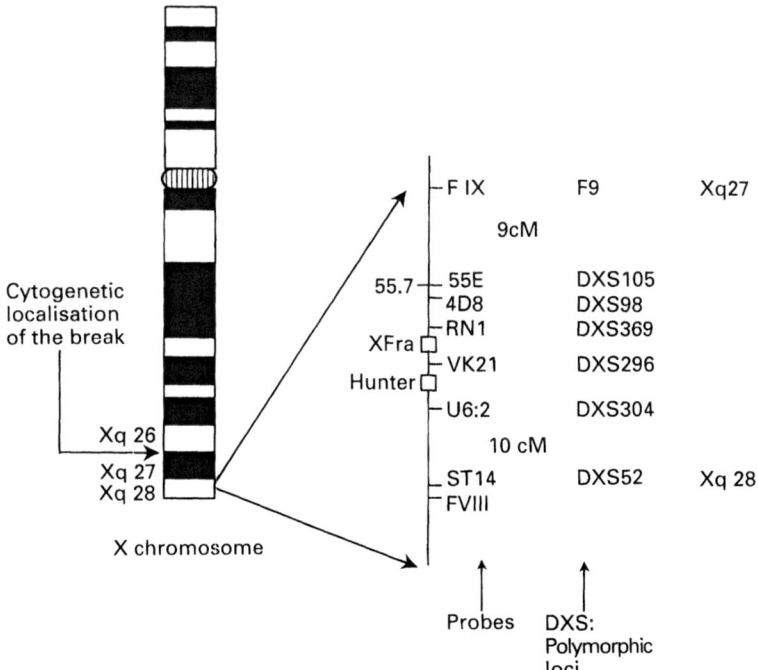

Fig. 5.5a Mapping of the Hunter disease gene and mental handicap associated with fragile X.

This is illustrated by the example of a family with Hunter disease (muco-polysaccharidosis type II) (Fig. 5.5b). In three generations, III, IV, V, 10 boys were affected. Prenatal diagnosis was proposed to all women who were obligate carriers or possible carriers. This has already resulted in the birth of six normal children from women in the fourth generation. Also, a daughter was revealed to be a potential carrier when prenatal diagnosis for her mother's (IV.8) fourth pregnancy detected an affected fetus, after three normal pregnancies.

Possible carrier females in the fifth generation were able to benefit from pre-natal diagnosis by chorionic villus sampling from the time of their first preg-nancy without knowing if they were carriers; two (V.2, V.4) had affected fetuses and are therefore carriers. One (V.1) had three girls and it could not be determined whether she was a carrier. Very recently, the gene for Hunter dis-ease has been better localized and the availability of polymorphic markers surrounding the gene has opened possibilities for carrier detection in this family. We now know that V.1, V.5, and V.6 are carrier females (Leguern *et al.* 1990).

Congenital adrenal hyperplasias

21-Hydroxylase deficiency

21-Hydroxylase deficiency is responsible for 90 per cent of congenital adrenal hyperplasia, an autosomal recessive disorder. The deficiency results in insufficient synthesis of cortisol, an increase in the secretion of ACTH which

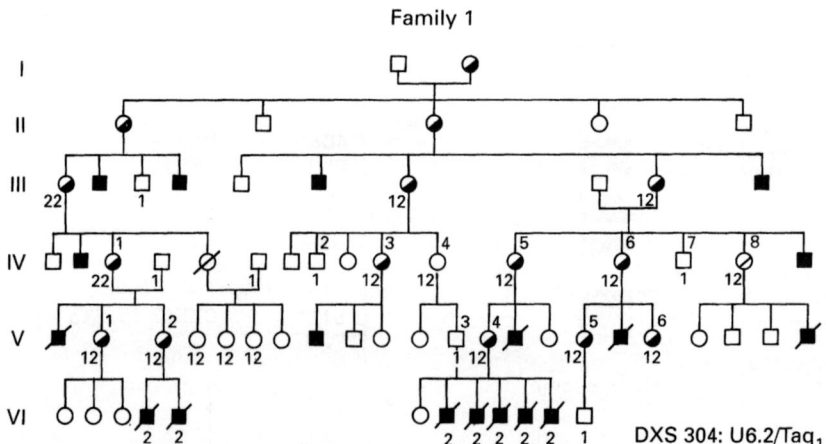

Fig. 5.5b Pedigree of a Hunter disease family using results from V6.2 probe analysis. All affected males carry allele 2, all unaffected males carry allele 1. Carrier status was determined by haplotype association to mutant genes using several probes.

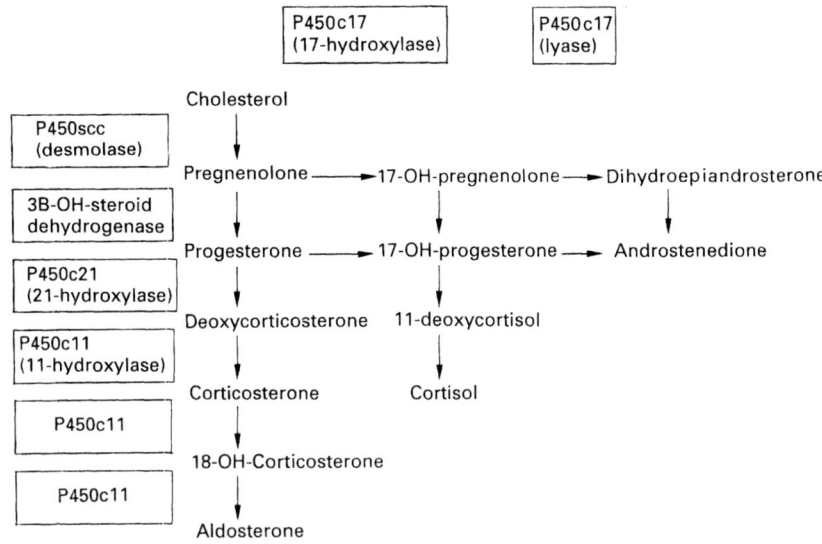

Fig. 5.6 Biosynthesis of steroid hormones.

is responsible for adrenal hyperplasia, an accumulation of the precursor 17-hydroxyprogesterone before the enzyme block, and excessive production of androgens (Fig. 5.6).

In the classical congenital form, we observe in girls different degrees of virilization resulting from the abnormally increased amount of androgen during fetal development. In approximately one-third of cases the biosynthesis of aldosterone is perturbed, resulting in a salt-losing syndrome which can be observed in boys and girls homozygous for the deficiency.

Along with this severe congenital form, which justifies prenatal diagnosis, there are other milder forms which are expressed by later virilization and hirsutism, and some completely asymptomatic forms which are only brought to light by biochemical analysis during family studies. In these milder forms there is only a partial enzyme deficiency and the secretion of cortisone may be sufficient, at the expense of an adrenal hyperplasia. Now that we have a better understanding of all forms of 21-hydroxylase deficiency, we are led to believe that this is one of the more common genetic diseases. For the congenital form alone, neonatal screening has shown that the incidence is between 1/500 and 1/15 000.

Classical genetics   There is close linkage between the gene of the major histocompatibility complex (HLA) on the short arm of chromosome 6 and the 21-hydroxylase gene (Fig. 5.7), and family studies have closely mapped the

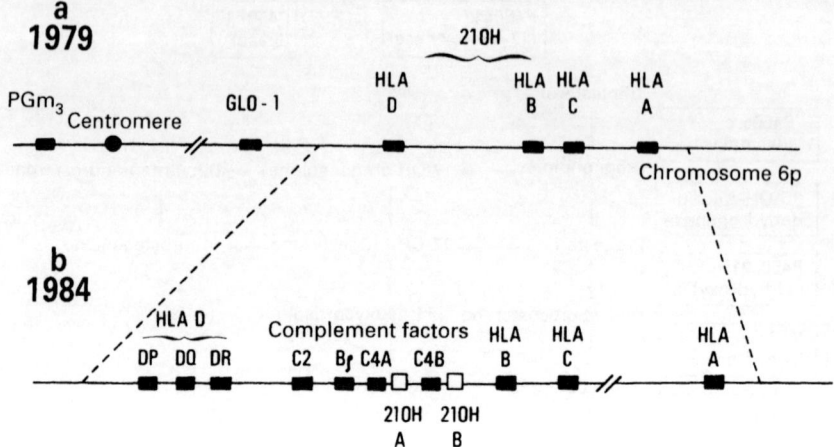

Fig. 5.7 *HLA* and *21-OH* genes on the short arm of chromosome 6. *a*, mapping in 1979; *b*, mapping of *21-OH* gene in 1984.

21-hydroxylase gene to HLA-B. It is an example of classical linkage, where two genes are physically linked on the same chromosome and remain linked during their genetic transmission. The serological HLA polymorphism can serve as a marker for the 21-hydroxylase gene and allows for segregation studies within families because the two HLA haplotypes are expressed co-dominantly.

In terms of the autosomal recessive transmission, each parent of the affected child is an obligate carrier and transmits an HLA haplotype linked to the 21-hydroxylase deficiency locus. Brothers and sisters having the same two HLA haplotypes as the index case are also homozygotic for the disease. Those having

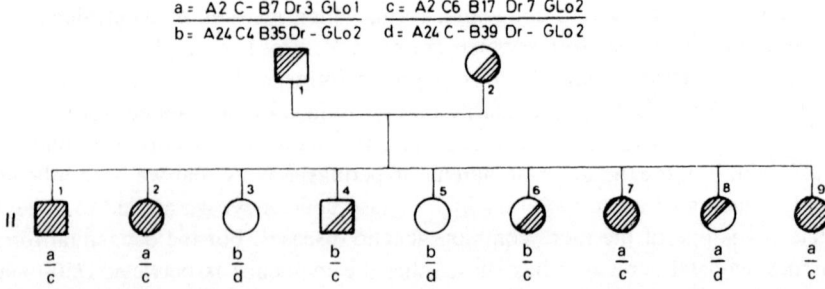

Fig. 5.8 Pedigree for family D. Affected children II. 1, 2, 7 and 9 are carriers of the same *HLA* haplotypes, a: *A2CB7 DRw3 GLO1* and c: *A2 Cw6 B17 DRw7 GLO2*. Knowing these haplotypes identifies children 3 and 5 as homozygous normal, children 4 and 6 as heterozygous for the defect inherited from the mother, and child 8 as heterozygous for the defect inherited from the father.

only one identical HLA haplotype are heterozygotic (Fig. 5.8). Family members having no common HLA haplotype are homozygous normal.

The mutation responsible for 21-hydroxylase deficiency can be linked to any HLA-B serotype, and the distribution of various antigens linked to the deficiency is the same as the distribution in the general population. This shows that mutations must have been very frequent and could have occurred randomly and close to any HLA-B serotype.

There are some exceptions: B47 haplotype is found in 10–15 per cent of patients with 21-hydroxylase deficiency; in these cases there is an absence of C4B, one of the C4 antigens. (In a normal person there are two genes, coding for C4A and C4B respectively.) Serotype B8 is rarely linked to 21-hydroxylase deficiency (2.8 per cent), but is frequent (8.3 per cent) in the general population, and in these normal people there is an absence of antigen C4A.

Genetic linkage, first made evident for the early-onset form, was subsequently shown to exist in the late-onset form. In the latter form, the link is with HLA B14 and is observed in 70 per cent of affected cases. In normal subjects 11 per cent also carry HLA B14; this association demonstrates a founder effect with simultaneous transmission of B14 haplotype and the late-onset 21-hydroxylase mutation. Study of antigen C4 demonstrates a duplication of C4B.

Molecular genetics of 21-hydroxylase 21-Hydroxylase is one of the four enzymes using cytochrome P450 which are necessary for the conversion of cholesterol to cortisol. DNA probes for the 21-hydroxylase gene were used to demonstrate the existence of two loci, *21-OH-A* and *21-OH-B*, situated in tandem and close to the *C4* genes, *C4A* and *C4B*, the reading sequence being the same (Fig. 5.9). The two genes, *21-OH-A* and *21-OH-B*, are of similar structure.

The existence of deletions or duplications in these genes has allowed progress in the understanding of the respective importance of each of these loci coding for 21-hydroxylase.

1. Homozygotes for haplotype *HLA B47* and showing the classical form of early-onset 21-hydroxylase deficiency have a homozygous deletion of genes *21-OH-B* and *C4B*, and fragments *21-OH-A* and *C4A* are intact.

2. Healthy subjects having the *HLA B8* haplotype have a deletion mutation of both *21-OH-A* and *C4A* without demonstrating a 21-hydroxylase deficiency.

3. Those affected with a late-onset 21-hydroxylase deficiency are carriers of the *HLA B14* haplotype and have a duplication of the *21-OH-A* gene.

There are therefore two genes, *21-OH-A* and *21-OH-B*, which code for cytochrome P450, specific for 21-hydroxylation. The B gene is definitely functional, because once the deletion has been demonstrated, early-onset 21-hydroxylase deficiency is observed. The B gene function alone is adequate as B8 normal individuals can have a deletion of the other gene, *21-OH-A*.

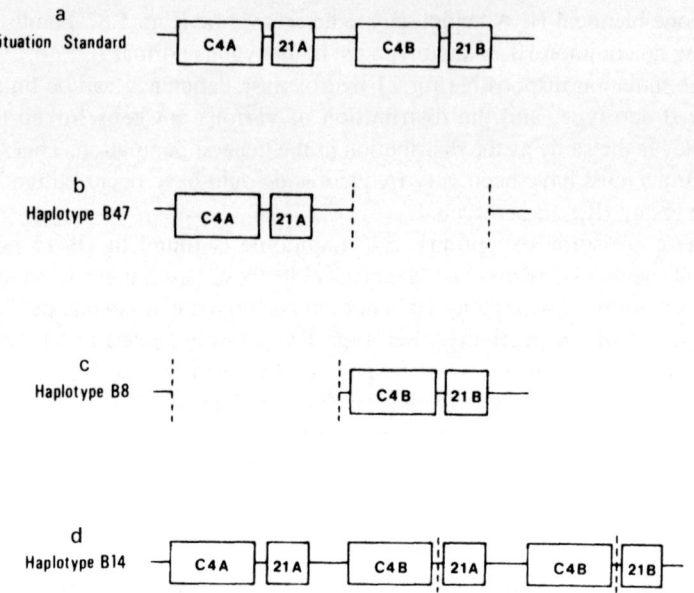

Fig. 5.9 Examples of deletions and duplications of *C4* and *21-OH* genes associated with certain *HLA* haplotypes. *a*, normal situation; *b*, haplotype *B47*; *c*, haplotype *B8*; *d*, haplotype *B14*.

In most individuals affected with the late onset form there is no gene deletion, but in recent studies a mutation in *21-OH-B* has been observed after sequencing of this gene. Some of these mutations correspond to the changes observed in the *21-OH-A* gene, which rendered it non-functional. There must have been gene conversion involving these two genes. Recent studies of the different mutations responsible for 21-hydroxylase deficiency have demonstrated that, in caucasian populations, 20 per cent were deletions, 60 per cent of the seven known mutations were due to gene conversion, and 20 per cent were of a mutation not yet identified. This means that in most affected cases the deficit is a result of two different mutational events. In practice, this excludes all possibility of diagnosis by direct analysis of the gene.

Methods of prenatal diagnosis   Prenatal diagnosis can be done in the first and second trimester using two complementary tests: description of the fetal genotype and demonstration of the enzymatic deficiency.

The fetal genotype can be established indirectly by using polymorphic markers. Segregation of the 21-hydroxylase gene in a family can be followed by using its close linkage to the HLA locus. Three techniques can be used:

1. *Typing of HLA antigens on fetal cells.* Common HLA antigen typing techniques on blood cells have been adapted to fetal cells obtained at amniocentesis and cultured *in vitro*, because a large number of cells is required.

HLA typing on fetal cells is done using cytotoxicity or microabsorption techniques. When some cases present technical difficulties (cross-reaction, antigens difficult to identify in culture), analysis of the following results permits internal control: two parental HLA haplotypes should be identified in the fetus and the other two should be excluded. Despite the great number of HLA polymorphisms, it is possible that the parents have common antigens or are homozygous, so that the number of markers is reduced.

The risk of genetic recombination (by crossing-over) between *HLA-A* and *21-OH* likely to lead to a misdiagnosis is about 2 per cent, and much less with *HLA-B*.

2. *Study of DNA markers using probes specific to HLA genes*: transfer of concepts used in HLA typing to the field of molecular biology. DNA probes for HLA class I (*HLA A, B, C*) and class II (*HLA*-D) genes are available. Serologically, there are a large number of *HLA* polymorphisms, and on the molecular level, the number is even greater. Some of the gene polymorphisms correspond to the serological polymorphisms.

In order to study the parent's and the proband's DNA using the restriction fragment length polymorphisms obtained with class I and class II probes, the diagnosis requires preliminary family studies using serological HLA polymorphisms and a choice of endonucleases according to these serological markers. The wealth of polymorphisms makes diagnosis of this disease reliable. The diagnosis of 21-hydroxylase deficiency is illustrated in Fig. 5.10.

In the light of current experience, one can simplify this protocol: serological typing in a family is not an absolute requirement, and use of the probes for class I alone is sufficient as, after studying several families, no crossing-over between *HLA B* and *21-OH* has yet been described.

3. *Direct diagnosis with probes for the 21-OH gene*. This is much more appealing theoretically, but it can only rarely be applied. In fact, only in families where the deletion is homozygous in the affected child, can a direct diagnosis be made. With the exception of *B47/B47* cases, detection of the deletion requires long family studies which are impossible in practice.

Steroid levels in amniotic fluid Observation of an increase in 17-dihydroxyprogesterone in amniotic fluid from pregnancies leading to the birth of child with 21-hydroxylase deficiency has allowed the measurement of this product for prenatal diagnosis.

Study of the levels of 17-dihydroxyprogesterone throughout pregnancy demonstrates a progressive decrease in both normal and abnormal levels. On amniotic fluids sampled between 16 and 18 weeks of gestation, the difference between an affected and unaffected fetus is clear; this method is the one largely used.

More recently, measurements of 17-dihydroxyprogesterone on amniotic fluids drawn earlier, at 10–11 weeks' gestation, have demonstrated that a diagnosis was possible as early as this, because the differences between normal and abnor-

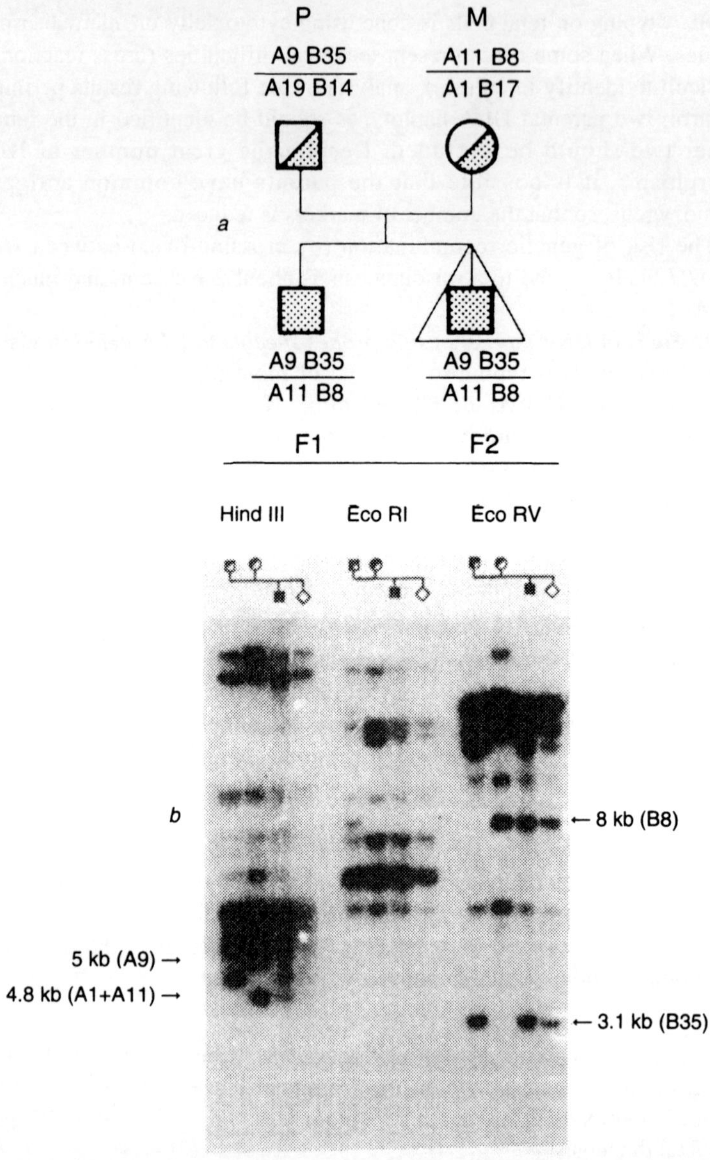

Fig. 5.10 Prenatal diagnosis of 21-hydroxylase deficiency. DNA from both parents from the proband, and from chorionic villi, are obtained. (*a*), pedigree and *HLA* haplotyping of the family using serological techniques; (*b*), results obtained with class I *HLA* (the order of the four tracks is, from left to right, father, mother, proband, and villi. With *EcoR5* one can identify band *B8* in the mother, the proband, and the villi, and band *B35* in the father, the proband, and the villi. The results are confirmed using *Hin*d III, which demonstrates bands *A9* and *A11* in the DNA of the villi. It is obvious that with each of the three enzymes the same band distribution is observed in the proband and the villi, demonstrating that they have the same genotype.

mal values are large enough at this time. Figure 5.11 shows data obtained by Raux-Demay (personal communication) and collaborators. 21-Deoxycortisol can be measured at the same time as 17-dihydroxyprogesterone.

In practice Prenatal diagnosis of 21-hydroxylase deficiency rests on two complementary methods: on one hand the fetal genotype for 21-hydroxylase, and on the other the biochemical expression of the disease. These techniques can be performed in either the first or second trimester.

Methods chosen as determined by family studies The following factors must be taken into account:

1. *Family structure.* To determine fetal genotype one must know the genotype of the index case. If the index case is deceased or sampling could not be done, this method of diagnosis is excluded.

2. *Gestational age at the time of referral.* Does it allow HLA typing and DNA analysis of parents and proband prior to fetal sampling?

3. *Parent's attitude should an affected fetus be diagnosed*:

- the parents decide to continue the pregnancy, with the desire for treatment to prevent masculinization of a female fetus. This treatment must be considered from the 5th week of pregnancy. In these cases, we do not have reliable 17-dihydroxyprogesterone levels; the diagnosis of the fetus will therefore be made on DNA obtained from chorionic villi;

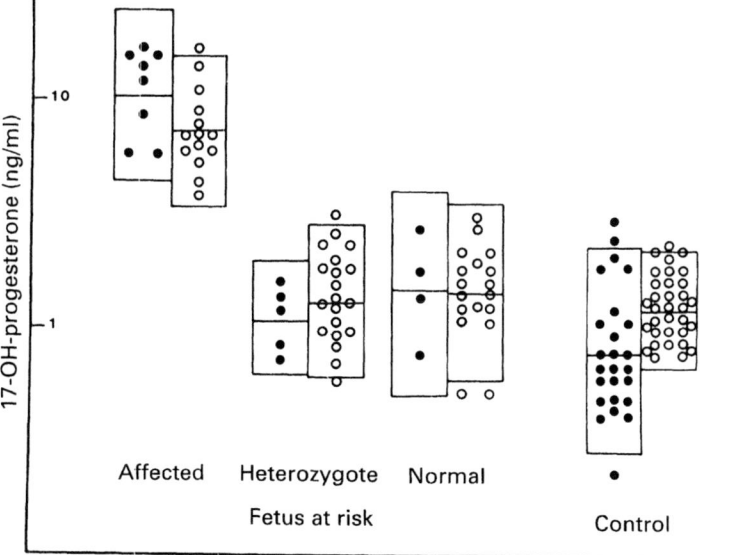

Fig. 5.11 Levels of 17-hydroxyprogesterone observed in amniotic fluid. ●, 11 weeks of gestation; ○, 16–17 weeks of gestation. From M. Raux-Demay, personal communication.

- the parents wish to terminate the pregnancy: (a) only in the case of an affect-ed female fetus, so one must determine fetal karyotype by chorionic villi; (b) in an affected fetus regardless of sex; then fetal karyotype is not important and an early amniocentesis to measure 17-dihydroxyprogesterone is all that is necessary for diagnosis.

Methods determined by the practicalities of techniques used   The following factors should be taken into account:

1. *Sampling conditions and their risks.* At the 11th week, simultaneous amniotic fluid sampling and chorionic villus sampling does not seem to present more risks than chorionic villus sampling alone, if the procedures are carried out by physicians with expertise. Once the pregnancy is beyond the 11th week the risk of chorionic villus sampling rises and at 12–16 weeks, it is preferable to limit testing to amnio-centesis for measurement of 17-dihydroxyprogesterone, along with fetal sexing. HLA typing on fetal cells should be done for fluids sampled beyond 16 weeks.

2. *Laboratory facilities.* Molecular studies depend on a laboratory having probes for 21-hydroxylase and HLA. A family study must be done, and a result should be obtained 10–15 days later. Measuring 17-dihydroxyprogesterone requires a radioimmunology laboratory with established norms from control fluid samples; results should be available 2–4 days later.

11-β-Hydroxylase deficiency

Much less frequent (in approximately 5 per cent of congenital adrenal hyperplasia cases), the 11-β-hydroxylase deficiency results in a deficiency in the conversion of 11-deoxycortisol to cortisol and of 11-deoxycorticosterone to corticosterone. This is an autosomal recessive disorder, not linked to HLA, located on 8q, and for which the gene has recently been sequenced (Mornet *et al.* 1989). Prenatal diag-nosis can be done by measurement of tetrahydro-11-deoxycortisol and of dioxy-cortisone, but this diagnosis still has its limits.

Cystic fibrosis

Cystic fibrosis is the most common single-gene mutation in northern European and North American populations, affecting 1/2000 to 1/2500 births. It is an auto-somal recessive disorder, and in the general population 1/20 to 1/25 people are carriers of the mutant gene.

Our knowledge of the disease has evolved gradually. At the clinical level the heterogeneity in each of its manifestations, and their lack of specificity, explains firstly why the disease was not fully described until 1938 and secondly the difficulty of determining the frequency of the disease in populations where mortal-ity of small children related to infection still exists (for example, North Africa).

Clinically, there is no biochemical assay specific for the disease, and the sweat test remains the only diagnostic test. Fundamentally, the biochemical

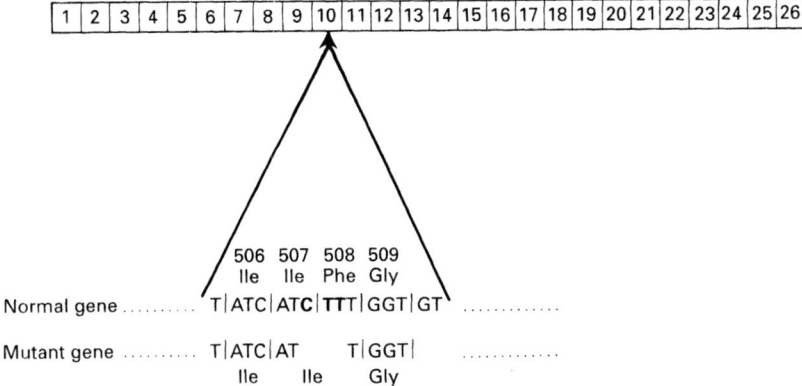

Fig. 5.12 Cystic fibrosis transmembrane regulator (CTFR). 1480 amino acids. Coding gene approximately 6500 bp, 26 exons. Total DNA length approximately 250 000 bp (exons + introns).

mechanisms have not been defined, but genetic progress has been spectacular. In September 1989 the gene was identified and characterized (Rommens *et al.* 1989). It is a long gene of 26 exons coding for a 1480 amino acid protein, the full length of DNA (exons and introns) being 250 000 base pairs (Fig. 5.12).

Clinical manifestations of cystic fibrosis are a result of an alteration in permeability to chlorine ions on the epithelial mucous membrane. The structure of the chloride channels is not modified; it is the regulatory mechanism for their function which is disturbed.

Discovery of the protein coded by the cystic fibrosis gene is important, because the cystic fibrosis transmembrane regulator (CFTR) is homologous in structure to a family of transmembrane proteins which plays an important role in ATP-dependent transport. One must elucidate the physiological role of this protein, as well as abnormalities in its function in cystic fibrosis.

Difficulties in basic analyses of cystic fibrosis have held back the development of diagnostic methods: specific diagnosis of disease in the child, neonatal and prenatal diagnosis, and the identification of heterozygotes. Research on prenatal diagnosis was disappointing until 1983, when David Brock demonstrated a deficiency of intestinal enzymes in amniotic fluid of pregnancies resulting in the birth of an affected child. Molecular genetic studies opened new doors. In 1985 a number of teams were able to map the gene for cystic fibrosis to the long arm of chromosome 7 at band 7q31. Two-allele polymorphisms were revealed by molecular probes corresponding to DNA segments surrounding and in close proximity to the gene (Fig. 5.13). Initially, only four probes *(Met D, Met H, 7C22, and J3.11)* were available. The family structure of those requesting prenatal diagnoses limited the possibility of identifying polymorphisms associated to the mutant gene: the affected child was often the only child. Then, new mol-

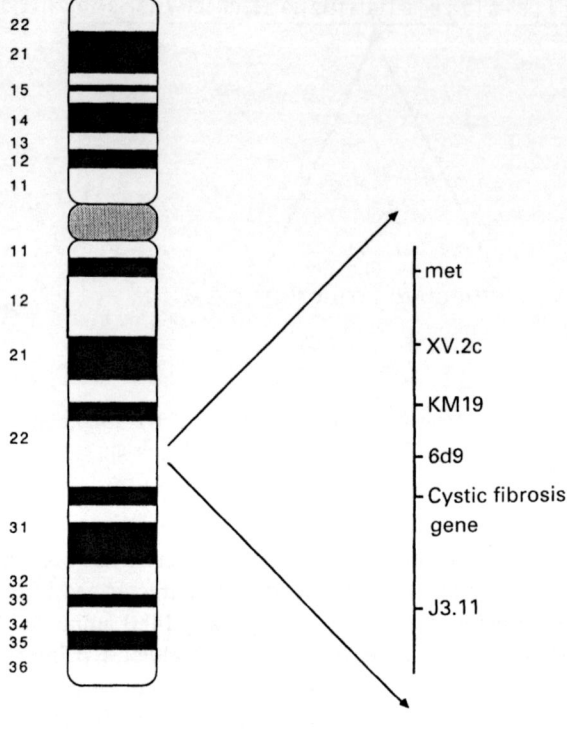

CHROMOSOME 7

Fig. 5.13 Chromosome 7.

ecular probes *XV2C* and *KM19* were found to be mapped very close to the gene. In addition, the distribution of the two allelic forms of these markers on the chromosomes of children affected with cystic fibrosis was different to that in those chromosomes not carrying the mutant gene; this is known as haplotype analysis and can be useful in assessing a risk for a chromosome to carry a cystic fibrosis gene.

Studies of families with an affected child have shown that haplotype B (*XV2C* allele 1/*KM19* allele 2) was found in 80–87 per cent of carriers of cystic fibrosis and was present in only 10–15 per cent of non-carrier subjects (Table 5.9). With the help of these two markers and the presence of strong linkage disequilibrium, the possibility of prenatal diagnosis could be extended to a large number of families.

In September 1989, at the time of the characterization of the gene, Rommens *et al.* (1989) showed the existence of a main mutation consisting of a 3 deletion in the tenth exon, contributing to the loss at the protein level of phenylalanine in position 508, hence the name of the mutation Δ*F508* (Fig. 5.12)

Studies on hundreds of affected children in northern Europe and North America show that 70–75 per cent of chromosomes carrying the disease have this mutation: 50 per cent of these children are homozygous for $\Delta F508$, 40 per cent are compound heterozygotes for $\Delta F508$ and another mutation, and 10 per cent are homozygous for other mutations.

A close international collaboration (The Cystic Fibrosis Genetic Analysis Consortium 1990) permitted, in a very short time, the establishment of the frequency of $\Delta F508$ in each country and the identification of many other mutations for cystic fibrosis (Table 5.10). So far over 350 mutations have been described, but these are still rare and can complicate the identification of non-$\Delta F508$ chromosomes carrying the mutant gene.

Gene isolation and discovery of many more mutations have extended the possibility of diagnosis in families having a child affected with cystic fibrosis. This diagnosis can be based on direct analysis of the gene or, if not, by indirect analysis of segregation of the gene, with markers *KM19* and *XV2C*.

Available techniques

Molecular techniques for diagnosis

Direct methods   A direct diagnosis is possible since the discovery of the $\Delta F508$ and other mutations. The diagnosis of the mutation is achieved by amplifying the DNA segment surrounding the mutation using primers on either end by the polymerase chain reaction (PCR), and by using the allele-specific oligonucleotide (ASO) method. Dot blot visualization uses two synthetic oligonucleotides labelled with radioactive phosphorus, one recognizing the normal sequence and the other the mutant sequence (see p. 73). This direct method for $\Delta F508$ alone would be possible in 60 per cent of cases if the frequency of $\Delta F508$ in the population is close to 80 per cent, 50 per cent if the frequency is 70 per cent, and 25 per cent if the frequency is 50 per cent (see Table 5.10).

Indirect diagnosis   This uses the classical method of analysing the segregation of the mutant gene in a family using polymorphic markers close to the gene. The PCR method is not always applicable, and one must rely on Southern blotting, which takes much longer and requires a larger amount of DNA. In addition, because the diagnosis is based on linkage between the gene and the polymorphic markers, one must first do a family study where the proband is investigated in order to assess the informativeness of the markers. One must first make use of the two markers, *KM19* and *XV2C*, which are informative alone or in association with each other in about two-thirds of families. In other cases other markers can be used. Overall, prenatal diagnosis will be possible in 9/10 families.

In our experience, after assessing informativeness, prenatal diagnosis was possible using only one informative marker in 61 per cent of cases, two markers in 38 per cent of cases, and three markers in 1 per cent of cases.

Table 5.9 Frequency of the different haplotypes in normal and in cystic fibrosis (CF) chromosomes in two studies (Beaudet et al. 1989, in the USA; INSERM U73 in France) and frequency of the ΔF 508 mutation associated with the different haplotypes. The numbers in brackets are the numbers of cases studied

Haplotype	KM-19 allele	XV-2C allele	Percentage of normal chromosomes with haplotype		Percentage of CF chromosomes with haplotype		Percentage of CF chromosomes with ΔF 508		without ΔF 508	
			USA	France	USA	France	USA	France	USA	France
			(425)	(222)	(425)	(171)	(326)	(171)	(99)	(51)
A	1	1	32.3	44.1	4.9	4	0.3	0.6	20.2	15.7
B	2	1	14.7	15.3	87.3	81.5	96.3	92.4	57.6	45.1
C	1	2	38.7	29.3	3	4.9	0	0.6	13.1	19.6
D	2	2	14.2	11.2	4.7	9.4	3.3	6.4	9	19.6

Table 5.10 Geographic distribution of the Δ*F 508* mutation. Data from the Cystic Fibrosis Genetic Analysis Consortium: the most important series have been selected

Country	Percentage of CF chromosomes with Δ*F 508*
Denmark	85.3
United Kingdom	
Manchester	79.8
London	74.4
Germany	77
France	
Britanny	80.8
Paris	73
South	62.8
Switzerland	
Basel	69.5
Spain	
Barcelona	64.8
Madrid	51.2
Italy	
North	54.9
South and Central	44.9
USA	75
Canada	
Toronto	70.8

Diagnosis by enzyme analysis of amniotic fluid   This type of diagnosis relies on the interpretation of digestive enzyme activity in the fluid: gamma glutamyl transpeptidase (GGT), leucine aminopeptidase (LAP), total alkaline phosphatase (PAL), and especially those isoenyzmes which are assessed by measure of the residual activity of alkaline phosphatase after action of various inhibitors:

- L-phenylalanine, which inhibits the intestinal form and the placental forms (the intestinal form makes up 80 per cent of total alkaline phosphatase activity in the amniotic fluid);
- L-homoarginine or, better, bromotetramisole which inhibits the kidney–liver–bone form;
- L-phenylalanine-glycyl-glycine, which inhibits only the placental form. This form is usually absent in amniotic fluid, and its presence may interfere with results.

As this diagnosis is based on a measure of the modification of normal values in amniotic fluid, it is essential to precisely determine the normal value for each enzyme, the normal variation, and the evolution with gestational age. It is easier to discriminate when the amniocentesis is done at 17–18 weeks of gestation, the bi-parietal diameter being 40 ± 2 mm at ultrasound.

Prenatal diagnosis   Two different situations are possible: a couple having had a child affected with cystic fibrosis, or a couple with a family history of cystic fibrosis.

1. *Families with a 1/4 risk*: that is, a couple where at least one child has been born with cystic fibrosis. The method of prenatal diagnosis will depend on molecular studies of the child and the family.

(a) The affected child is alive and family studies have identified both of the child's mutations. The parents are therefore heterozygous for this mutations, and a direct prenatal diagnosis by chorionic villus sampling at around 11 weeks can be proposed.

(b) The affected child is alive and family studies have shown that the child has only known mutation (*M*), the child being *M/X.*, or the child has unknown mutations: *X/X*. The second gene or the two genes responsible for the disease have an X mutation not yet identified. Study of other markers close to the mutant gene allows prenatal diagnosis by chorionic villus sampling if the family studies have shown that the markers are informative. This is no longer a direct prenatal diagnosis but an indirect one by linkage with other markers. Nevertheless, because the recombination frequency between the gene and these two important markers is small, the diagnosis is reliable (Fig. 5.14).

(c) The affected child is deceased. Until September 1989 it was not possible to offer prenatal diagnosis at 11 weeks of gestation by molecular techniques, in this case for one-third of couples referred for this diagnosis. Today if parental studies show that they are heterozygous for known mutations it is possible to offer early prenatal diagnosis; for the Δ*F508* mutation this is observed in about half of the cases arising in the northern European population, and less frequently in southern European populations (Table 5.10).

(d) Families non-informative for either known mutations or markers *KM19* and *XV2C*. It is possible to study informativeness using other markers more distant from the gene, *Met* and *J3.11*. The risk of recombination is higher and the chances of informativeness become very small. Study of amniotic fluid at 18 weeks becomes necessary. The fetus affected with cystic fibrosis has, at around 18 weeks of gestation, a digestive block which is manifested as a decline of digestive enzymes normally found in amniotic fluid.

2. *Low-risk families*. Progress in methods of diagnosis, and information given to high-risk families, has created an increasing demand from low-risk families: remarriage, couples having one affected relative (brother, sister, nephew, or niece). Discovery of the Δ*F508* and other mutations has dramatically changed the strategy for these families. We can distinguish between two major alternatives:

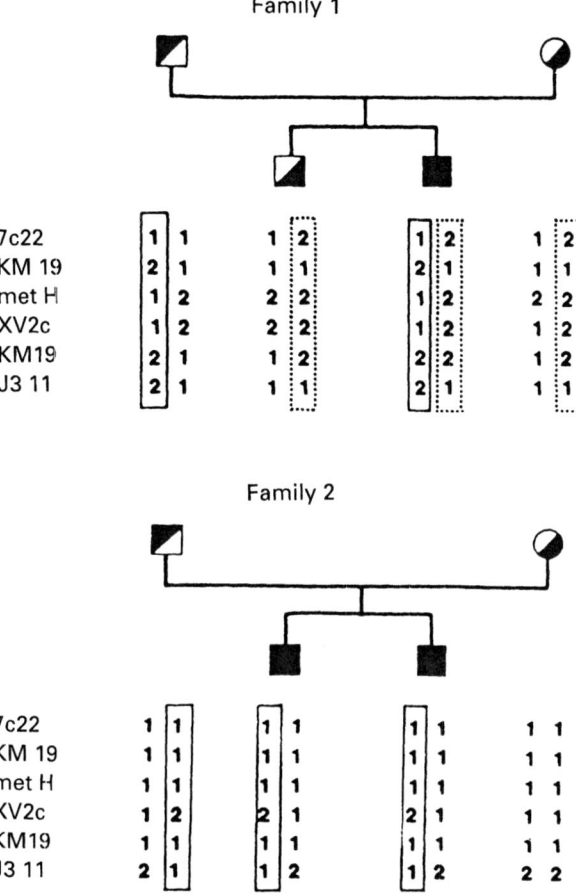

Fig. 5.14 In family 1, determination of alleles with six molecular probes permits the identification in the affected child of the two chromosomes 7 carrying the mutation and therefore determining the segregation in the family. The first child is heterozygous, having received the healthy chromosome from his father and the mutant chromosome from his mother; early prenatal diagnosis would be possible. In family 2, it is only possible to identify the mutant chromosome 7 of paternal origin, the mother being homozygous for the six probes. Prenatal diagnosis would only exclude the risk should the fetus inherit the healthy chromosome 7 from the father. If he has inherited the mutant paternal chromosome 7, the two maternal copies of chromosome 7 cannot be distinguished to show whether the fetus is heterozygous or homozygous affected. Amniocentesis for enzyme analysis must be done. In this case molecular biology is not really valuable because, even if there is reason to terminate the pregnancy, the intervention will be late. From E. Mornet and B. Simon-Bony.

(a) The affected child has been studied on the molecular level, and the parents are informative for either the known mutations or for markers (*KM19* and *XV2C* in particular). It is then possible to determine, in a couple where one spouse is related to the affected child, whether the related person is a carrier of the mutation responsible for the disease.

Once the heterozygosity has been determined in one spouse, one then has to assess the risk for this couple after studying the other spouse. Of course, this occurs in every case where a parent of an affected child remarries. This study is often done solely to look for the Δ*F508* mutation.

Demonstrating the presence of Δ*F508* in the spouse confirms that he or she is a carrier of cystic fibrosis and that this couple has a 1/4 risk of an affected child. Absence of the Δ*F508* mutation does not exclude the possibility that this spouse is heterozygous for another mutation, but it does dramatically reduce the estimated risk with respect to the frequency of Δ*F508* in the population from which this couple originates. The varying frequency of Δ*F508* in different populations can be seen in Table 5.10. It is not feasible to look randomly for all other mutations responsible for cystic fibrosis, however it is possible to examine the most likely common mutations by knowing the ethnicity or haplotype for the person in question.

(b) The child affected with cystic fibrosis could not be studied molecularly, therefore one must rely on a probability estimate of heterozygosity. For a brother or sister of an affected child it is 2/3, and for an uncle or aunt it is 1/2. The Δ*F508* mutation must be looked for in the two members of the couple. If the Δ*F508* mutation is found in a relative of the affected child, that relative is therefore carrying the gene for cystic fibrosis: the situation is as described in the paragraph above.

If Δ*F508* is absent in both spouses, one can evaluate the risk of having an affected child. If the Δ*F508* mutation is found only in the unrelated spouse the risk can also be evaluated (Table 5.11a, 11b).

How does one foresee prenatal diagnosis in cases where risk assessment justifies the procedures and where only one member of the couple is a carrier of a known mutation?

Diagnosis by exclusion can be considered by looking for the mutation on fetal DNA: absence of the mutation excludes the risk for the child. Should the mutation be carried by the fetus, fetal intestinal enzymes in amniotic fluid should be studied. In this case, the theoretical risk evaluated for the particular couple should be compared to the false positive rate observed with this method of diagnosis. If the fetal mutation was observed after chorionic villus sampling, one must be aware of the woman's anxiety in waiting for confirmation on amniotic fluid.

It seems preferable to do all this testing on the amniotic fluid, as study of DNA and intestinal enzyme study then can be done simultaneously.

When a low-risk couple has a risk of less than 1 per cent of having an affected child, it is not reasonable to do prenatal diagnosis based exclusively on enzyme

Table 5.11 In these pedigrees, subjects A and D are not related to the affected child; they are part of the general population. B is the sister of an affected child and C is his uncle. Tables (a) and (b) give for each member of couples AB and CD the probability of each being a carrier of cystic fibrosis and subsequently the risk of giving birth to an affected child. In the calculations it is assumed that mutations represent 4 per cent of the population, of which 2.8 per cent carry the $\Delta F\ 508$ mutation and 1.2 per cent (1/85) carry all the other mutations. This corresponds on average to the total French population

(a)

	Subject B		
	Not tested (or undeterminable) (2/3)	Tested (carrier) (1)	Tested (non-carrier) (0)
Subject A Not tested (1/25)	1/150	1/100	0
Tested (carrier) (1)	1/6	1/4	0
Tested (non-carrier) (1/85)	1/510	1/340	0

(b)

	Subject D		
	Not tested (or undeterminable) (1/2)	Tested (carrier) (1)	Tested (non-carrier) (0)
Subject C Not tested (1/25)	1/200	1/100	0
Tested (carrier) (1)	1/8	1/4	0
Tested (non-carrier) (1/85)	1/680	1/340	0

study of the amniotic fluid. None the less ultrasound results at 18 weeks of gestation may change this policy. Intestinal obstruction characteristic of cystic fibrosis in the fetus at this gestational age can be visualized ultrasonographically as a hyperechogenic abdominal mass with pseudocalcification of the right iliac fossa. This ultrasound picture should lead to intestinal enzyme determination, which will confirm the intestinal obstruction; hyperechogenic masses other than those associated with cystic fibrosis are not rare, but in a couple with a greater than 1 per cent risk, this should be seriously evaluated.

Towards population screening

Until recently, prenatal diagnosis of cystic fibrosis could only be offered to couples who already had an affected child. Discovery of the *ΔF508* and other mutations will allow carrier determination in relatives of an affected child, avoiding the birth of a first affected child in those relatives where a high risk could be established by studying the couple's DNA (see above).

Might this heterozygote screening be applied to all pregnant women by DNA testing for the *ΔF508* mutation on maternal blood, thereby identifying a heterozygous woman? Study of the spouse would then be undertaken, permitting prenatal diagnosis if both members of the couple were found to be carriers of the mutation.

The correlation between *ΔF508* mutation and cystic fibrosis means that only about 70 per cent of heterozygous women can be detected. It is difficult to propose screening where 30 per cent of carriers would not be picked up. Discovery of other mutations causing cystic fibrosis is progressing at a good pace, but preliminary results indicate a large number of mutations which are each responsible for only 1 per cent or less of cystic fibrosis cases. As in other single-gene disorders, a specific mutation may be found but only in an individual family. There are reservations about such a screening programme until more is known about the presence of other mutations.

Haemoglobinopathies

Haemoglobinopathies are undoubtedly the most common hereditary diseases (Table 5.12). They affect Mediterranean people, Africans, and Asians with variable frequency from one area to the other, mostly areas where malaria is or used to be endemic.

In France there are West Indian and African black populations, for whom the risk is of sickle cell anaemia and, with lesser frequency, certain forms of thalassaemia. β-Thalassaemia is also found in immigrants coming from regions bordering the Mediterranean. Unlike sickle cell anaemia, where the causal mutation is unique, β-thalassaemia is caused by any one of a group of usually single-gene mutations, which result in a decrease or absence of synthesis of β-globin. More than 50 have been identified; each population contains its own spectrum of mutations, the knowledge of which is useful for certain antenatal diagnosis approaches. Unlike the inherited X-linked disorders, there are practically no *de novo* mutations, molecular heterogeneity being the rule.

α-Thalassaemias are indications for prenatal diagnosis only when the risk of fetal hydrops due to a total absence of α genes exists. This risk is of concern primarily for couples of Asian origin, because in this population α-thalassaemia is caused by a more or less extensive deletion of α globin genes. The WHO (1983)

Table 5.12 Frequency (in percentages) of sickle cell anaemia and β-thalassaemia carriers (heterozygotes) in Africa and the Mediterranean

Sickle cell anaemia		β-Thalassaemia	
West Indies	8.9	Italy	3–4
Africa		Sardinia	15
Gabon, Nigeria, and		Algeria	2
Central African Republic	24	Corsica and	
Senegal	15	Provence	
North Africa	1	(primarily in minority groups)	1–2

estimates that annually in Europe there are 2500 births of children severely affected with a haemoglobinopathy, of which about 100 have sickle cell anaemia. In France, the demand for prenatal diagnosis for this indication is 100–150 cases a year, 3/4 of them being for sickle cell anaemia.

Screening for carriers of sickle cell anaemia and thalassaemia is simple. It relies on a complete blood count and haemoglobin electrophoresis, testing which should automatically be made available to all couples of either prenuptially or prenatally.

Genes coding for α- and β-globin have been cloned and analysed in detail using molecular biological techniques. These studies have permitted an understanding of their function and, for a significant number of them, an understanding of the nature of the mutation which alters their expression. Parallel to these methods, study of the genome has progressed rapidly and the biologist now has available a panoply of powerful tools permitting a diagnosis by studying the gene, rather than its product, when at all possible. Genes which code for α- and β-globin make up a family of sequences in series on chromosome 11 (for the β genes) and chromosome 16 (for the α genes) (Fig. 5.15). Expression of the gene products during ontogenesis is described in Fig. 5.16. It can be seen that the adult globins are already present in the fetus at 10 weeks of gestation, which allows the study of their structure or synthesis as soon as it is possible to obtain blood *in utero*. Globin genes are small, and this greatly facilitates the study of their DNA sequences.

Diagnosis at the level of globin gene expression

The first approach, introduced by Kan *et al.* (1974), was analysis of fetal blood *in utero*. This is now used only when circumstances prevent study of DNA. Fetal blood is sampled from the cord either by ultrasound guidance or by optic guidance (fetoscopy) and analysed using appropriate techniques (electrofocusing, high-pressure liquid chromatography) allowing a qualitative study of fetal haemoglobin (presence or absence of variant haemoglobins F, C, or E) or a quantitative study (capacity of fetal reticulocytes to synthesize β-globin chains *in vitro*). Sampling can only take place from the 18th week of pregnancy, but results are quickly available (same day or following day).

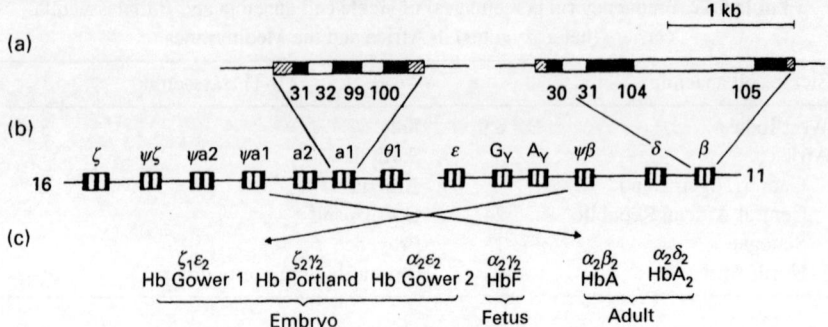

Fig. 5.15 *a*, Structure of α and β globin genes. ■, exons; □, introns; □ regions that are transcribed but not translated. *b*, organization of α and β globin gene complexes. *c*, structure of various haemoglobins expressed during ontogenesis.

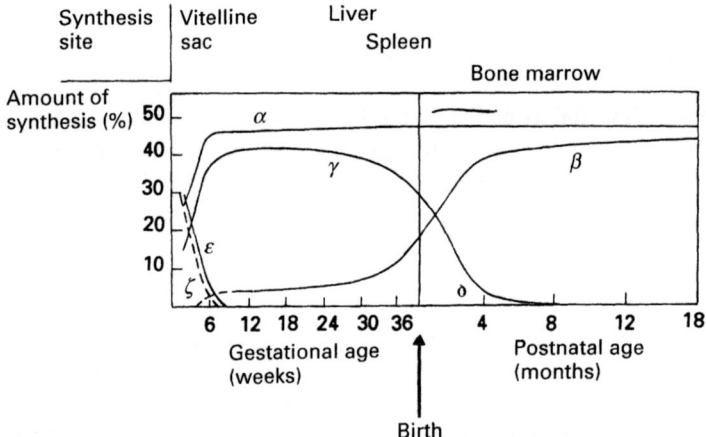

Fig. 5.16 Ontogenesis of haemoglobin subunits.

Diagnosis at the gene level

Direct analysis

Mutation by deletion or a large gene rearrangement.   These are easily detectable by the Southern method, a deletion resulting in complete disappearance of some DNA fragments for which the presence is normally recognized by a specific DNA probe. Mutations that completely alter the restriction map being studied are very rarely observed in practice (Table 5.13).

Single-gene mutations   Direct detection of a point mutation is greatly facilitated if the nature of the mutation is understood. With this in mind, knowing whether

Table 5.13 Mediterranean β-thalassemia mutations. Associated haplotypes and direct methods of detection

Mutations	Haplotypes	Direct detection
β^+ Thalassaemias		
– 88C → T	Na	Oligonucleotide
– 87C → G	VIII	Avr II(–)
-30 T → A	VII	Oligonucleotide
Codon 29 GGG → GCT	II	Oligonucleotide
IVS1 nt5 G → C	Va, IX	Oligonucleotide
IVS1 nt5 G → T	I, Va	Oligonucleotide
IVS1 nt5 G → A	C	EcoR V (+)
IVS1 nt6 T → C	VI, VIIIa, X	Sfa N I(+)
IVS1 nt110 G → A	I, II, IX	Oligonucleotide
IVS2 nt745 C → G	VIIa	Rsa I (+)
IVS2 nt843 C → G	D	Mnl I (–)
β^0 Thalassaemias		
Frameshift 6 GAG → G-G	I, Va, IX	Mst II (–)
Frameshift 8 AAG → - - G	IV	Oligonucleotide
IVS nt1 G → A	Va, G	Oligonucleotide
IVS nt2 T → G	IX	Oligonucleotide
Codon 39 CAG → TAG	I, II, V, VIIb, IX, E, F, H	Mae I (+)
Frameshift 44 TCC → TC-	ND	Oligonucleotide
IVS nt1 G → A	III, Vb	Hph I (–)
β^0 or β^+ Thalassaemias		
Codon 30 AGG → ACG	I	Oligonucleotide
IVS1 nt116 T → G	I	Mae I (+)
IVS2 nt705 T → G	ND	Oligonucleotide

Notes
1. Theoretically all mutations can be characterized using oligonucleotides.
2. (+) indicates that the restriction site is created by the mutation.
3. (–) indicates that the restriction site is destroyed by the mutation.
4. Detection of the mutation C → G in –87 requires a double digestion Avr II/Hind III.
5. Detection of mutation IVS1 nt6 T → C by the Sfa NI enzyme results in restriction fragments whose length is a function of the frameshift mutation.
6. ND indicates that the haplotype has not been determined.

the phenotype is β^0 or β^+ has a predictive value in determining the types of mutations possible, and a number of approaches can be adopted:

1. *Identification of mutations by restriction enzyme analysis.* Certain substitutions remove a restriction site and others introduce one (Table 5.13): they

are therefore easily identified by Southern methods as a change in a restriction fragment length. This type of analysis is best illustrated by the test used to detect sickle cell anaemia. The A to T substitution at codon 6, which changes glutamic acid to valine in the protein, alters the recognition site for *Mst* II (CCTNAGG). Loss of the cleavage site at this codon results in a 1.4 kb fragment instead of the normal 1.2 kb fragment (Figs. 5.17a, b).

2. *Detection of mutation using oligonucleotides.* Most of the time the mutation can only be detected by hybridizing the patient's DNA with short nucleotide sequences (oligonucleotides) homologous to the mutated region, synthesized *in vitro* and radiolabelled. The genomic DNA–oligonucleotide hybrid formed by complementary strands alone is much more stable than the heteroduplex resulting from pairing of the normal sequence with the oligonucleotide of the mutant form, so under these selected experimental conditions they are the only ones detectable (Fig. 5.18). This approach has rarely been used in clinical practice, because of the difficulty in implementation. These obstacles are circumvented by recent development of a technique allowing *in vitro* enzymatic amplification of the DNA sequence containing the mutation (Fig. 5.19).

Amplified DNA-dot blots are fixed onto a nylon membrane, before being hybridized to an oligonucleotide probe which is specific for the allele being looked for (Fig. 5.20). This simple and rapid technique is superseding all other approaches to the study of point mutations (even detection of restriction fragment length polymorphisms produced by nucleotide substitution), so much so that one can in certain cases visualize the amplified sequence and, if not, the restriction fragment length polymorphisms produced by the cutting enzyme avoiding use of a marker probe.

Sickle cell anaemia and haemoglobin C are easily detected using specific oligonucleotides hybridized to the amplified DNA. Because of the heterogeneity of the mutations responsible for β-thalassaemia, a prior knowledge of the molecular defect transmitted by the parent makes detection easier. The simplicity and efficiency of amplification of DNA now reduces the necessity for this. In practice, it is sufficient to know the nature of a few mutations predominating in the population from which the subject or the at-risk couple originate. It is enough to have available the corresponding oligonucleotides and to hybridize the amplified DNA samples with the various sequences, either successively (three or four mutations can be tested in one day) or in parallel. A further simplification of technique is that isolation of medium-life isotopes (such as sulfur-35) permits the use of a longer-lived probe (2–3 months) and amplification of gene sequences containing the mutation, because it permits the use of a sensitive detection system perhaps along with the use of non-radioactive probes which are more easily handled in an analytical laboratory.

Indirect analysis: detection of abnormal genes by genetic linkage analysis. Analysis of the DNA region containing the set of β-globin genes revealed the existence of restriction fragment length polymorphisms (absent or present

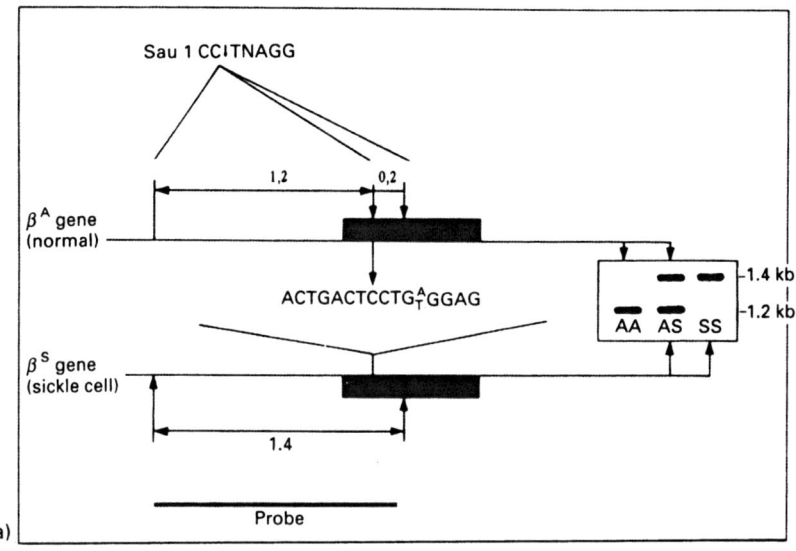

(a)

(b)

Fig. 5.17a+b Detection of mutations by restriction enzyme analysis. *a*, the Sau 1 enzyme (Boehringer Mannheim) is used to determine the existence of β^s. When this is present, the CCTAGG sequence, the restriction site, is modified and the restriction fragment is not cut. The restriction fragment is longer, and this difference in length can be detected by a radioactive cDNA probe using Southern blotting. *b*, results of DNA analysis using the Sau 1 enzyme. Tracks 1, 2 and 4 are normal AA DNA, track 3 is heterozygous AS DNA, and tracks 5, 6 and 7 are DNA from an SS homozygous fetus.

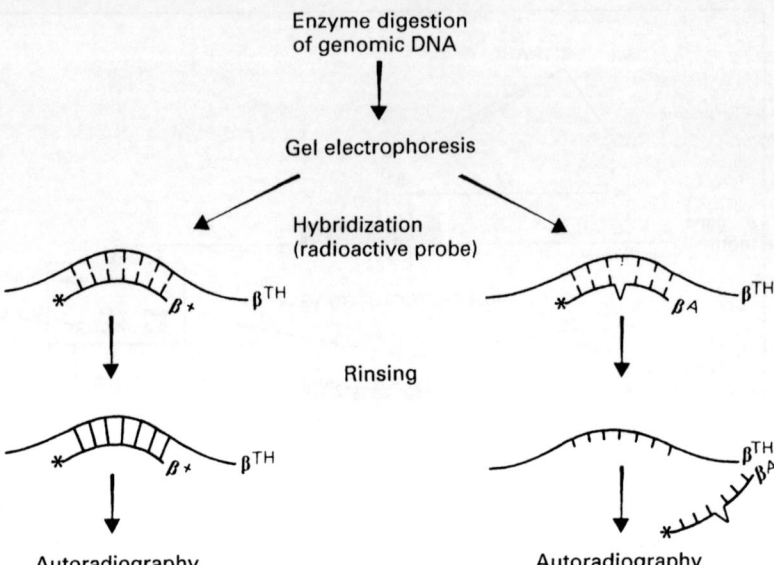

Fig. 5.18 The use of synthetic oligonucleotide probes to search for point mutations. The restriction fragments of genomic DNA are separated by agarose gel electrophoresis. The β^+ probe corresponding to the β-thalassaemia sequence hybridizes perfectly with the β-thalassaemia gene (β^{th}), but the normal probe (β^A) mispairs. The hybridization and washing conditions ensure that mispaired hybrids dissociate, while the perfect hybrids are stable. The probes are radioactively labelled, so the hybrids can be revealed by autoradiography.

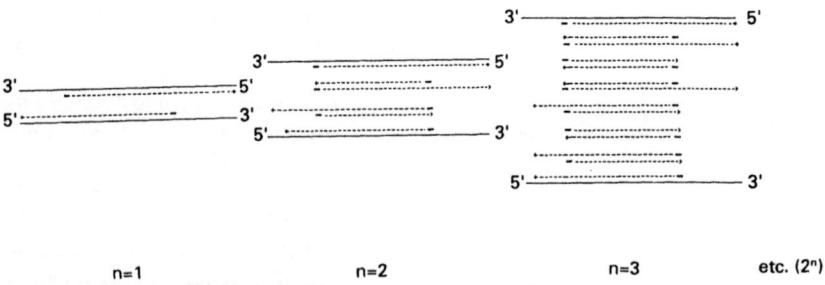

Fig. 5.19 Principles of the PCR amplification reaction.

according to the individual and to the different chromosomes in the same individual) which are DNA markers for that particular locus (Fig. 5.21). The number of possible arrangements of these sites in a particular order on a chromosome (or haplotype) is theoretically large (2^n for n polymorphic sites), but in reality a limited number of haplotypes have been identified. This shows

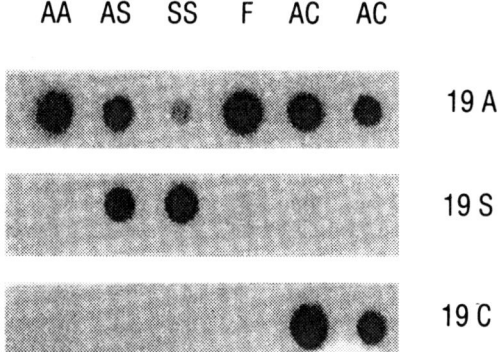

Fig. 5.20 Autoradiography showing the prenatal exclusion of the S/C genotype by analysis of amplified β-globin using allele-specific oligomers 19A, 19S, and 19C. F is the fetal sample; AA, AS, SS, and CC are controls

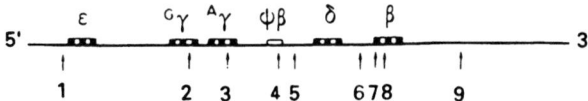

Fig. 5.21 Restriction site polymorphisms in the β gene group. Sites are numbered as follows: 1, *Hinc II*; 2 and 3, *Hind III*; 4 and 5, *Hinc II*; 6, *Hinf I*; 7, *Hgi AI*; 8, *Ava II*; 9, *Bam HI*.

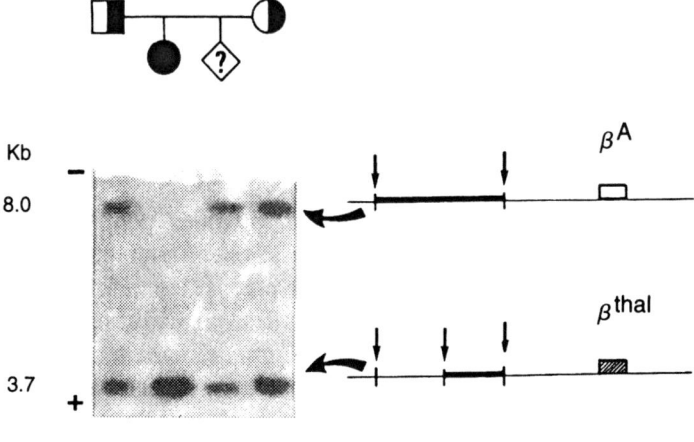

Hinc II, ε probe

Fig. 5.22 Linkage analysis using a probe complementary to the ε globin gene and detecting a restriction polymorphism *Hinc II*. This analysis shows that the fetus is heterozygous for the thalassaemia gene.

that polymorphic sites are not associated to each other randomly. The distribution of haplotypes among populations and ethnic groups, as well as their preferential association with particular mutations, has been the subject of numerous extensive studies.

With respect to prenatal diagnosis of the thalassaemias, the restriction polymorphism sites are of use only if they can be used as gene markers (Figs. 5.22, 5.23). As stated earlier, the success of linkage analysis relies on the informativeness of the marker or markers used as well as the informativeness of the family with respect to these markers; it is also dependent on examination of the proband or a healthy child of the couple. It is at times necessary to use several markers, which renders testing long, difficult, and costly. According to the population studies, these analyses are possible in only 70–80 per cent of cases; when it is not possible to identify informative markers, it is necessary to test fetal blood.

Antenatal diagnosis of haemoglobinopathies can be done using a battery of tests, of which the testing chosen is determined by the circumstances in which diagnosis must be made (early or late referral), the nature of the abnormality,

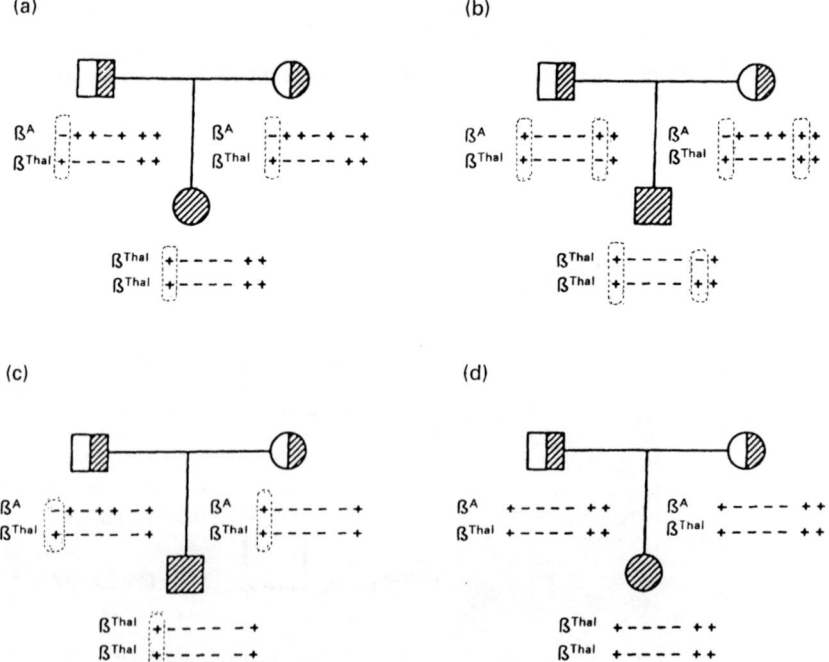

Fig. 5.23 Analysis of four families, illustrating the different possibilities for prenatal diagnosis. *a*, diagnosis using one enzyme; *b*, diagnosis using two enzymes; *c*, diagnosis possible in 50 per cent of cases; *d*, diagnosis impossible.

and the possible laboratory techniques. These tests are all extremely reliable when they are done by a specialized laboratory with experience in all methods.

The best situation is when the couple at risk is seen before pregnancy, especially in the case of thalassaemia where several members of the family must be studied, either to characterize the causal mutations, or to identify DNA markers that are linked to them.

In practice
Diagnosis of sickle cell anaemia in the fetus   This does not impose any particular problem. The mutation is unique, and detection tests are easy to use, very reproducible, and highly reliable.

Diagnosis of β-thalassaemia   This is more complicated. Once the couple already has an affected child, study of this patient's phenotype can give an idea of the nature of the mutation involved (β^0, β^+ thal). This information, added to the other elements (ethnic or geographic origin) are useful in choosing the oligonucleotides to be used. When there is no index case one must rely on ethnic or geographic origin to make this choice, and it is hoped that enough time will be available to type both parents. This typing should be done before the initiation of pregnancy.

Haemophilias

The haemophilias are conditions of X-linked recessive inheritance, resulting in haemorrhaging due to a deficit in clotting factors VIIIC (haemophilia A) or IXC (haemophilia B). The incidence is 1/10 000 male births (85 per cent haemophilia A, 15 per cent haemophilia B), regardless of ethnic group, giving an estimate of 5000 haemophiliacs in France, of whom two-thirds are severely affected. (Factor VIIIC or IXC deficiencies account for less than 1 per cent). Simultaneous determination of clotting activity and the presence of antigen allows the identification of two different major groups based on the existence (CRM+) or absence (CRM–) of a protein (known as cross-reacting material) detected by immunological reactions.

Severe haemophilia is a crippling disease of the joints because of repeated bleeding episodes (haemarthroses). It requires frequent plasma transfusions with their inherent problems — risk of B or non-A and non-B hepatitis, AIDS, risk of production of antifactors VIII and IX — all constituting a major drawback to the efficiency of transfusion.

Genes coding these factors have been cloned and sequenced (Fig. 5.24). The gene for factor VIIIC, found on chromosome X q28 is 18.6 kb long (0.1 per cent of chromosome X). It contains 26 exons, and almost 95 per cent of its length is made up of introns. The mRNA is 9 kb long and codes for a 2351 amino acid protein (the mature protein has 2332 amino acids). The gene for factor IX,

Haemophilia A Factor VIIIC	Haemophilia B Factor IX
Xq28	Xq27
186 kb, 26 exons	34 kb, 8 exons
9 kb mRNA	2.8 kb mRNA
2332 amino acids	415 amino acids

Fig. 5.24 Cloning and sequencing of genes coding for factor VIIIC and factor IX.

located in the q27 region of the X chromosome, is 35 kb long. It contains eight exons, and almost 95 per cent of its length is made up of introns. The mRNA is 2.8 kb long and codes for a 461 amino acid protein (the mature protein has 415 amino acids).

Detection of haemophilia carriers is an indispensable first step to prenatal diagnosis. It is provided by pedigree analysis (allowing for identification of obligate carriers and potential carriers) and biological data (clotting activity of VIIIC or IXC coupled to immunological measure VWFAg or IXAg). Women heterozygous for the mutation (the homozygous state being extremely rare) theoretically present levels 50 per cent of normal. But because of random X inactivation, lyonization, this is not constant and only a portion of the carriers are detected by analysis of clotting factors (70–80 per cent for haemophilia A, 60 per cent for haemophilia B). Risk of being a carrier is established by applying Bayes' theorem which take into account the genetic and biological data. With this, 'normal' results in a potential carrier do not allow for any definitive conclusion with respect to her carrier status. This study is complicated even further by the fact that one-third of haemophiliacs are due to new mutations. We must be aware that even in the absence of a known family history, a woman may give birth to an affected boy (sporadic cases). There are two possible reasons: a woman, although she has inherited a mutant gene from her mother, may be unaware of her genetic status either because the boys in her family have been spared or there are too few of them; or the child's condition may be the result of a new mutation. These women are carriers if the new mutation occurred in their mother's or father's gamete (the mutation affecting their whole genome). They are unlikely to be carriers if the new mutation occurred in one of their own gametes.

Introduction of DNA techniques has rendered possible the detection of carriers who are biologically normal as well as the study of sporadic cases of haemophilia.

Diagnosis at the level of expression of the genes coding for VIIIC and IX

Perfected in 1979, analysis of fetal blood remains indispensable, despite the introduction of DNA techniques. Contamination of fetal blood samples by maternal blood, or more by amniotic fluid, can activate thromboplastic activity and result in diagnostic error. To detect amniotic fluid contamination, it is necessary to determine the level of the clotting factor concerned and of factors V and

II, and to ensure that the values obtained are in accordance with reference values previously determined in normal fetuses of the same gestational age.

The sampling is done from the 18th week of pregnancy, and results are obtained on the same day.

Diagnosis of haemophilia A is possible by assay of VIIIC, VWAg, or VIIIAg, VC, and IIC. Measure of VIIIAg is not possible in CRM+ variants, which are rare in major haemophilia A (less than 5 per cent). Diagnosis of haemophilia B is more difficult when considering the low levels of factor IX. (Physiologically a fetus has four times less factor IX than factor VIII, and in these conditions the comparison with other vitamin K-dependent factors, factors II, VII, and X are of the greatest importance.) Also, measure of IXAg cannot be used in CRM+ cases which represent more than one third of the total.

Diagnosis at the gene level

Two strategies are possible.

Direct analysis of the mutation As far as the haemophilias are concerned, this approach is only possible for deletions (5 per cent of mutations), or when there is a specific type of point mutation, both associated with a change in the restriction fragment length. Thus, restriction enzyme TaqI which contains in its recognition site the dinucleotide CpG (T↓CGA) is used to identify certain mutations. In fact, CpG dinucleotides are 'hot spots' for mutations because C residues of CpG dimers are methylated in mammals in 90 per cent of cases. Methylcytosines, being unstable, often undergo deamination resulting in transition of C to T. When the dinucleotide CpG belongs to a CGA codon (arginine), this transition results in a stop codon (TGA) or a glutamine codon (CAA), and destroys the TaqI recognition site. There are five TaqI sites of this type for factor VIII and three for factor IX. In haemophilia A this mutation frequency is about 5 per cent (Figs. 5.25, 5.26).

Direct analysis is rarely used, because of:

- rarity of deletions;
- great heterogeneity of point mutations;
- frequency of new mutations (1/3 of haemophilic cases are due to new mutations);
- size of the genes (by comparison more than 50 different point mutations forming the basis of β-thalassaemia have been identified in the β-globin gene which is only 1.6 kb in size and contains three exons).

Indirect detection of mutations using RFLPs When direct analysis is not possible, the alternative is to use DNA polymorphisms present in or close to the gene being studied as genetic markers. This strategy is possible even when the mutation is not known.

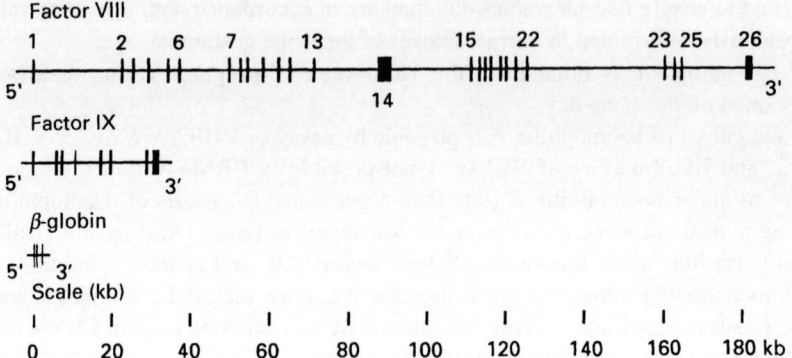

Fig. 5.25 Comparative lengths of genes coding for coagulation factors VIIIC and IXC and β-globin.

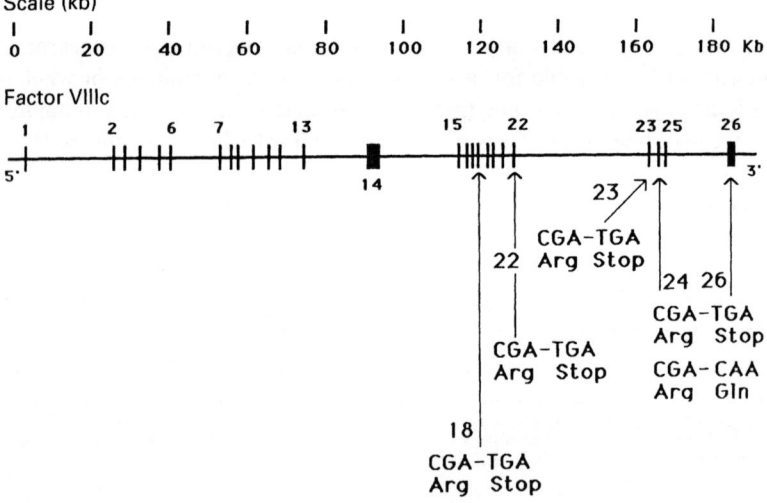

Fig. 5.26 Mutations of the factor VIII gene can be shown using Taq I endonuclease.

Regardless of the type, the restriction fragment length polymorphisms (RFLPs) are codominant markers, both alleles being detectable simultaneously in the heterozygote.

Use of RFLPs is possible only under certain conditions:

- the carrier must be informative for the marker;
- family study is required to determine which allele is linked to the mutated gene; success is dependent on the informativeness of the family for the marker.

In the context of carrier screening, it is important to determine the allele carried by the father's X, marker of the normal chromosome.

Indirect analysis of the mutation can be accomplished using two kinds of RFLPs:

- RFLPs detected by a gene-specific probe, intragenic RFLPs;
- RFLPs detected by a non-specific probe, often anonymous and linked to the mutant gene, extragenic RFLPs.

Intragenic RFLPs   These consist primarily of restriction site polymorphisms. The main drawback of such bi-allelic markers is their low informativeness. The advantage is that the rate of recombination between marker and mutation is negligible and therefore results are unambiguous.

This type of polymorphism has been described in the genes for factors VIIIC and IV.

1. *Gene coding for factor VIIIC (Figs. 5.27, 5.28).* A polymorphism is detected with the enzyme Bcl 1, of which the informativeness is 32 per cent.

Four other polymorphisms, detected with Hind III enzymes, *Xba* I, *Bgl* I, *Msp* I have been described. *Hind*III, *Bgl* I, and *Msp* I are in very strong linkage disequilibrium with the *Bcl* 1 polymorphisms, which does not allow for an increase in informativeness. The *Xba* I polymorphism seems more informative: 30–40 per cent of women homozygous for *Bcl* 1 are heterozygous for *Xba* I, which raises its informativeness to 50 per cent.

2. *Gene coding for factor IX (Fig. 5.29).* The first polymorphism was detected with Taq I and gave 40 per cent informativeness. Three other poly-

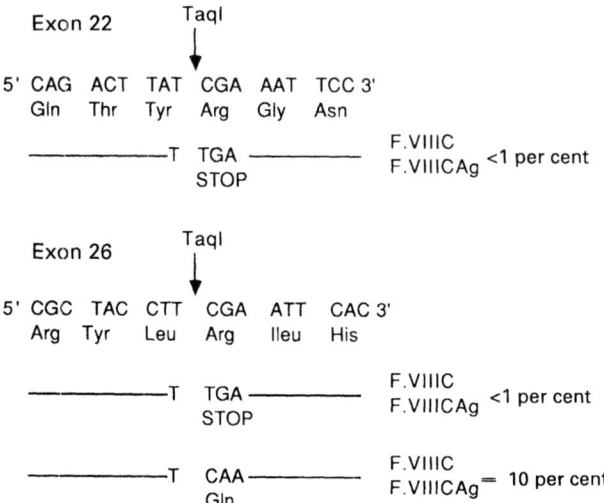

Fig. 5.27 Mutations occurring at a restriction site of the Taq I enzyme (factor VIII): mechanisms.

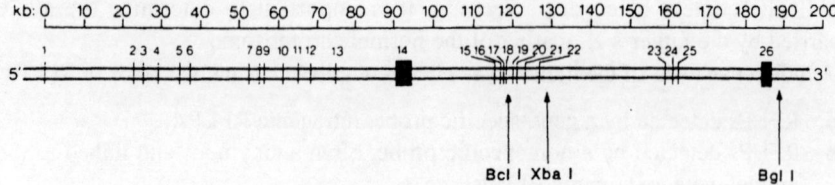

Fig. 5.28 Restriction site polymorphisms in the gene coding for factor VIII.

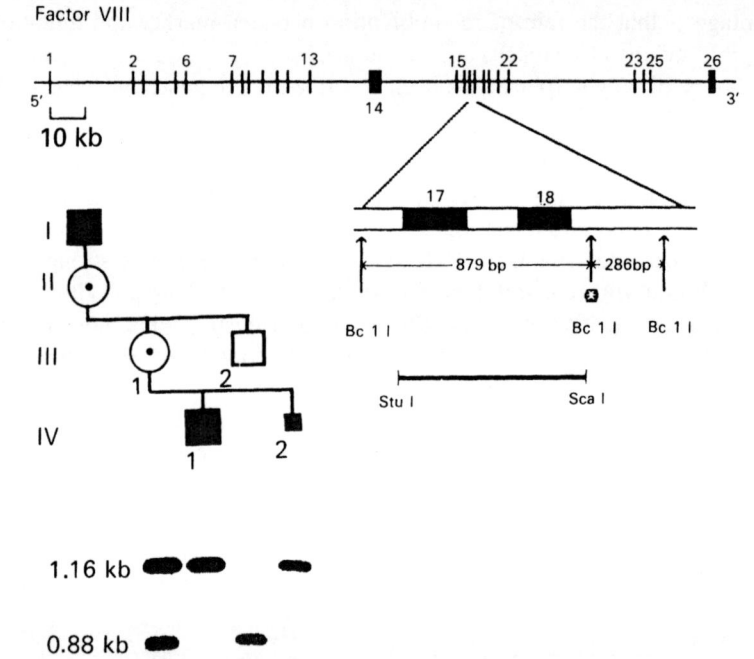

Fig. 5.29 The *Bcl* restriction site and its importance in the diagnosis of haemophilia A.

morphisms, *Msp* I, *Xmn* I, *Bam* HI, give little information or are in strong linkage disequilibrium with *Taq* I. Informativeness is not notably increased. The last polymorphism detected with enzyme Dde I increases informativeness to more than 60 per cent. Its use is sensitive. The two alleles differ by only 50 bp. This type of polymorphism corresponds to an insertion or deletion of 50 bp.

Extragenic RFLPs   When direct or indirect analysis with intragenic RFLPs does not provide any information, it is possible to use extragenic RFLPs in genetic linkage with the disease locus. If the marker is too close to the disease locus there will generally be co-segregation. However, a meiotic recombination event can occur by a crossing-over between homologous chromosomes with a frequency as large as the physical distance (unknown) between the marker and the mutant gene. Physical and genetic distance are not usually superimposed, mainly because of the existence of 'hot spots' in the genome where recombination seems more common. Despite this, we can establish the following correlation: 1 per cent of recombination (1 cM) corresponds in man to a physical distance of 1000 kb.

When the marker or markers are close to the gene but still far enough away that the frequencies of recombination are not negligible, their usefulness in prenatal diagnosis is diminished because of the risk of error this entails. These markers are, nonetheless, helpful tools in the diagnosis of carrier status, when conventional measures are uninformative.

The possibility of recombination between marker and disease locus can be the cause of error in diagnosis. The following points are important in minimizing the risk:

1. *Do as extensive a family study as possible*. It can be demonstrated that the risk of error in diagnosis changes according to whether the phase is known or not (alleles associated with the chromosome carrying the mutation in the mother).

2. *Use markers surrounding the locus (flanking markers)*. In fact if there is no recombination between flanking markers during meiosis there is not likely to be recombination between markers and the disease gene since this would imply a double recombination event between markers, a rare event whose probability is equal to the product of the recombination probability between each marker and the mutant gene.

3. *Take into account, for carrier screening, all aspects of data collected on the family* (pedigree, biological measures, and RFLP segregation) in order to evaluate the genetic risk.

This type of polymorphism has been described surrounding genes coding for factors VIIIC and IX.

1. *Factor VIIIC*. A polymorphism resulting from deletion or insertion has been identified on q28 of chromosome X: polymorphism Taq I detected by an anonymous probe St14 (DXS52). The main advantage of this multiallelic polymorphism is its informativeness, which is of the order of 85 per cent. The rate of recombination between factor VIIIC and St14 is estimated at 3–5 per cent.

A restriction site polymorphism (Bgl II) revealed by the anonymous probe *DX13 (DXS15)* has also been found linked to the gene coding for factor VIIIC. The informativeness of this polymorphism is 50 per cent and the rate of recombination in relation to factor VIIIC is of the order of 3–5 per cent.

The genetic distance between *St14* and *DX13* is of the order of 3 per cent of recombination; however, it has been recently demonstrated that the physical distance between these two markers is less than 100 kb. This demonstrates that in this region of chromosome X 'hot spots' of recombination exist and *St14* and

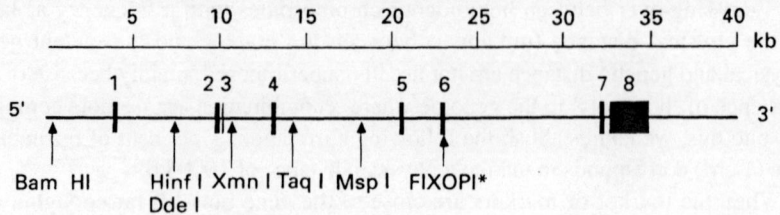

Fig. 5.30 Restriction site polymorphisms in the gene coding for factor IX.

DX13 are on the same side of the gene coding for factor VIIIC, although we cannot pinpoint their position as being centromeric or telomeric (Fig. 5.30).

2. *Factor IX.* Some restriction length polymorphisms have been described surrounding the gene coding for factor IX. They are:

- cX38.1 (*DXS102*): informativeness 25 per cent, rate of recombination 2 per cent;
- 52A (*DXS51*): informativeness 50 per cent, rate of recombination 5 per cent;
- pX58C (*DXS99*): informativeness 50 per cent, rate of recombination 5–10 per cent.

These three markers are on the same side (centromeric) in relation to the gene coding for factor IX. Other markers have recently been localized surrounding genes coding for factors VIIIC or IX, but the results of linkage studies are not yet sufficient to allow their use in the diagnosis of haemophilia.

Indirect analysis has limitations: homozygosity for the marker, linkage disequilibrium between markers limiting the informativeness of the haplotype, possible recombination with extragenic markers, and the need for complete family studies including analysis of the index case.

Gene analysis is now an important tool for the genetic study of haemophiliac families (Table 5.14, Fig. 5.31). This analysis, at least, must be done prior to any pregnancy. Prenatal diagnosis does not pose any problem when the mutation is characterized on when an informative intragenic marker is available. In cases when only an extragenic marker is informative there are two possibilities. When the diagnosis performed during the first trimester is an affected male, it is legitimate to propose pregnancy termination because the risk of error is low. On the other hand, when a healthy boy is diagnosed our policy has been to offer a verification by analysis of fetal blood. This analysis remains the only means of diagnosis when the family is uninformative (Fig. 5.32).

For carrier screening, DNA analysis is an irreplaceable tool. In fact, we have studied 65 potential haemophilia A carriers: 43 seem in all likelihood not to be carriers after DNA analysis. This result is important as in the absence of DNA study, these potential carriers would have had to undergo a prenatal diagnosis by analysis of clotting factors in fetal blood. Finally, diagnosis of new mutations is

Table 5.14 Advantages and disadvantages of conventional methods and methods involving DNA analysis

Conventional methods	
Advantages	Easily accomplished
	Applicable in all situations
Disadvantages	Lyonization
	De novo mutation
	Late diagnosis (18–20 weeks)
DNA analysis	
Advantages	Screening for female carriers
	regardless of lyonization
	Early diagnosis (9–11 weeks)
	Study of new mutations possible
Disadvantages	Not applicable in all genetic cases
	Heterogeneity in defects at the molecular level
	Complicated technology

Probe	Locus	Rate of recombination	
cX38,1	DXS102	F9-DXS102	1–2 per cent
767	DXS115	F8-DXS115	Physical linkage
St14	DXS52	F8-DXS52	3–5 per cent
DX13	DXS15	F8-DXS15	3–5 per cent

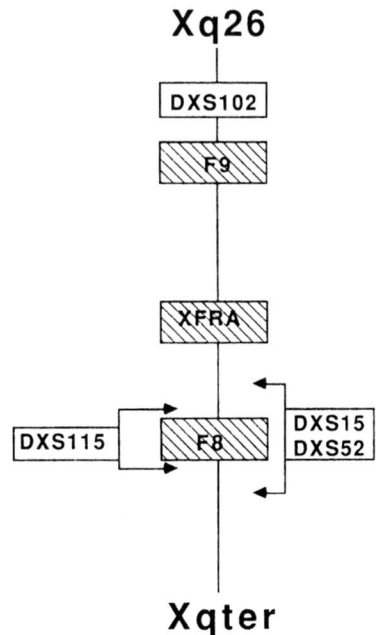

Fig. 5.31 Mapping of molecular probes useful in the diagnosis of haemophilia A and B.

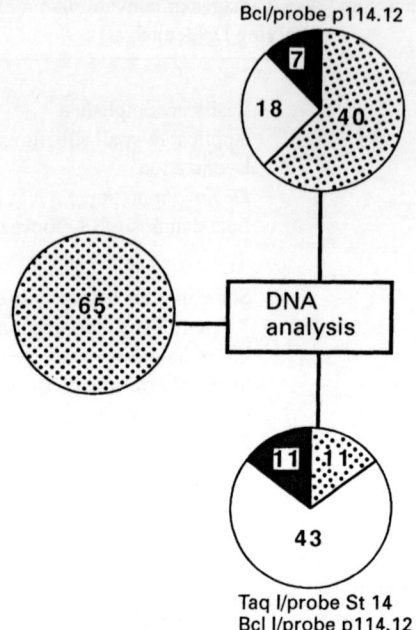

Fig. 5.32 Screening of 65 potential carriers of haemophilia A by DNA analysis. □, potential carriers; □, non-carriers; ■, carriers.

important in genetic counselling of members of haemophiliac families where there is a sporadic case of haemophilia, because it permits the reassurance of members in the branch of the family that is not implicated.

Duchenne and Becker muscular dystrophies

Duchenne muscular dystrophy (DMD) is an inherited disease, transmitted in the X-linked recessive mode. This form of myopathy, which is the most frequent and most severe, manifests itself as a progressive degeneration of the skeletal muscles and affects 1/3500 males. A less severe form, Becker's myopathy (BMD) corresponds to a mutation of the same gene mapped on Xp21. The 2000 kb gene whose alteration or absence is responsible for these disorders has recently been isolated (Monaco and Kunkel 1987), mostly by the work of L. Kunkel's team in Boston as well as by several other groups (Fig. 5.33).

Much progress in understanding the gene and its product has now been made, including the demonstration of a 14 kb mRNA and a protein called dystrophin (molecular weight about 400 000 daltons) absent in affected males or in MDX mice.

Use of an increasing number of probes covering almost all of the gene, and particularly more recent use of cDNA probes, have revealed a larger number of deletions than had been predicted, as a deletion of variable size and position has been found in about 70 per cent of DMD cases studied with the help of pulsed-field gel electrophoresis. It is likely that the number of cases with a deletion will increase as an increasing number of new probes, particularly for the distal part of the gene, are identified.

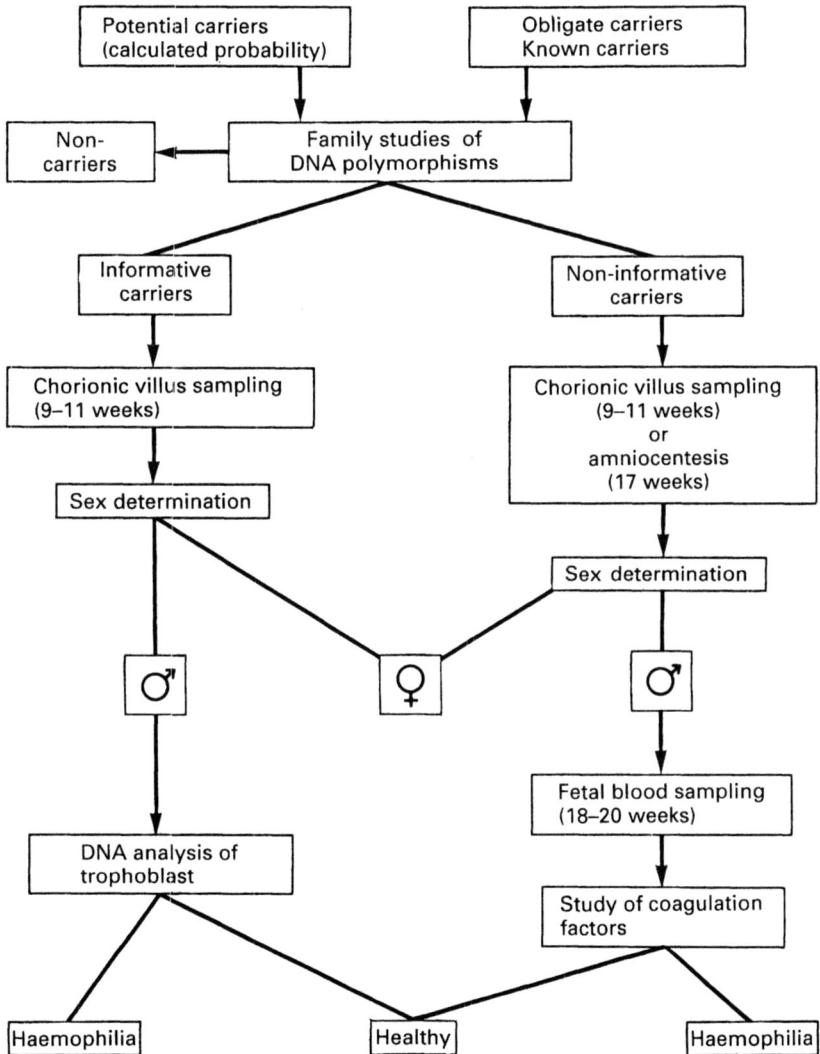

Fig. 5.33 Study of haemophiliac families.

Other studies have demonstrated a clustering of deletions on certain exons in both DMD and BMD subjects. Also, it seems that an apparently identical deletion of size and position can be translated into the same disorder with variable severity within the same family.

At present we have no data to explain the presence, in some children, of an associated mental retardation. Dystrophin, which represents only 0.002 per cent of muscle protein, has been found in trace quantities in the brain.

The mutation rate at this locus is high (10^{-4}) and one-third of cases are the result of a new mutation. There does not seem to be a significant difference between the sexes. There are a few cases, of which five have been published, demonstrating transmission by unaffected females or males. These examples, probably due to the existence of germ cell mosaicism, increase the difficulty of interpreting results and genetic counselling.

As the gene is located on the X chromosome, detection of the heterozygous females is rendered difficult by random inactivation of one of the two X chromosomes. An increase in the level of creatine kinase in serum, measurable in cord blood at birth, is pathognomic in boys, but is found in only two thirds of obligate carriers. As with all X-linked disorders, study of DNA is indicated every time specific biological measurements show normal activity in a woman at risk. Prenatal diagnosis can none the less be done on at-risk male fetuses due to the large number of polymorphic markers which cover the length of the dystrophin gene and its surrounding areas, and because of the possibility of family studies.

Family study: screening for female carriers

Risk assessment The majority of women asking for genetic counselling are not necessarily carriers. Before carrying out DNA studies one must first establish their *a priori* risk, keeping in mind biological and genealogical factors. It is in fact useless to carry out such DNA studies if the risk is less than 1 per cent.

Estimation of risk can be done using the computer program LINKAGE, or by means of Bayes' theorem or its simplified form. In any case, the information obtained in the family history and the creatine kinase levels are taken into consideration.

Importance of creatine kinase The value of measuring creatine kinase remains controversial for those who doubt its usefulness. This enzyme can be abnormally elevated in normal women, which leads to error in interpretation of female carrier status. Also, the measure of this enzyme's activity is variable from one laboratory to another without any difficulty in the actual measurement of the enzyme. It is therefore imperative to know laboratory norms and to repeat measurements at different time periods if the first measurement shows an increase in enzyme activity. Nevertheless, knowing that serum enzyme activity is increased in two-thirds of carrier females plays a significant role in evaluation of risk when using Bayes' theorem. It seems, therefore, that its advantages far outweigh the inconveniences (with the exception of false positives).

Study of levels of creatine kinase in a normal population and in a population of obligate carriers permits an estimate of the probability of a woman's being a carrier or not for any particular creatine kinase value. The LINKAGE program allows the use of this quantitative variable for an estimation of risk.

Bayesian methods   For any individual's *a priori* risk of being a carrier of the gene, along with the probability that a second condition is present (for example, creatine kinase values and the pedigree), it is possible to establish the risk.

The *a priori* risk of a mother of a sporadic case being a carrier is two thirds, because one third are new mutations. The probability of a woman's being a carrier is equal to the probability of her daughter's being a carrier multiplied by 2. Otherwise stated, the probability of a woman's being a carrier is the probability of her mother's being a carrier multiplied by ½.

The conditional probability of having a normal creatine kinase level and being a carrier is one-third, and the conditional probability of having a normal son and being a carrier is one half.

Use of Bayes' theorem implies first calculating the risk of being a carrier by measuring creatine kinase, which will give a new *a priori* risk. This value will then be used to determine carrier status, taking into consideration the pedigree and the existence of one, two, three, ..., normal sons.

The *simplified version* of Bayes' theorem has the advantage of reducing to one operation per individual, however many conditional probabilities must be considered:

$$T = 1 + (T_0 - 1)\, r_1 \times r_2 \times r_3 \times r_n$$

T is 1/risk, T_0 is 1/*a priori* risk, and r_1, r_2, r_3, r_n are 1/conditional probability.

Examples:

- for one normal son, $r = 2$
- for one normal creatine kinase level, $r = 3$

It is equally possible, with this formula, to insert the real creatine kinase value, the value of r varying from 1 to 6. It also is possible, without complicating the calculations, to consider the existence of normal daughters themselves having a normal son and/or normal creatine kinase levels: obviously a daughter having many normal sons is less likely to be a carrier and this then diminishes her mother's risk of being a carrier. The value of r tends to 2.

LINKAGE program   This software is IBM-PC compatible. The first stage is to enter pedigree information (using the PED POINT program) and characteristics of the locus concerned, i.e. the mode of transmission (here, X-linked recessive)

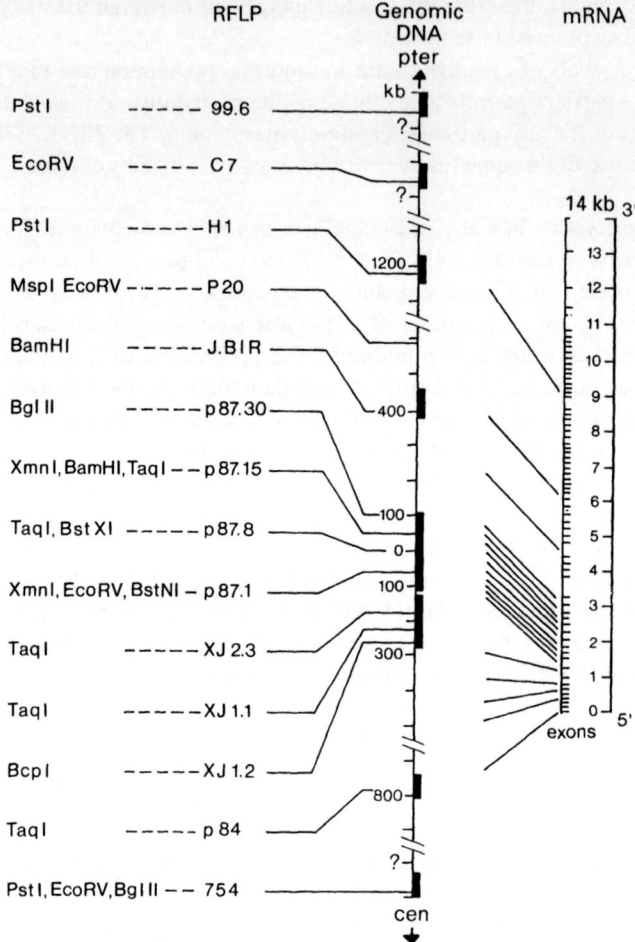

Fig. 5.34 Map of the *DMD* gene and markers. The position of the markers (RFLP) on the gene or in the flanking regions is indicated by the restriction enzyme detecting a restriction site polymorphism. Some probes detect several polymorphisms, for example p87.1 with enzymes XmnI, EcoRI, and Bst NI. The *DMD* gene is approximately 2000 kb long and consists of about 100 exons and introns. The splicing of the introns results in a 14 kb mRNA.

the frequency of alleles, the penetrance with respect to sex and age, a quantitative value such as creatine kinase level, and finally, the order and distance of markers from the studied locus (using PRELINK). This then permits the calculation of different parameters using three other programs: MLINK, ILINK, and LINKMAP. This enables us to:

• reject or confirm linkage between an unknown locus and known marker;
• estimate the order of different markers and their genetic distance;

● calculate the probability, for an individual to be a carrier of the mutant gene, in other words calculating the error risk.

As for all programs of this type, one must be particularly attentive to the possibility of error in the coding of families or other parameters. A correct estimation of risk is strictly dependent on this.

Choice of key individuals to be studied: strategy
Pregnant obligate carrier women (risk = 1) One must identify which X chromosome has the mutation. The requirements, in order of priority, are as follows:

1. Find an intragenic probe for which the woman is heterozygous. The minimal risk of recombination is variable, according to different sources (3–6 per cent). Theoretically, the number and informativeness of available DMD probes should allow for an informative probe for each woman tested. In practice, for about 10 per cent of cases, it is impossible to find the appropriate probe in a reasonable time period.

2. Find flanking probes for which the mother is heterozygous: the risk of error rises with the distance between these markers and the locus.

3. Identify the mutant X by a family study: phase can be determined with minimal risk if the maternal grandfather of the fetus can be studied. If only the maternal grandmother of the fetus is available, she would have to be homozygous for the markers studied. If the grandparents cannot be studied, phase can be determined by studying other members, but the risk of error will increase in function with an increase in meiotic recombination, the further back in the pedigree one must go. It will decrease as a larger number of individuals are studied and are concordant, determining phase with greater certainty.

In practice the pregnant woman's DNA can be digested by four restriction enzymes, and the corresponding blots hybridized with six probes, permitting analysis of nine RFLPs. Should these markers prove uninformative, other digestions can be initiated for analysis using other markers.

Pregnant women for whom creatine kinase values are normal (risk maximum of 0.4; minimum 0.0002).

One must know whether the woman is a carrier or not. It is reasonable to anticipate prenatal diagnosis for a risk above 0.01. In practice, a majority of cases studied have had a risk between 0.4 and 0.5.

1. If it is a familial case, one would choose the key individual, an obligate heterozygous for the mutation. The closest is usually the maternal grandmother of the hypothetical child or the affected child. The goal, in the case of an obligate carrier, is to quickly find an intragenic marker for which she is heterozygous; then, by family study or study of normal and affected sons, to identify the

mutant X. If the affected or normal sons cannot be studied, one must not ignore the information which can be obtained from their sisters (identification of paternal X being possible in this way).

In practice, the maternal grandmother's DNA is studied after digestion by two enzymes, which allows identification of five polymorphisms using four probes. If these probes are not informative, other markers will be studied.

2. If it is a sporadic case in the family, one may suspect a new mutation. With a family study, it is sometimes possible to recognize the individual in whose gametes the mutation occurred, and in this way evaluate the risk for a pregnant woman from her place in the pedigree (Fig. 5.34). There are four possibilities:

(a) The mutation linked to allele A1 is carried by the maternal grandfather's normal X chromosome. One can say that the mutation occurred in the grandfather's gamete if the mother's creatine kinase value is elevated or if she has two affected sons. If the creatine kinase value is normal and there is only one affected son, it is not possible to determine. The consequence is that for the rest of the family, the risk for another woman being a carrier is around the mutation rate.

(b) The mutation is linked to allele A_2 carried by the maternal grandmother's chromosome. As in the previous case, the mother is necessarily a carrier if she has a raised creatine kinase or if she has two affected children. If she and her mother have normal levels of creatine kinase it is impossible to determine risk, but consequences for the rest of the family are different. Bayes' theorem allows evaluation of risk for the rest of the family taking into consideration the pedigree and creatine kinase values.

(c) The mutation has occurred in the mother's gametes. A normal son and affected son both have the same allele. Then, the mutation has occurred in the mother. None the less, the small risk of recombination should not be ignored.

(d) The affected son has a deletion while his mother is heterozygous. Theoretically, all future children of these women should be healthy regardless of the chromosome inherited. In fact, there are rare cases where the birth of a second child having the same mutation has been observed. There are two possible explanations: either the woman is a carrier of a chromosomal anomaly (chromosome inversion) producing a deletion on that chromosome at meiosis, or the mutation occurred at an early stage of oogenesis resulting in germinal mosaicism involving only the gametes. In practice, it is appropriate, by use of markers flanking the deletion, to identify the mutant chromosome.

The woman is not pregnant   This is the best situation, as after study of the key person with the necessary number of markers, it permits recognition of female carriers and non-carriers with the minimum number of markers (generally one or two). Contrary to when the woman is pregnant, it is not necessary to study the key individual closest to the pregnant woman. In fact, a key individual at a distance in the pedigree will provide information for many more women at risk.

In practice, key individuals from a number of similar families are studied in series for the same markers. A second marker will only be used for those cases where women are homozygous for the first marker: a third and fourth marker will be used if necessary, until all key individuals are heterozygous for any one marker. This marker will then be used to study the entire family.

Carrier women, or those at high risk of being carriers, will be studied with flanking markers until they are informative with a proximal and distal marker. This strategy is less wasteful of RFLPs.

1. If the woman is not a carrier with the DNA markers studied, then fetal DNA is not required.

2. If the woman is a carrier, the steps are those taken for pregnant obligate carrier women.

3. If it is not possible to recognize the carrier status, but the paternal X can be identified, prenatal diagnosis is possible. One must then, depending on the risk, look for informativeness with flanking markers.

4. If the paternal X cannot be identified, prenatal diagnosis cannot be done: sexing must be considered. This is still done in 10 per cent of cases. New markers should reduce this number. However, there is an ethical issue to be considered: what is the number of probes which should be used before stopping testing? Gestational age, cost of the analyses, lack of resources, and the increasing number of incomplete family studies are as good arguments as any other to consider here.

Prenatal diagnosis

Prenatal diagnosis is carried out by chorionic villus sampling, at 11 weeks of pregnancy. The karyotype is analysed directly on mitoses of chorionic villi. Diagnosis of sex is obtained within a day.

If it is a male fetus, DNA of the villi will be extracted in the presence of urea or guanidine. The quantity of DNA varies depending on the weight of the sample, 10–100 μg. If the amount of DNA is too small to study intragenic and flanking markers, a second sampling can be done. It is clear that, if an informative marker is already known from a previous family study and DNA study shows the fetus is affected, a second sampling could be avoided.

Prenatal diagnosis in optimal conditions requires a previous family study. Discovering that a woman is not a carrier after the 15th or 16th week means that one could have avoided the one or two chorionic villus samplings, which have a significant risk of spontaneous abortion, which is even more difficult to accept had it been a healthy fetus.

Interpretation of results   An estimate of the risk of being carrier or non-carrier is relevant to a woman (diagnosis of carrier) as well as to a male fetus at risk of being affected (prenatal diagnosis).

Error at the time of diagnosis of non-carrier is as serious as an error at prenatal diagnosis, and therefore should not be neglected. There are causes of error, other than technical ones, and these should be taken into account in risk evaluation.

Non-paternity   Determination of phase between studied markers and the mutant allele is a prerequisite for successful prenatal diagnosis. Identification of this chromosomal region can be done in various ways, depending on accessibility of different members of the family. As seen above, identification of the maternal grandfather's haplotype implies a minimum risk, and in many cases allows a prenatal diagnosis even if the affected child is deceased. When the grandfather is the only available relative it is therefore indispensable to verify paternity with the use of polymorphic markers, for example HLA or hypervariable sequences such as mini-satellites, the same ones we use for 'fingerprinting' by DNA analysis. If doubt persists, it is preferable to look for markers similar to the situation described in Fig. 5.35. The grandmother of the fetus at risk must be homozygous and the mother heterozygous for this marker.

New mutations   The frequency of new mutations at the DMD locus is estimated to be $7–10 \times 10^{-5}$. Recent work has shown that there is no difference in estimated and observed mutation rates between the sexes.

   The old notion that one-third of DMD cases represent a new mutation is still applicable in estimating the risk that the mother of an affected case is a carrier. This is true with DMD, as there is no case of transmission through a male. On the other hand, with Becker's muscular dystrophy the lifespan of an affected male is variable and they can reproduce. This raises substantially the number of cases of both sexes carrying the mutation, compared to cases where a new mutation has occurred (Fig. 5.34).

Germinal mosaicism   Discovery of a new mutation occurring in an individual's gametes excludes the risk of having a second affected child. Examples of this are known, however, and the explanation is that as for factor VIII there is germinal mosaicism, a mutation occurring at one of the mitoses in oogenesis. Figure 5.35 shows a germinal mutation in the female (A) and in the male (B). Proof of a new mutation, as in the case in the diagram, demonstrates that the mother of the affected child has a significant risk of being a carrier. With new probes, the possibility of detecting an increasing number of deletions should permit a more precise diagnosis in third pregnancies. Also, prenatal diagnosis should be considered for all mothers of isolated cases and non-carriers (in their lymphocytes) of the deletion found in their affected son. Study of the deletion should also be done for the affected child's sisters.

Meiotic recombination   Estimated incidence of meiotic exchanges within the Xp21 region, which represents 2×10^6 bp, is common, as shown in 25 studied

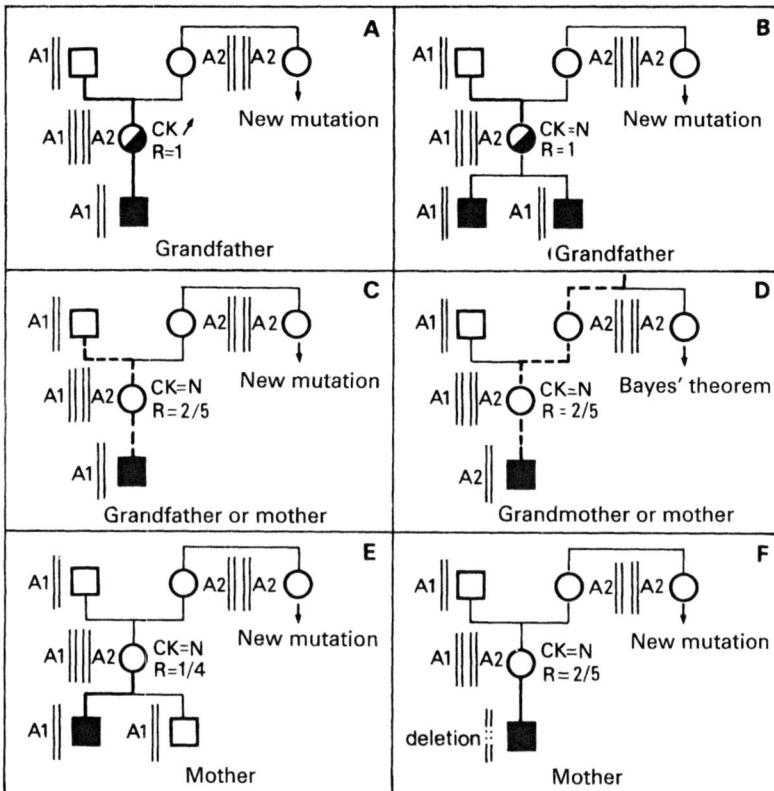

Fig. 5.35 Identifying the origin of new mutations. The heavy line shows the origin of the mutation when the individual in whose gametes it occurred could be identified (A,B grandfather; E,F mother). The dashed line indicates that it is impossible to identify the origin of the mutation. R is the *a priori* probability of being a carrier.

families. Also, linkage studies done on 31 families of DMD and BMD (41 informative meioses), using *pERT* and *XJ*, have shown the absence of recombination between these two loci as well as linkage disequilibrium between the three RFLPs detected with the XJ probe. These data do not favour a hot spot for recombination. However, meiotic recombination with unequal crossing-over could explain the unusually high rate of mutation at the DMD locus, because in four of eight cases of new mutations identified in women, a recombination between *pERT* and a flanking marker has been observed. We have observed, in one family, a situation demonstrating a reverse phenomenon: possible influence of a mutation on recombination (Fig. 5.36).

Probes currently used for diagnosis are positioned on different regions of the gene, and there is therefore the possibility of recombination on either side of the probe, making contiguous, on the same chromatid, the mutated region and

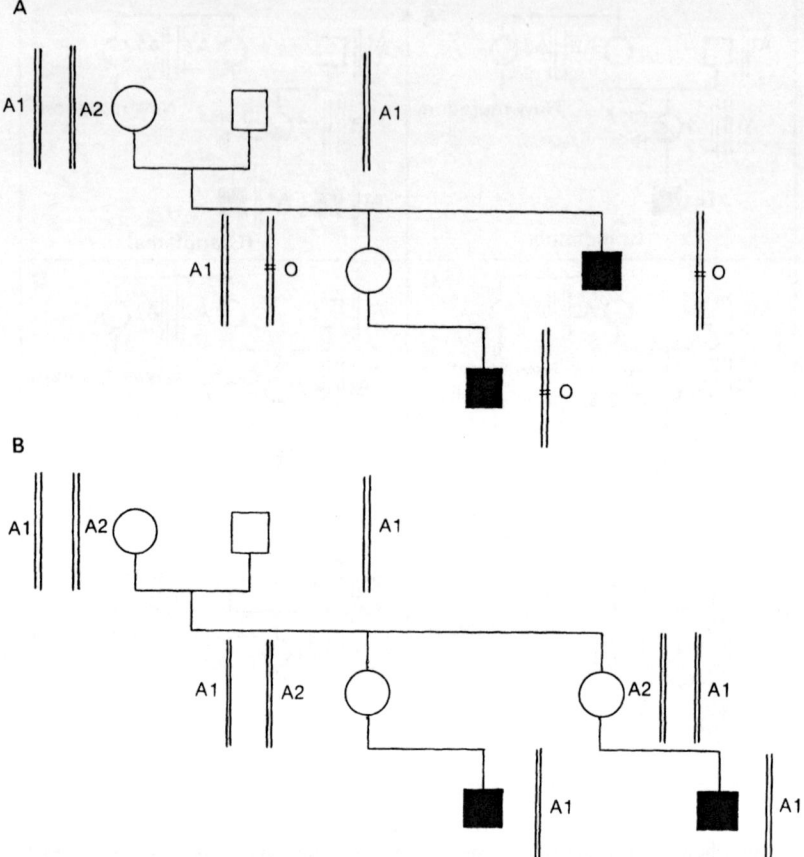

Fig. 5.36 Germinal mosaicism. *A* In the mother. The grandmother's lymphocytes show two different alleles A1 and A2. The grandfather carries allele A1. This couple's daughter had given birth to an affected boy having a deletion demonstrated with a probe for A alleles. This deletion is also found in the couple's son, who is also affected. This indicates that there are three populations of maternal gametes: one with Xs carrying a deletion, another with Xs carrying allele A1, and a third with Xs carrying allele A2. *B* In the father. The two affected cousins have inherited allele A1 found on a chromosome carrying the mutation. As this chromosome comes from the healthy grandfather, it seems that he has two populations of gametes, one having normal Xs and the other with mutant Xs.

the marker allele which was initially in phase with the gene's normal allele (Fig. 5.36).

In this example the informative marker A is found above the mutation, but it could be below. The difficulty in interpretation would be the same. It is not possible, even with flanking markers T and C, to differentiate between possibilities 1 and 5 on the one hand or 2, 3, and 4 on the other. The gene for the myopathy, which is over 200 kb long, is found at a genetic distance of at least 10 cM from the extragenic surrounding markers.

Risk calculation after DNA analysis   Risk calculation for the fetus is necessary when the mother is a carrier. Even though it is possible, with some experience, to estimate the risk intuitively, taking into account the markers used and their position and distance from the DMD locus, it is always preferable to calculate it.

Ideally one needs flanking markers at the centromeric and telomeric region, but in reality the situation is often different. Additionally, the precise position of each mutation is unknown in a majority of cases, and in fact it may be that the intragenic marker is on the same side as the flanking extragenic marker (Fig. 5.37).

In this case only the closest marker (intragenic) will be taken into account for the calculation, and the flanking marker becomes useless. The minimum risk is around that of the rate of mutation (4 per cent in the example shown in the figure) instead of the 0.47 per cent expected.

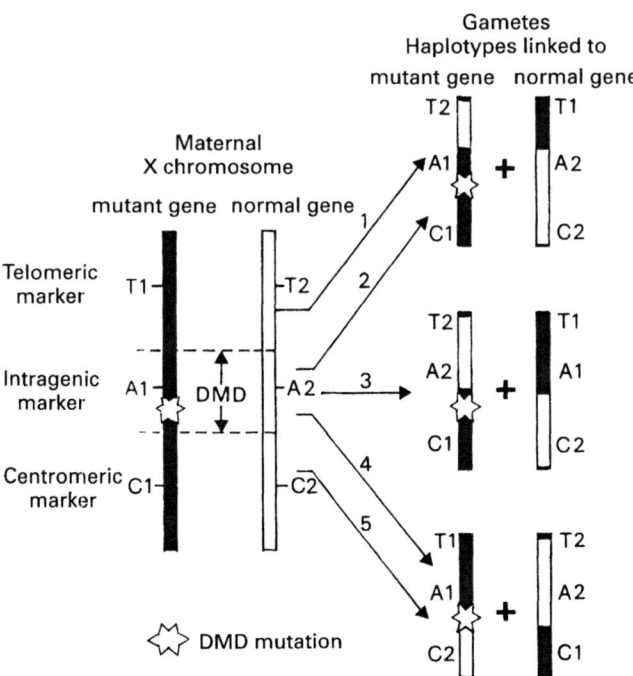

Fig. 5.37 Meiotic recombination. Possible haplotypes with respect to points of crossover and mutation sites. Situations 1 and 5 correspond to recombination occurring outside the gene; situations 2, 3, and 4 represent recombination occurring within the gene.

The LINKAGE program (see above) permits 'simulations' of different orders and distances for loci studied, which can be useful when the site of the mutation is unknown relative to the markers used.

Conclusions and future directions

Since the first evidence of linkage between polymorphic markers and the DMD locus in 1982, prediction of possible diagnosis of carriers and of prenatal diagnosis using this methodology has been realized; not only for DMD and BMD but also for other X-linked diseases (haemophilia A and B, fragile X syndromes, etc).

Between 1982 and 1985, several markers surrounding the DMD locus as well as pERT probes were used to study families: it turned out that about 20 intragenic markers were informative for almost every woman studied.

Once a woman is informative for one of these extragenic markers, be it centromeric or telomeric, precision is high and minimum risk can be hoped for. As seen previously, the risk of a double recombination still exists although we cannot anticipate the exact risk of this or the precise site in any one individual. Ideally, one would like to have flanking markers next to the gene itself, but studies of polymorphisms must continue in order to make them informative for all women. The prospect of identifying the protein responsible for DMD leads one to hope that future prenatal diagnosis will not be on the study of DNA, with the risk of recombination previously pointed out, but rather on the protein itself. Present data point to a large dystrophin gene, and also a large protein, with multiple opportunities for mutation. This may sometimes be difficult to recognize, particularly since it is still not known whether this protein is expressed in fetal tissue.

For the same reasons one should not expect the method of carrier determination to change, especially considering that in addition there is random inactivation of one X chromosome. As one-third of obligate carriers do not express the mutation, our study indicates that approximately two-thirds of at-risk women with a normal creatine kinase were not carriers. For these women study of DNA will remain the only technique available for detection of this disorder, as it will for a large majority of X-linked diseases subject to the same constraints.

Southern blotting, available since 1975, is still the basic technique. Its high cost can be partially reduced by replacing radioactive probes with non-radioactive ones. But the difficulty of the technique, which may require several weeks (sometimes months), depending on the family's informativeness, remains the major obstacle to its application to a large group of families and diseases. Attempts at automation are still disappointing. Only an attempt at rationalization might improve the present situation, when there are long months of waiting before a family can be studied. In fact, demand for prenatal diagnosis from families not studied prior to pregnancy is too high, and greatly limits the possibility of studying families in a rational way. An attempt to rationalize would oblige one to educate those families at risk. Outside a pregnancy, family studies require that healthy as well as affected members accept testing. This is essential for the study to be done in the best possible circumstances, resulting in information for a greater number of women at once, and the risk as small as possible.

Finally, the nature of the technique used implies a clinical diagnosis of the disease, without any possible error. Only a competent geneticist who has up-to-date knowledge of progress in molecular biology and epidemiology (and particularly of what is technically possible or impossible) can counsel a family. The geneticist must take into consideration clinical aspects as well as ethnic background and family history, which can, particularly in cases of myopathy, make one suspect an autosomal recessive form of disease, as seen in the North African populations (where there is consanguinity), where these techniques would not be applicable.

Steinert myotonic dystrophy

Steinert myotonic dystrophy is a common muscular dystrophy characterized in the adult by progressive muscular deficiency and atrophy associated with a myotonic phenomenon. Prevalence of the disease varies from 2.4 to 5.5 in 100 000. Incidence of the mutation is higher than its prevalence and is about 13/100 000 births.

Steinert myotonic dystrophy is autosomal dominant and virtually 100 per cent penetrant. About 50 per cent of affected subjects present with symptoms at about 20 years of age, but a significant number of patients show clinical signs only around the age of 50.

A congenital form of this myopathy (neonatal myotonic dystrophy) has been described, and the serious forms of these neonatal disorders are now well known: polyhydramnios in the latter part of the pregnancy, a severe hypotonia, including disturbance of postural tone and reduction of spontaneous movement, a respiratory abnormality, often associated with diaphragmatic abnormalities, facial anomalies, suction difficulties, constant swallowing difficulties, as well as frequent joint anomalies. These neonatal forms are found exclusively in babies of affected mothers. This suggests an environmental factor whose effect superimposes itself on expression of the mutation itself. The abnormal increase in the number of affected children in the descendants of affected women does not accord with an autosomal dominant mode of inheritance, and this leads one to believe that another non-genetic factor is involved in the occurrence of this neonatal form of the disease. It is estimated that a woman with myotonic dystrophy has a 6 per cent risk of giving birth to a child affected with neonatal myotonic dystrophy, but if the mother has already had a child affected with a neonatal form, this risk increases to 30 per cent for the next child.

A number of hypotheses suggesting maternal factors and/or parental imprinting have been proposed to explain the unusual genetics. As in Huntington's disease, it had been suggested that there existed a mechanism of anticipation which could explain the earlier onset of more severe symptoms from generation to generation. Indeed, it is not infrequent to observe a progression over three generations: a grandfather practically asymptomatic, with baldness or cataracts of late onset not particular to the diagnosis of myotonic dystrophy, then a mother with typical muscle involvement (myotonia, characteristic muscle fibre), and finally, in the third generation, a child presenting with the severe congenital form.

Chromosome mapping

Classically, Steinert's myotonic dystrophy had been considered as a single entity resulting from a single mutation. Linkage studies based on protein polymorphisms showed that the locus for this disorder belongs to a linkage group found on chromosome 19 consisting of the locus for the Lutheran blood groups as well as the ABH secretor system, the Lewis blood groups, C3 complement factor, and the peptidase D enzyme.

Localization of the gene to chromosome 19 has been possible because of molecular markers mapped to chromosome 19. The closest proximal markers are the genes coding for apolipoprotein C_2 and the gene coding for creatine kinase CKMM. It should be pointed out that the rate of recombination of these markers with the myotonic dystrophy locus differs according to sex.

Cytogenetic studies so far carried out on myotonic dystrophy patients have not resulted in the detection of chromosomal anomalies (e.g. chromosomal deletion).

In 1992, several groups simultaneously cloned the gene and determined its sequence. The unstable sequence is due to a triplet repeat $(CTG)_n$ located in the 3' untranslated region of a gene whose predicted product is a member of the protein kinase family. The expansion in fragment length seen in myotonic dystrophy patients is caused by an increase in the copy number (n) of the CTG repeat: in normal individuals n is between 5 and 27, but in affected individuals it ranges from about 50 to 2000 or more (Harley *et al.* 1992).

The finding of hereditary unstable DNA in patients with myotonic dystrophy helps to explain anticipation and variable manifestations among patients with this condition. (Fig. 5.38).

Diagnosis

This new data alters genetic counselling. The fastidious search for mutations for each individual will no longer be necessary in a considerable majority of families (approximately 70 per cent). Henceforth, carrier detection should be by direct testing, and no longer by indirect family study often resting on an uncertain diagnosis as a result of variability in expression and difficulty of interpretation of clinical or laboratory tests. However, as with all single-gene disorders, for which there is no preventative treatment, one can question the value of informing an individual of the results of genotype analysis outside of the context of prenatal diagnosis.

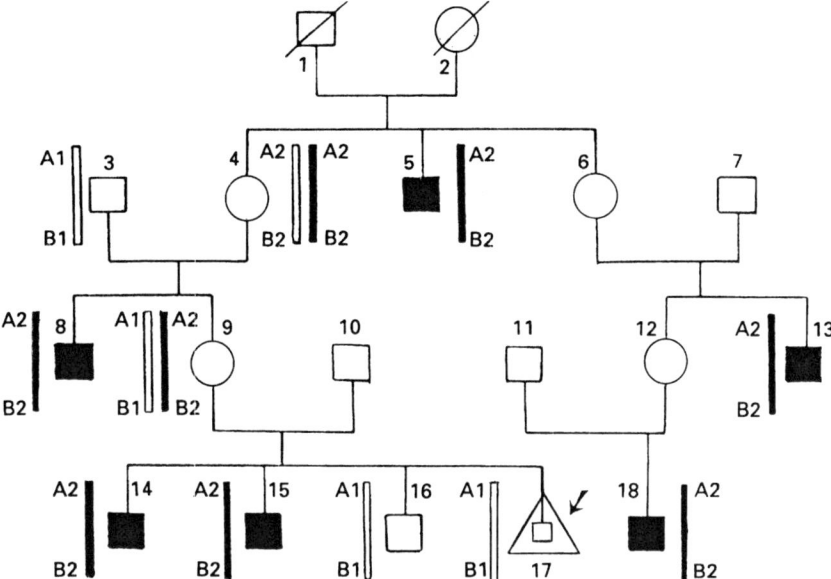

Fig. 5.38 Phase determination. Evaluation of risk of error for an at-risk fetus (indicated by an arrow) taking into consideration the availability of family members as well as the distance and position of informative markers. In this example marker A is above the disease locus at 4 per cent recombination (probe *pERT-DMD*) and marker B is below the disease locus at 10 per cent recombination. Using a single marker leads to a minimum risk of recombination of 4 per cent, increasing rapidly as the family members available to determine a phase become more distant. Using two markers, one on either side of the locus, allows for a minimum risk of 0.5 per cent if the second marker B is at 10 per cent recombination distance from the locus.

Fanconi's anaemia

Fanconi's anaemia is autosomal recessive, expressed by a progressive pancytopaenia, death occurring at a young age by haemorrhage, infection, or leukaemia or other types of cancer. Other anomalies which are often associated are growth retardation, abnormal pigmentation, skeletal anomalies (radial aplasia), and malformations of the kidney and heart.

The molecular defect is unknown: the disorder falls into the category of syndromes resulting from defects in DNA repair mechanisms. It is diagnosed cytogenetically by observing an increase in spontaneous chromosome breaks in the cultured lymphocytes and fibroblasts of these patients.

The rate of chromosome breaks is increased by certain agents such as mytomycin C, diepoxybutane, or caryolysine. Characteristic radial configurations of the chromosomes are also observed in cultured cells.

Adaptation of this cytogenetic technique to fetal cell culture of the amniotic fluid and chorionic villi allows a prenatal diagnosis of this disorder. The best technique is that done on chorionic villus cultures by study of spontaneous chromosome breaks and radial configurations (Fig. 5.39); it allows for a diagnosis at 12–13 weeks of gestation. The rate of spontaneous breaks is high enough (on average one per observed mitosis) to leave little ambiguity in diagnosis. Cord blood sampling at 20 weeks' gestation is justified where interpretation is difficult or when the woman has presented late in pregnancy.

Use of agents such as caryolysine on fetal blood is necessary to demonstrate specific chromosome rearrangements and breaks. Diagnosis is reliable, but late.

We have performed about 20 prenatal diagnoses of Fanconi's anaemia and found five affected fetuses; most testing was done on chorionic villi. We have used fetal blood sampling to determine the reliability of this testing only at the time of termination, once a diagnosis has already been established.

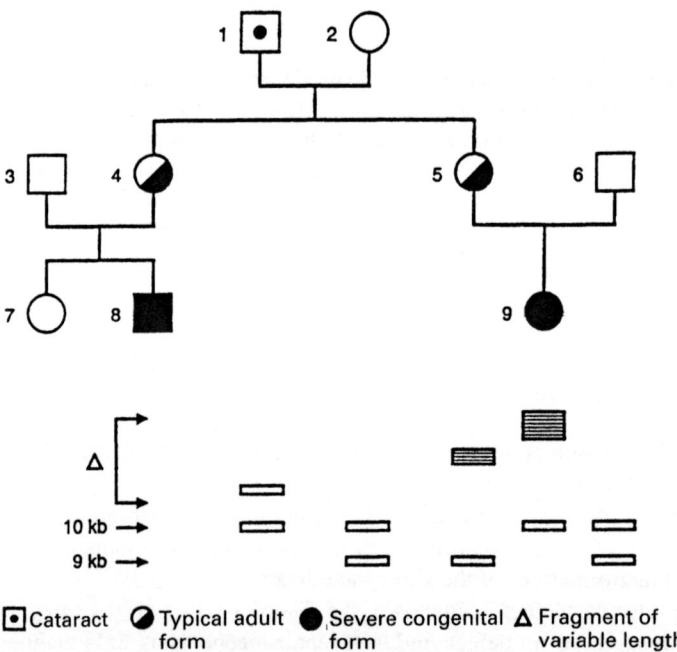

Fig. 5.39 The anticipation phenomenon in Steinert's myotonic dystrophy. Southern blot from a family using K. Johnson's cDNA 25 probe. This case of two affected sisters (4 and 5) both giving birth to children affected with the congenital form (8 and 9) is common. Is there a point of no return: a certain increase in sequence length such that the affected woman will systematically have a severely affected child?

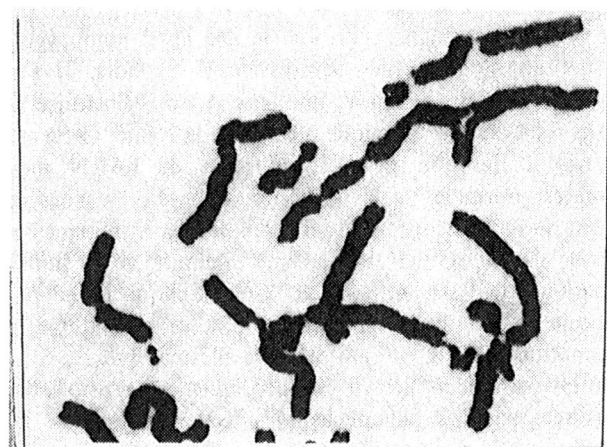

Fig. 5.40 A metaphase showing structural chromosomal anomalies in Fanconi's anaemia: triradials, breaks. From Boué and Deluchat .

Phenylketonuria

Phenylketonuria, an autosomal recessive disease, is caused by deficient activity of phenylalaninehydroxylase. Neonatal screening of all newborns by Guthrie testing has demonstrated an incidence of 1/16 000 and has allowed dietary management to prevent consequences of the deficiency on mental development.

The phenylalaninehydroxylase gene was isolated and, in using cDNA for the genes as a molecular probe, DNA polymorphisms were identified. A large number of families are informative with these polymorphisms (about two-thirds) and it is therefore possible to offer prenatal diagnosis. Risk of recombination is extremely low. Substitution of one base was identified in two mutant phenylalaninehydroxylase alleles frequent in northern European populations (Rey *et al.* 1987). Oligonucleotides specific for these mutants could be used to detect carriers of the mutant gene in the general population.

Alpha-1-antitrypsin deficiency

The gene coding for α-1-antitrypsin has been mapped to the long arm of chromosome 14 (14q3). This gene contains seven exons, and 65 allelic variants are recognized and are inherited co-dominantly. A large number of these alleles result in production of a normal protein. A homozygote Z allele, *Pi ZZ*, is responsible for the severe form of the disease. It is caused by a point mutation in exon V, where a G to A substitution results in glutamine rather than lysine. This substitution does not alter production of mRNA, and glycosylation is normal, but the mutation results in a slowing down of tertiary folding leading to a clumping of the molecule in the Golgi apparatus and therefore an extreme deficiency of plasma levels of antitrypsin. This explains both the local accumulation and its effect on liver function, and also a reduction in the antiprotease activity in plasma.

Having identified the mutation, it is theoretically possible to make a direct diagnosis using oligonucleotides, as this method does not require study of parents or index case.

Indirect diagnosis is based on the existence of linkage disequilibrium with a DNA polymorphism. Using a genomic probe (coding for the gene and the flanking region at the 3' end) and Ava III endonuclease, it was demonstrated that the same haplotype exists in all ZZ cases so far tested. Theoretically this single marker can be used without a prerequisite family study. However, if all families studied appear to have the same mutation (which originated in Scandinavia) it is preferable, before offering prenatal diagnosis, to control for the existence of this haplotype in the parents and index case, particularly if the family is from another region. Most recently, a technique has been proposed using amplification of a DNA segment at the polymorphic site shown on exon 3, with endonuclease Mac III.

Immunodeficiencies

Almost 100 immunodeficiencies are known. Most are rare but severe, resulting in morbidity and mortality in the early years of life.

The patients are referred to specialized centres where an understanding of the disease present in the index case can allow for an appreciation of the best strategies to follow in offering the parents prenatal diagnosis for future pregnancies.

A majority of these diseases result from a specific immunodeficiency determined by B or T lymphocytes. Others result from a non-specific immunodeficiency determined either by a defect in the granulocytic function or by a defect in a complement factor.

Transmission of these diseases is X-linked recessive in more than half of all cases, and autosomal recessive in other cases (Table 5.15). Prenatal diagnosis is possible either on fetal blood, demonstrating cellular anomalies present in the newborn, or on chorionic villi by study of the enzyme when the enzyme deficiency is known, or by molecular biological techniques for those X-linked forms for which the gene has been mapped and polymorphic markers exist.

Hereditary skin disease

Prenatal diagnosis may be imminent for some hereditary skin diseases that either have a poor prognosis for life or, in the absence of successful treatment, have consequences which affect physical development and the social life of those affected. These patients are referred to a specialized service which can provide a precise diagnosis and information on the availability of prenatal diagnosis.

Table 5.15 Specific and non-specific immune deficiency.
AR denotes autosomal recessive, XR X-linked recessive

	Mode of transmission and gene map	Type of sample
Specific immune deficiency		
Severe combined immunodeficiency		
1. Inborn errors of purine metabolism		
Adenosine deaminase deficiency	AR	CVS
Purine nucleoside phosphorylase deficiency	AR	CVS
2. Absence of T lymphocytes		
Alymphocytoses with agammaglobulinaemia	AR or XR	Fetal blood
T lymphocyte precursor deficiency	XL (Xq11)	Fetal blood
Omenn's reticuloendotheliosis	AR	Fetal blood
Combined immunodeficiency with		
defective HLA expression		Fetal blood
X-linked agammaglobulinaemia (Bruton type)	XL (Xq21)	Fetal blood or CVS
Non-specific immune deficiency		
Chronic granulomatosis	XL (Xp21)	Fetal blood or CVS
Chediak–Higashi disease	AR	Fetal blood
Wiscott–Aldrich syndrome	XL (Xp11)	CVS CVS
Ataxia telangectasia	AR	Villus cells

These diagnoses rely on a histological study, usually of the ultrastructure of fetal skin.

The fetal skin biopsy is done using fetoscopy between 20 and 22 weeks of pregnancy; it is at this gestational age that keratinization begins and the dermal epidermic junction is established, allowing the diagnosis of abnormalities of keratinization, of pigmentation, and of epidermolysis bullosa (Table 5.16).

Using continual ultrasound guidance and the same principles as fetoscopy, avoiding the placenta, the stylet or trocar in its sheath is introduced into the amniotic sac and the ultrasound guided optic scouts the different area of the skin to be sampled. At each chosen site, the fetoscope is held firmly in place, securing the fetus, and the optic is replaced by biopsy forceps (1.2 mm) which will remove 1 mm^2 of skin. Several samples are taken, and the sites chosen are determined by the disease in question (scalp, back, and buttocks).

Risks are higher than that involved in simple fetoscopy, because sampling takes longer (abortion in 5–7 per cent of cases). At birth, the skin scars are generally limited to a depigmented area with small sclerotic scars; sampling should avoid the face, limbs, and feet.

Table 5.16 Genodermatoses. AR denotes autosomal recessive, AD autosomal dominant

Anomalies of the dermoepidermal junction	
Herlitz syndrome (epidermolysis bullosa lethalis)	AR
Hallopeau–Siemens disease (epidermolysis bullosa dystrophica)	AR
Dystrophic epidermolysis bullosa	AD
Disorders of keratinization	
Harlequin fetus	AR
Congenital ichthyosis (collodion baby syndrome)	AR
Sjögren–Larsson syndrome	AR
Pigmentary disorders	
Tyrosinase-negative albinism	AR
Chediak–Higashi syndrome	AR
Anhydrotic ectodermal dysplasia	AR
	(X-linked)

References and further reading

Inborn errors of metabolism

Emery, A. E. H. and Rimoin, D. L. (eds) (1983). *Principles and practice of medical genetics*, Vol. 1, pp. 57–8, Churchill Livingstone, Edinburgh.

Galjaard, H. (1980). *Genetic metabolic diseases. Early diagnosis and prenatal analysis*, pp. 657–65, Elsevier/North-Holland, Amsterdam.

Kleijer, W. J., Mancini, G. M. S., Jahoda, R. P. L., *et al.* (1984). First trimester diagnosis of Krabbe's disease by direct enzyme analysis of chorionic villi. *New Engl. J. Med.*, **311**, 1257.

McKusick, V. A. (1983). *Mendelian inheritance in man*, 6th edn. The Johns Hopkins University Press, Baltimore.

Mossman, J. and Patrick, A. D. (1982). Prenatal diagnosis of mucopolysaccharidosis by two dimensional clectrophoresis of amniotic fluid glycosaminoglycans. *Prenat. Diagn.*, **2**, 169–76.

Poenaru, L. (1987). First trimester prenatal diagnosis of metabolic diseases: a survey in countries from the European Community. *Prenat. Diagn.*, **7**, 333–41.

Poenaru, L., Kaplan, L., Dumez, Y., *et al.* (1984). Evaluation of possible first trimester prenatal diagnosis in lysosomal diseases by trophoblast biopsy. *Ped. Res.*, **18**, 1032–4.

Saudubray, J. M., Ogier, H., Hervé, F., *et al.* (1983). Diagnostic clinique des amino-acidopathies á révélation aigue tardive. In *Entretiens de Bichat*, pp.16–18, Exp. Sci. Fr, Paris.

Stambury J. B., Wyngaarden, B., Fredricksoin, D. S., *et al.* (1983). *The metabolic basis of inherited disease*, 5th edn. McGraw-Hill, New York.

Vanier, M. T., Revol, A., and Boué, A. (1979). Semimicrotechniques for the assay of sphingohydrolasc activity measured with natural labelled substrates. In *Proc. 3rd Eur. Conf. Prenat. Diagnosis* (ed. J. D. Murken), pp. 292–8, Eude, Stuttgart.

Prenatal diagnosis of X-linked genetic disease

Aubourg, P. R., Sack, G. H. Jr, Meyer, D. A., *et al.* (1987). Linkage of adrenoleuko-dystrophy to a polymorphic DNA probe. *Ann. Neurol.*, **21**, 349–52.

Boué, J., Oberle, I., Heilig, R., *et al.* (1985). First trimester prenatal diagnosis of adrenoleuko-dystrophy by determination of very long chain fatty acid levels and by linkage analysis to a DNA probe. *Hum. Genet.*, **69**, 272–4.

Kleijer, W. J., Van Diggelen, O. P., Janst, H. C., *et al.* (1984). First trimester diagnosis of Hunter syndrome on chorionic villi. *Lancet*, **ii**, 472.

Tonnesen, T., Horn, N., Songergaard, F. *et al.* (1985). Measurement of copper in chorionic villi for first trimester diagnosis of Menkes disease. *Lancet, i*, 1038.

Congenital adrenal hyperplasia

Boué, A., Mornet, E., and Couillin, P. (1987). Génétique moléculaire du déficit en 21 hydroxylase. *Ann. Endocrinol. (Paris)*, **48**, 24–30.

Couillin, P., Boué, J., Nicolas, H., *et al.* (1981). Prenatal diagnosis on congenital adrenal hyperplasia (21 OH deficiency type) by HLA typing. *Prenat. Diagn.*, **1**, 25–33.

Forest, M. G., Betuel, H., Couillin, P., *et al.* (1981). Prenatal diagnosis of congenital adrenal hyperplasia due to 21-hydroxylase deficiency by steroid analysis in the amniotic fluid of mid pregnancy. *Prenat. Diagn.*, **1**, 197–208.

Kuttenn, F., Billaud, L., Thalalabard, J. C., *et al.* (1987). L'hyperplasie congénitale des sur-rénales à révélation tardive pour déficit en 21 hydroxylase. *Actual. Gynecol.*, **18**, 271–80.

Mornet, L., Boué, J., Raux-Demay, M., *et al.* (1986). First trimester prenatal diagnosis of 21 hydroxylase deficiency by linkage analysis to HLA-DNA probes and by 17-hydroxyprogesterone determination. *Hum. Genet.*, **73**, 358–64.

Parry, S., Pollack, M. S., Lau, M., *et al.* (1985). Pitfalls of prenatal diagnosis of 21 hydroxylase deficiency congenital adrenal hyperplasia. *Ann. N. Y. Acad. Sci.*, **458**, 111–29.

Raux-Demay, M., Boué, J., Oury, J. F., *et al.* (1989). Early prenatal diagnosis of 21 hydroxylase deficiency using amniotic fluid 17 hydroxyprogesterone determination. *Prenat. Diagn.*, **9**, 457–66.

White, P. C., New, M. I., and Dupont, B. (1987). Congenital adrenal hyperplasia New *Engl. J. Med.*, **316**, 1519–24, 1580–6.

Prenatal diagnosis of cystic fibrosis

Beaudet, A.L., Feldman, G.L., Fernbach, S.D., Buffone, G.J., and O'Brien, W.E. (1989). Linkage disequilibrium, cystic fibrosis and genetic counselling, *Am. J. Hum. Genet.*, **44**, 319–26.

Boué A., Muller, F., Nezelof, C., *et al.* (1986). Prenatal diagnosis in 200 pregnancies with a 1-in-4 risk of cystic fibrosis. *Hum. Genet.*, **74**, 288–97.

Brock, D. J. (1983) Amniotic fluid alkaline phosphatase isoenzymes in early prenatal diagnosis of cystic fibrosis. *Lancet*, **ii**, 941–3.

Brock, D. J., Clarke, H. A, and Barron, L. (1988). Prenatal diagnosis of cystic fibrosis by microvillar enzyme assay on a sequence of 258 pregnancies. *Hum. Genet.*, **78,** 271–5.

Caskey, C. T., Kaback, M. M., and Beaudet, A. L., (1990). The American Society of Human Genetics Statement on Cystic Fibrosis Screening. *Am. J. Hum. Genet.*, **46**, 393–5.

Eiberg, H., Mohr, J., Schmiegelow, K., *et al.* (1985). Linkage relationships of para-oxonase (PON) with other markers. Indications of PON-cystic fibrosis synteny. *Clin. Genet.*, **28**, 265–71.

Estivill, X., Farall, M., Scambler, P. J., *et al.* (1987). A candidate for the cystic fibrosis locus isolated by selection of methylation-free islands. *Nature*, **326**, 340–5.

Farrall, M., Rodeck, C. H., Stanier, P., *et al.* (1986). First trimester prenatal diagnosis of cystic fibrosis with linked DNA probes. *Lancet*, **ii**, 1402–4.

Lemma, W. K., Feldman, G. L., Kerem, B., *et al.* (1990). Mutation analysis for hetero-zygote detection and the prenatal diagnosis of cystic fibrosis. *New Engl. J. Med.*, **322**, 291–3.

Mornet, E., Simon-Bouy, B., Serre, J. L., *et al.* (1988). Differences in genetic association between CF chromosomes and linked DNA markers for CF with or without meconium ileus. *Lancet*, **i**, 376–8.

Muller, F., Aubry, M. C., Gasser, B., *et al.* (1985). Prenatal diagnosis of cystic fibrosis: 2. meconium ileus in affected fetuses. *Prenat. Diagn.*, **5**, 104–17.

Rommens, J. M., Iannuzzi, M. C., Kerem, B., *et al.* (1989). Identification of the cystic fibrosis gene: chromosome walking and jumping. *Science* **245**, 1059–65.

Rommens, J. M., Buchanan, J. A., *et al.* (1989). Identification of the cystic fibrosis gene: genetic analysis. *Science*, **245**, 1073–80 (Correction 245, 1437).

Tsui, L. C., Buchwald, M., Barker, D., *et al.* (1985). Cystic fibrosis locus defined by a genetically linked polymorphic DNA marker. *Science*, **230**, 1054–7.

Diagnosis of haemophilias

Antonarakis, S. E., *et al.* (1985). Hemophilia A: Detection of molecular defects and of carriers by DNA analysis. *New Engl. J. Med.*, **313**, 842–8.

Gitschier, J., *et al.* (1985). Detection and sequence of mutations in the factor VIII gene of haemophiliacs. *Nature*, **315**, 427–30.

Graham, J. B., *et al.* (1985). Application of molecular genetics of prenatal diagnosis and carrier detection in the hemophilias: some limitations. *Blood*, **66**, 759–64.

Mattei, J. F. and Dumez, Y. (1986). Le diagnostic prenatal. *Progrés en pédiatrie* 1, Doin, Paris.

Weatherall, D. J. (1986). *The new genetics and clinical practice*, 2nd edn. Oxford University Press.

Duchenne and Becker muscular dystrophy

Bakker, E., van Broeckhoven, C. H., Bonten, E., *et al.* (1987). Germline mosaicism and Duchenne muscular dystrophy mutations. *Nature*, **329**, 554–6.

Burmeister, M. and Lehrach, H. (1986). Long range restriction map around the Duchenne muscular dystrophy gene. *Nature*, **324**, 582–5.

Den Dunnen, J., Bakker, E., Klein Breteler, E. G., *et al.* (1987). Direct detection of more than 50 per cent of the Duchenne muscular mutations by field inversion gels. *Nature*, **329**, 640–2.

Dorkins, J., Junein, C., Mandel, J. L., *et al.* (1985). Segregation analysis of a marker localized Xp21.2-Xp21.3 in Duchenne and Becker muscular dystrophy families. *Hum. Genet.*, **71**, 103–7.

Emery, A. E. H. (1986). *Methodology in medical genetics: An introduction to statistical methods*, 2nd edn. Churchill Livingstone, Edinburgh.

Fishbeck, K. H., Ritter, A. W., Tirschwell, D. L., *et al.* (1986). Recombination with pERT 87 198 (DXS 164) in families with X-linked muscular dystrophy. *Lancet*, **i**, 104.

Jeanpierre, M. (1987). Une méthode simple de calcul du risque dans les maladies liées à l'X. *Ann. Génet.*, **23**, 521.

Lathrop, G. M., Lalouel, J. M., Julier, C., *et al.* (1984). Multilocus linkage analysis in humans: detection of linkage and estimation of recombination. *Proc. Natl. Acad. Sci. (USA)*, **81**, 3443.

Monaco, A. and Kunkel, L. (1987). A giant locus for the Duchenne and Becker muscular dystrophy gene. *TIG*, **3**, 33–7.

Plauchu, H., Junien, C., and Maire, L., *et al.* (1982). Detection of carriers for Duchenne muscular dystrophy. Quality control of creatine kinase assay. *Hum. Genet.*, **61**, 205–9.

Steinert myotonic dystrophy

Bartlett, R. J., Pericak-Vance, M. A., Yamaoka, *et al.* (1987). A new probe for the diagnosis of myotonic dystrophy. *Science*, **35**, 1648–50.

Harley, H. G., Rundle, S. A., Reardon, W., *et al.* (1992). Unstable DNA sequence in myotonic dystrophy. *Lancet*, **i**, 1125–8.

Harper, P. S. (1979). Myotonic dystrophy. In *Major problems in neurology*, Vol. 9. W. B. Saunders, Philadelphia.

Shaw, D., Meredith, A., Sarfarazi, M., *et al.* (1986). Regional localisations and linkage relationships of seven RFLPs and myotonic dystrophy on chromosome 19. *Hum. Genet.*, **74**, 262–6.

Phenylketonuria

Dillela, A. G., Huang, W. M., Woo, S. L. C., *et al.* (1988). Screening for phenylketonuria mutations by DNA amplification with the polymerase chain reaction. *Lancet*, **i**, 497–9.

Rey, F., Berthelon, M., Munnici, A., *et al.* (1987). Dépistage prenatal de la phenylcétonurie dans deux familles à partir de biopsies de trophoblaste. *Arch. Fr. Pediatr.*, **44**, 565–8.

α-1 Antitrypsin deficiency

Abbott, C. M., McMahon, C. J., Whitehouse, D. B., *et al.* (1988). Prenatal diagnosis of alpha-1-antitrypsin deficiency using polymerase chain reaction. *Lancet*, **i**, 763–4.

Cox, D. W. and Mansfield, T. (1987). Prenatal diagnosis of α-1 antitrypsin deficiency and estimates of fetal risk for disease. *J. Med. Genet.*, **4**, 52–9.

Immune deficiencies

Durandy, A. and Griscelli, C. (1987). Diagnostic prénatal des deficits immunitaires graves et héréditaires. *Rev. Prat.*, **37**, 2634–41.

Goodship, J., Malcom, S., Lau, Y. L., *et al.* (1988). Use of X chromosome inactivation analysis to establish carrier status for X linked severe combined immunodeficiency. *Lancet*, **i**, 729–31.

Hirschhorn, R. (1986). Prenatal diagnosis of adenosine deaminase deficiency, purine nucleoside phosphorylase deficiency and severe combined immunodeficiency of unknown etiology. In *Genetic disorders and the fetus* (ed. A. Milunsky), pp. 419–25, Plenum, New York.

Malcom, S., de Saint Basile, G., and Arveiler, B. (1987). Close linkage of random DNA fragments from Xq21.3-22 to X-linked agammaglobulinamia (XLA). *Hum. Genet.*, **77**, 172–174.

Meusink, E. J. and Schurman, R. K. (1987). Immunodefficiency disease genes on the X chromosome. *Dis. Mark.* **5**, 129–40.

de Saint Basile, G., Arvieiler, B., and Oberle, I. (1987). Close linkage of the locus for X chromosome-linked severe combined immunodeficiency to polymorphic DNA markers on Xq 1I-q13. *Proc. Natl. Acad. Sci. USA*, **84**, 7576–9.

Genodermatoses

Blanchet-Bardon, C., Dumez, Y., *et al.* (1987). Diagnostic anténatal des génodermatoses par microscopie électonique. *Rev. Prat. (Paris)*, **i**, 729–31.

6 Diagnosis of neural tube defects

Neural tube defects lead to malformation for which the prognosis is severe (see p. 9). Anencephaly is incompatible with life and, despite progress in medical care, spina bifida remains serious as the Oxford prospective study (UK Collaborative Study 1982) demonstrates (Table 6.1).

In many countries the frequency of this malformation at birth remains high, but large variation is observed between regions and over time. The highest frequencies were observed several years ago by Carter (1971) in Scotland and Northern Ireland (6–8/1000). In western European countries and in North America the frequency remains at 1–3/1000 births, with equal proportions of anencephaly and spina bifida. In France, a high frequency has been reported in Brittany (2.7/1000 in the early 1970s). The frequency is much lower in the rest of France (less than 1/1000 births in most recent years).

In each region there are great variations over time; in recent years there has been a large drop in the number of these malformations. The birth prevalence of neural tube defects in England and Wales declined from 31.5 to 6.2/10 000 between 1964–1972 and 1986, based on official notifications of congenital malformations. Different surveys estimate that the number of terminations of pregnancy because of severe tube defects account for about half of the decline in the prevalence of births with these defects over this period; a similar trend has been observed in other regions, particularly in Ireland, where there has been no prenatal diagnosis.

Geographic and time variations must reflect variations in environmental factors which play an important role in the cause of these malformations, usually of classical multifactorial or polygenic inheritance. The many attempts to try and understand these factors have been disappointing. Genetic factors are suspected,

Table 6.1 Spina bifida diagnosed at birth, Oxford 1965–1972.
A five year study. Figures in brackets are percentages

	Open spina bifida	Closed spina bifida
Number of observations	163	50
Number surviving at 5 years	49 (30)	30 (60)
Handicap at 5 years		
None	3 (6)	9 (30)
Moderate	5 (10)	10 (33)
Severe	41 (84)	11 (37)

Table 6.2 Risk of recurrence for neural tube defects (United Kingdom data)

One affected child	5 per cent
Two affected children	10 per cent
One affected parent	5 per cent

as the incidence is higher in the Celtic population. For anencephaly there are a great number of affected females, and familial studies show an increase in frequency in relatives (Table 6.2).

The environmental factors are many and varied. It should be noted that the incidence is higher in lower social classes, and the hypothesis that nutritional factors play a role is substantiated by results of studies of multivitamin (including folic acid) supplements prior to conception, as a preventative measure, for high-risk women.

Finally, the teratogenic effect of certain antiepileptic drugs such as valproic acid has been recognized.

Diagnostic methods

In 1972, in Edinburgh, David Brock demonstrated a significant rise in alphafetoprotein in amniotic fluid, sampled at 17 weeks of pregnancy, when a fetus is shown to be affected with a neural tube defect (Brock *et al.* 1972). In the same year, in London, Campbell diagnosed anencephaly by ultrasound. In the following year, British workers showed that a raise in maternal serum alphafetoprotein is associated to the rise in amniotic fluid, and proposed screening of at-risk pregnancies by measuring AFP levels in maternal serum (Brock *et al.* 1973). In 1979, electrophoresis of amniotic fluid cholinesterase showed that the presence of acetylcholinesterase in fluid is associated with a neural tube defect (Collaborative Acetylcholinesterase Study 1981). Based on long experience, these techniques (ultrasound, alphafetoprotein, and acetylcholinesterase) remain the basis of diagnosis of neural tube defects.

Strategy

Screening for neural tube defects is based on the selection of groups of at-risk pregnancies by epidemiological and biological criteria, and on the possibility of systematic ultrasound surveillance in conjunction with amniotic fluid analysis.

Previous neural tube defect or other affected relative

Recurrence risks for abnormality based on family history were established (Carter 1971) based on data from the United Kingdom (Table 6.2).

Though these recurrence risks are useful, it must be kept in mind that they have been established in a population where the incidence of anomaly is raised. They should be modified with respect to the incidence of anomaly in the region from which the couple originates. From experience in French centres, for a woman having had an affected child (anencephaly or spina bifida) the observed recurrence risk is about 1–2 per cent (rather than 5 per cent as in the British series); but after the birth of a second affected child the recurrence risk is identical to British observations.

For mothers already having an affected child, ultrasound surveillance and amniocentesis at 16–17 weeks with acetylcholinesterase electrophoresis on amniotic fluid should be done.

All anencephalies, as well as many spina bifidas, should be detected early by a good detailed ultrasound examination, though some may be missed at 17 weeks. It may be important, where a neural tube defect is not detected, to check by amniotic fluid assay of acetylcholinesterase; amniocentesis is possible earlier, around 15–16 weeks.

In these situations, measure of alphafetoprotein in maternal serum is not indicated; experience in the United Kingdom shows that this screening is unreliable in 20 per cent of cases and so an amniocentesis with acetylcholinesterase assay is preferable.

Systematic screening for neural tube defects by measure of maternal serum alphafetoprotein

This strategy can be applied where the incidence is above 2/1000. Some important points should be considered.

Time of maternal blood sampling   The rapid change in normal serum alphafetoprotein values (Fig. 6.1) in the second trimester of pregnancy requires a very precise time for blood testing. Before 16 weeks of pregnancy, normal values have been observed where there was in fact a neural tube defect. After 18 weeks, any complementary testing required would lead to a late termination.

Cut-off value for determining at-risk pregnancies   Figure 6.2 shows an overlap between normal values and values observed when the fetus has anencephaly or spina bifida. Choosing the cut-off value relative to the median — 2 MoM, 2.5 MoM, or 3.0 MoM — determines the efficiency of screening and the number of false positives; that is, the number of women who must undergo further testing without considering the anxiety involved.

Timely follow-up of at risk women   The first step is to check for any possible errors: error in dating of pregnancy at the time of blood testing (advanced gestational age with higher alphafetoprotein value); twin pregnancy (serum alphafetoprotein at about 2.5 MoM); threatened abortion.

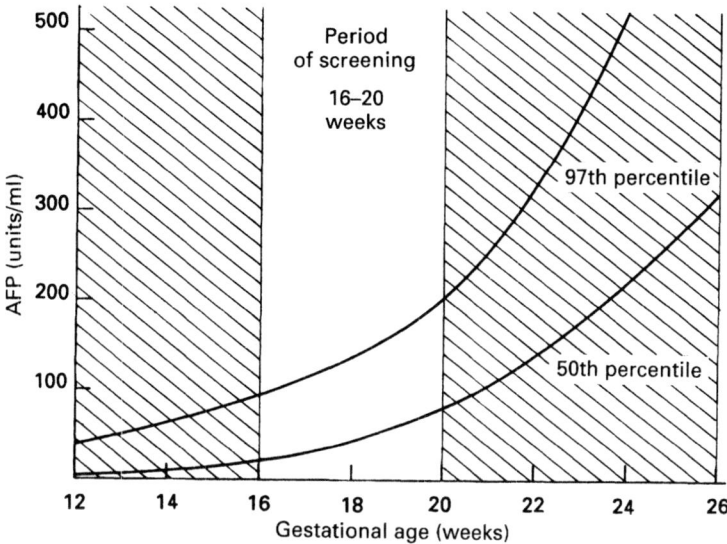

Fig. 6.1 Changes in maternal serum alphafetoprotein levels between 12 and 26 weeks of gestation, with median level (50th percentile) and the 97th percentile limit. From Ferguson-Smith (1983).

Once these causes of error have been excluded, it is important to confirm the value by a second blood test. If the raised value persists, a detailed ultrasound examination should be carried out to look for a neural tube defect, an amniocentesis to measure amniotic fluid alphafetoprotein, and particularly acetylcholinesterase electrophoresis. In many cases, the patient would find it hard to accept that a karyotype should not be done, again increasing the financial burden of such testing. The cut-off value for maternal serum alphafetoprotein in any one population should be such that only 1 per cent of cases result in amniocentesis. In high-incidence areas for neural tube defects the introduction of such a strategy has proved its importance. In Scotland, of 14 000 pregnancies, confirmed raised levels of maternal serum alphafetoprotein have led to amniocentesis in 0.86 per cent of pregnancies, permitting diagnosis of 97 per cent of anencephalies and 72 per cent of spina bifidas.

Table 6.3 shows the value of doing acetylcholinesterase electrophoresis in amniotic fluid as acetylcholinesterase has been positive in almost all cases of anencephaly and spina bifida. Those cases that are apparently false positive are either multiple malformations, easily observed on ultrasound, or fetal deaths.

Maternal serum alphafetoprotein or ultrasound surveillance? Figure 6.3 shows results of the prenatal diagnosis of neural tube defects in England and Wales in 1985.

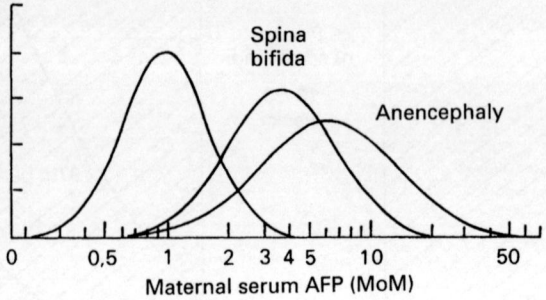

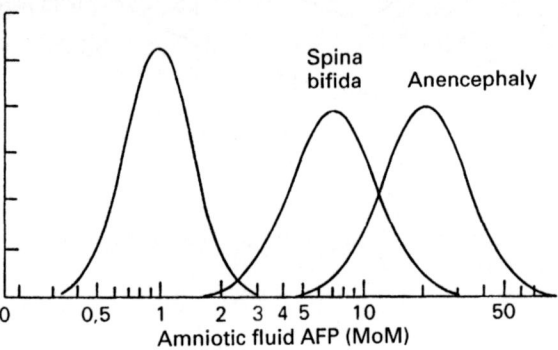

Fig. 6.2 Distribution of alphafetoprotein levels in maternal serum and amniotic fluid at 16–18 weeks' gestation in relation to the state of the fetus — normal, anencephalic, or spina bifida. Alphafetoprotein levels are expressed in MoM (multiples of the median). The proportion of false positives and false negatives varies, depending on whether the value chosen is 2 or 3 MoM. From UK Collaborative Study (1982).

An estimated 534 pregnancies associated with anencephaly were terminated and an estimated 445 pregnancies associated with spina bifida (but without anencephaly) were terminated. Most (63 per cent) of the anencephalic pregnancies were first suspected from an ultrasound examination; 57 per cent of the spina bifida pregnancies were first suspected from a positive maternal serum alphafetoprotein test, 35 per cent by ultrasound, and the remaining 8 per cent by other means.

Given the miscarriage risk of amniocentesis, some authors have questioned the need for serum alphafetoprotein measurements compared to the possibility of detection simply using a good ultrasound, but there is still some controversy.

Is it practical to do testing for neural tube defects on all amniotic fluids sampled for other reasons?

In areas where population maternal serum screening is not justified, one might consider searching for a neural tube defect on amniotic fluid sampled for a cyto-

Table 6.3 Effectiveness of AChE electrophoresis (collaborative acetylcholinesterase study 1981) Amniocentesis after discovery of raised maternal serum AFP. Figures in brackets are percentages

Pregnancy outcome	Number of tests	Acetylcholinesterase positive
Anencephaly	478	476 (99.6)
Open spina bifida	335	333 (99.4)
Multiple malformation (omphalocoele)	88	54 (61)
Fetal death	73	34 (47)
Normal child	125	8 (6)

Analysis of 125 normal outcomes

Characteristics of amniotic fluid	Number of samples	Acetylcholinesterase positive
Very bloody	34	5
Fetal blood		
Maternal blood	19	
Unknown	6	2
Clear	59	1
No information	7	

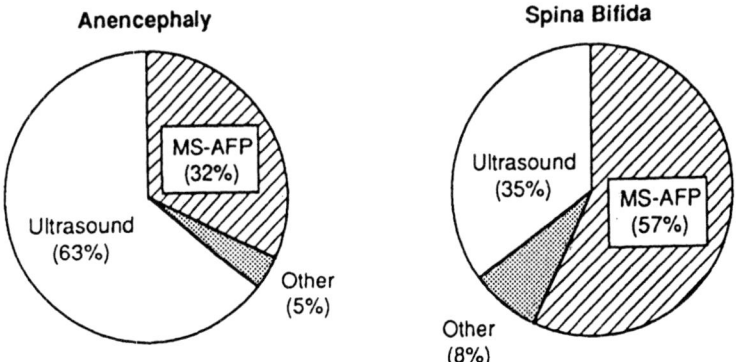

Fig. 6.3 Results of prenatal diagnosis of neural tube defects in England and Wales in 1985 (Cuckle *et al.* 1989)

genetic analysis (maternal age) or other reasons. In practical terms, only alphafetoprotein measurement is feasible on a large number of samples. Figure 6.2 shows that there is a minimal overlap between normal values and those observed in the case of anomaly. There are also raised values because of the presence of fetal blood. Therefore, acetylcholinesterase electrophoresis should be done to verify all abnormal alphafetoprotein values.

Such a strategy can be justified where the incidence is 1–2/1000, thereby selecting all samples where the alphafetoprotein value is more than 2.0 MoM for acetylcholinesterase electrophoresis. This was demonstrated in California where the incidence was 1.5/1000 in those samples of amniotic fluid drawn for advanced maternal age. In France, a similar strategy can be considered in the northwestern regions. Experience in the Paris region has shown an incidence of 1/4000, which resulted in discontinuation of this strategy.

It must always be borne in mind that a large number of anencephalies and spina bifidas will be picked up early by ultrasound.

Why acetylcholinesterase electrophoresis may be preferred over amniotic fluid alphafetoprotein, a simpler test

Until acetylcholinesterase electrophoresis became available, alphafetoprotein in amniotic fluid permitted the diagnosis of many neural tube defects, but its interpretation remains difficult. A rise in amniotic fluid alphafetoprotein is not specific to neural tube defects; it is also found with omphalocele, gastroschisis, intestinal atresias, and nephrotic syndromes.

There are many false positives due to amniotic fluid contamination with fetal blood. Alphafetoprotein produced by the fetal liver is present in fetal serum in 1000 times greater amounts than in fluid. This is why the slightest blood contamination, sometimes difficult to prove, will affect the fluid alphafetoprotein value considerably.

There are also false negatives: in our series 16 cases of neural tube defects had a normal AFP value (less than the 95th percentile); they included one anencephaly, seven spina bifidas (meningocoeles covered by skin), seven spina bifida aperta, and one myelomeningocoele covered by an encapsulated angioma. Finally, the alphafetoprotein level in amniotic fluid varies with gestational age, and beyond 20 weeks of gestation the reliability of AFP measurement is disputable.

In 125 pregnancies leading to the birth of a normal child, the level of maternal serum alphafetoprotein was raised. Electrophoresis was positive in eight cases, but in seven of them the amniotic fluid was extremely bloody, explaining the presence of the second acetylcholinesterase band. It was only in one observation that a false positive acetylcholinesterase was observed (representing, in the study, only 1/1000).

References and further reading

Brock, D. J. H. (1989). Towards the prevention of neural tube defects. *Clin. Genet.*, **36**, 339–47.
Brock, D. J. H., Sutcliffe, R. G. (1972). Alpha-feroprotein in the antenatal diagnosis of anencephaly and spina bifida. *Lancet*, **ii**, 197.

Brock, D. J. H., Bolton, A. E., Monoghan, J. M. (1973). Prenatal diagnosis of anencephaly through maternal serum alpha-feroprotein measurement. *Lancet*, **ii**, 923.

Carter, C. O. (1971). Genetics of common malformations. In *Recent advances in paediatrics* (ed. D. Gairdner and D. Hull), p. 527. Churchill Livingstone, London.

Collaborative Acetylcholinesterase Study (1981). Amniotic fluid acetylcholinesterase electrophoresis as a secondary test in the diagnosis of anencephaly and open spina bifida in early pregnancy. *Lancet*, **i**, 321.

Crandall, B. F. and Matsumoto, M. (1986). Routine amniotic fluid alpha-fetoprotein assay: experience with 40 000 pregnancies. *Am. J. Med. Genet.*, **24**, 143–9.

Cuckle, H. S., Wald, N. J., and Cuckle, P. M. (1989). Prenatal screening and diagnosis of neural tube defect in England and Wales in 1985. *Prenat. Diagn.*, **9**, 393–400.

Dulard, E., Boué C., Muller, F., Boué J., *et al.* (1988). L. électrophorèse des cholinestérases du liquide amniotique dans le diagnostic prénatal des défauts de ferme-ture du tube neural. *J. Gynecol. Obstet. Biol. Reprod. (Paris)*, **17**.

Ferguson-Smith, M. A. (1983). The reduction of anencephalic and spina-bifida birth by maternal serum alpha-foetoprotein screening. *Br. Med. Bull.* **39**, 365–72.

Tidy, J. (1989). A study of the value of measuring maternal serum alpha-fetoprotein for the antenatal diagnosis of neural tube defects. *Arch. Gynecol. Obstet.*, **244**, 133–6.

UK Collaborative Study. (1982). Fourth report. *J. Epidemiol. Community Health*, **36**, 87–95.

Wald, N. J. and Cuckle, H. S. (1984). Neural tube defects: screening and biochemical diagnosis. In *Prenatal diagnosis* (ed. C. H. Rodeck and K. H. Nicolaides), pp. 219–41, Wiley, New York.

PART III   NO PREDICTABLE RISK OF ANOMALY

7 Ultrasound indications for laboratory testing

Fortuitous finding of anomaly on ultrasound examination is a frequent indication for laboratory analyses which are increasingly indispensable in the appropriate management of cases.

In terms of diagnosis, the indication may be for diagnosis of cause (e.g. chromosomal anomaly), or for more precise diagnosis (e.g. acetylcholinesterase for neural tube defect).

In terms of prognosis, for a pregnancy in progress, laboratory testing may provide a better appreciation of the disorder (e.g. renal function). Mainly, however, the concern is to establish recurrence risks for future pregnancies (e.g. identification of chromosome translocation).

Ultrasound diagnosis may permit the identification of abnormalities of fetal development, either an apparently single malformation or multiple congenital malformations. These malformations may be associated with a change in the volume of amniotic fluid, oligohydramnios or polyhydramnios, and/or intrauterine growth retardation. In other cases, the only sign will be a change in volume of amniotic fluid or severe fetal growth retardation; these signs should lead to a detailed ultrasound examination looking for other malformations before determining that the initial sign is isolated.

Given these ultrasound findings, there are two questions: which laboratory analyses to request and what method of sampling to use?

Laboratory analyses

Fetal karyotype

This should always be requested. The value of abnormal ultrasound findings as an indication of a chromosomal anomaly has been known since 1982 (Boué *et al.* 1982): first by observation of phenotypic features characteristic of chromosomal anomalies (the hand findings associated with trisomy 18), and also by study of pregnancies where ultrasound findings had led to an amniocentesis. Nine chromosomal abnormalities were observed in 38 cases studied (24 per cent).

To establish better indications, a collaborative study was initiated on 1 October 1985, lasting until 30 June 1987, and involving 42 French laboratories in prenatal diagnosis centres (Boué *et al.* 1988). This study of 7982 diagnoses clearly shows the importance of such studies (Table 7.1). Overall the study

Table 7.1. Frequency of chromosome anomalies with respect to abnormal ultrasound findings. A study by the Association française pour le dépistage et la prévention des maladies et des handicaps de l'enfant and the prenatal centres of Amiens, Angers, Bordeaux, Boulogne, Brest, Caen, Chambéry, Clermont-Ferrand, Dijon, Grenoble, Lille, Lyon, Marseille, Montpellier, Nancy, Nîce, Nimes, Paris, Reims, Rouen, Strasbourg, Toulouse, Tours

Ultrasound signs	Number of Observations	Chromosomal anomalies n	%		
Single malformation (4362)					
isolated	2984	263	8.8	9.6	10.5
associated with: oligo/polyhydramnios	988	117	11.8		
IUGR	216	38	17.6	20.0	
IUGR + oligo/polyhydramnios	174	40	23		
Multiple malformations (1242)					
isolated	667	140	27	22.8	26.2
associated with: oligo/polyhydramnios	395	102	25.8		
IUGR	85	40	47.1	46.1	
IUGR + oligo/polyhydramnios	95	43	45.3		
Oligo/polyhydramnios	1142	40	3.5		
IUGR	709	37	5.2		
IUGR + oligo/polyhydramnios	527	39	7.5		
Total	7982	899	11.3		

shows an 11 per cent frequency of chromosomal anomalies, of various types. When an isolated malformation is found, a chromosomal anomaly is found in about 10.5 per cent of cases, but this frequency rises once the abnormality is associated with intrauterine growth retardation (20 per cent). Those syndromes with multiple malformations are the ones most often associated with a chromosomal anomaly: 26.2 per cent overall, with a rise in number (46.1 per cent) if there is intrauterine grown retardation. In those cases where ultrasound has shown intrauterine growth retardation, isolated or in association with a change in amniotic fluid volume, the frequency of chromosomal anomalies is about 5–7 per cent. The frequency is at its lowest (3.5 per cent) for isolated poly- or oligo-hydramnios and one must consider whether amniocentesis is indicated in the absence of other ultrasound signs.

Table 7.2 shows data on the most frequent types of chromosomal anomalies; trisomies 18 and 21, and monosomy X. The table also shows figures obtained in recent years on results of women 38 years and over tested because of advanced maternal age.

Table 7.3 shows the frequency of different types of chromosomal anomalies identified by different types of abnormal ultrasound findings. It is interesting to note the frequency of trisomy 21 in association with a single malformation.

Table 7.2 Types of chromosomal anomalies detected after ultrasound indications, and those observed in women over 38 years of age. Figures in brackets are percentages

Chromosomal anomaly	Detected on ultrasound (7982 diagnoses)	Maternal age indication (36 754 diagnoses)
Trisomy 21	251 (3.2)	559 (1.5)
Trisomy 18	242 (3.0)	147 (0.4)
Trisomy 13	90	35
45X	140	17
47XXY, 47XXX	12	118
Triploidy	67	3
Other anomalies	27	58
Total	899 (11.3)	937 (2.55)

Table 7.3 Frequency and types of chromosomal anomalies detected by whether single or multiple malformations are observed on ultrasound examination (French Collaborative study). Figures in brackets are percentages

Chromosomal anomaly	Single malformation	Multiple malformations
Trisomy 21	168 (41.2)	63 (19.4)
Trisomy 18	92 (22.5)	120 (37.0)
Trisomy 13	35 (8.6)	46 (14.2)
45 X	42 (10.3)	37 (11.4)
47 XXY	9 (2.2)	4 (1.2)
Triploidy	20 (4.9)	23 (7.1)
Structural anomalies	42 (10.3)	31 (9.6)

These observations are confirmed by our results when diagnosis was made based on an intestinal abnormality (Table 7.4). All these data illustrate well the necessity of fetal karyotyping when an abnormality is observed on ultrasound. More extensive studies are needed to confirm further details.

1. *Indications using particular criteria for measuring intrauterine growth retardation* — biparietal diameter, abdominal circumference, femur length, etc. A dissociation of these parameters may be a diagnostic criteria: for example, in trisomy 18, where there is a dissociation between biparietal diameter and abdominal circumference.

2. *Frequency of chromosomal anomalies in relation to certain types of malformations*, for example cardiac malformations. A large study conducted by Fermont (Table 7.5) shows on the one hand the overall frequency of chromosomal anomalies in ultrasound-diagnosed cardiac malformations (20 per cent), and on the other hand the particular attention that should be paid to certain cardiac abnormalities such as the atrioventricular canal defect, often associated with trisomy 21 (Fermont, personal communication).

Table 7.4 Frequency and types of chromosome anomalies associated with digestive tract malformations detected on ultrasound examination

Ultrasound diagnosis	Chromosome anomaly	Frequency
Oesophageal atresia (8 cases)	Trisomy 18 (1 case) Trisomy 13 (1 case)	2/8 (25 per cent)
Duodenal stenosis (22 cases)	Trisomy 21 (7 cases) Trisomy 18 (1 case)	8/22 (36 per cent)
Intestinal dilatation (7 cases)	Trisomy 18 (2 cases)	2/7 (28 per cent)
Total (37 cases)	Trisomy 21 (7 cases) Trisomy 18 (4 cases) Trisomy 13 (1 case)	12/37 (32.5 per cent)

Table 7.5 Chromosomal anomalies in cardiac malformations detected on ultrasound examination. (L. Fermont, 300 diagnoses from 1 January 1983 to 1 January 1988)

Ultrasound diagnosis	Chromosomal anomalies		
	Trisomy 21	Trisomy 18	Trisomy 13
Atrioventricular canal			
complete	34	4	–
associated	5	3	1
Tetralogy of Fallot	2	7	–
Interventricular communication	5	3	1
Hypoplasia of left ventricle	–	2	1
Tricuspid atresia	2	1	3

Biochemical assays

The tests to be run are determined by the types of abnormalities observed on ultrasound examination; consultation between the biochemist and the ultrasonographer is imperative before the choice of sampling is made and before any analyses are performed.

Qualitative analyses   Of all possible analyses, acetylcholinesterase electrophoresis of amniotic fluid is the most important biochemical assay to consider.

Cholinesterase electrophoresis must be done on all amniotic fluids sampled as a result of ultrasound finding of a central nervous system malformation. It allows confirmation of all open neural tube defects diagnosed on ultrasound, and reveals neural tube defects when the indication for amniocentesis was not a neural tube defect, such as hydrocephaly, for example. In some of these, a repeat ultrasound directed by acetylcholinesterase findings will find the neural tube defect. Should ultrasound not find a neural tube defect, a repeat amniocentesis should be done to confirm the first acetylcholinesterase result.

Table 7.6 shows results for 146 acetylcholinesterase electrophoreses performed on amniotic fluid sampled as a result of ultrasound findings of central nervous system malformations. For anencephaly, the need for an acetylcholinesterase electrophoresis to confirm findings may not be necessary because all studies have demonstrated a perfect correlation. For spinal defects, acetylcholinesterase electrophoresis is an important complementary test either to confirm extensive leaking of cerebral spinal fluid (for which the prognosis is poor) or the presence of a skin-covered spina bifida defect (with a better prognosis). In some cases, absence of acetylcholinesterase in the fluid will reverse the original false ultrasound diagnosis. Results of biochemical assays on amniotic fluid after ultrasound finding of isolated hydrocephalus illustrates the use of these tests.

Table 7.6 Results of acetylcholinesterase electrophoresis on amniotic fluid sampled after abnormal ultrasound findings

Ultrasound diagnosis	Number of samples	Acetylcholinesterase positive		Acetylcholinesterase negative	
Central nervous system disorders					
Suggesting a neural tube defect					
Anencephaly	31	30	29 anencephalies		
			1 amniotic band	1	1 amniotic band
Encephalocoele	7	6	6 encephalocoeles	1	1 neuroblastoma
Meningoencephalocoele	17	6	6 meningo-encephalocoeles	11	9 meningo-encephalocoeles (skin normal)
					1 multiple pterygium
					1 normal
Spina bifida	24	22	22 spina bifida	2	2 meningocoeles (skin normal)
Others					
Microcephaly	5	3	1 encephalocoele		
			2 spina bifida		
Ventricular dilatation	62	8	8 spina bifida		
Other anomalies					
Omphalocoele + laparoschisis	46	1	1 spina bifida		
oligo/polyhydramnios	149				
IUGR	73	0			
Urinary tract malformation	91				
Other (digestive, cardiac)	68				

On 64 amniotic fluid samples examined, 10 chromosomal abnormalities (15.6 per cent) and 7 spina bifidas (11.6 per cent), previously undetected, were picked up. Figure 7.1 shows the gestational age when these tests were performed. Amongst the 20 analyses done before the 25th week of pregnancy, eight chromosomal anomalies (40 per cent, including three trisomy 18 associated with a spina bifida) and one spina bifida were detected. Amongst the 32 analyses done after 28 weeks of pregnancy, two chromosomal anomalies and six spina bifidas were picked up. It should be noted that three of seven spina bifidas were not detected even on detailed ultrasound after acetylcholinesterase measurement. The biochemical detection of open neural tube defect associated with hydro-cephalus is important as, because of the leaking of spinal fluid, hydrocephalus does not progress and may not appear to be of such great concern.

Must acetylcholinesterase electrophoresis be done on all amniotic fluids drawn after ultrasound detection of an abnormality? On 427 samples drawn after various ultrasound indications, other than central nervous system malformations, acetylcholinesterase electrophoresis revealed only one case of open neural tube defect, an undetected spina bifida, where the ultrasound indication was an omphalocoele (1 of 46 cases). Other indications were oligo/polyhydramnios (149 cases), intrauterine growth retardation (73 cases), urinary tract malformations (91 cases), cardiac and digestive tract malformations (68 cases).

The difficulty in interpreting acetylcholinesterase electrophoresis in these cases should be considered. A second non-specific band can be confused with the characteristic second band of acetylcholinesterase, particularly in cases of omphalocoeles, and sometimes when fluids are drawn after 32 weeks.

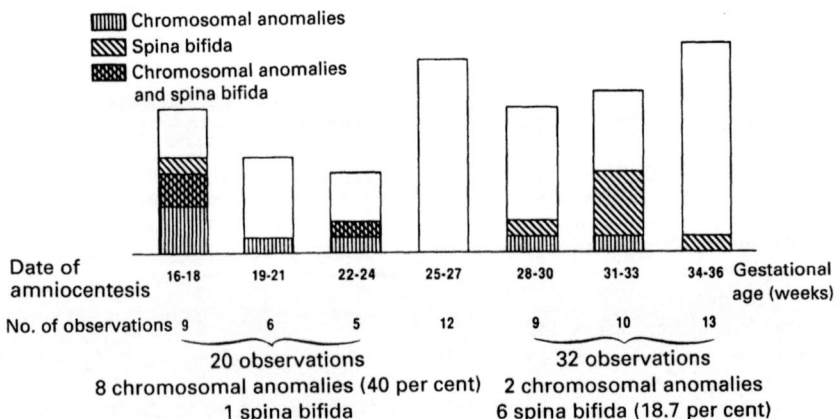

Fig. 7.1 Fetal karyotype and cholinesterase electrophoresis results from amniotic fluid drawn after detection of hydrocephaly by ultrasound examination.

Quantitative analyses   These analyses evaluate variations in normal constituents and are therefore difficult to interpret. This is the case with alphafetoprotein assay. Large variations in its level have been observed, in particular after the 20th week of gestation, and the frequency of false positives and false negatives is well known. This gives preference to acetylcholinesterase measurements, which is a qualitative test not varying with gestational age.

Gastrointestinal malformations   An assay of digestive enzymes can be made in amniotic fluid. Figures 7.2 and 7.3 illustrate situations where these measurements contribute to a diagnosis. Biliary atresia may be suspected in the absence of gammaglutamyl transpeptidase of hepatic origin (Figure 7.2A). This result can be confirmed by measurement of 5'-nucleotidase, an enzyme produced by the liver and absent in these cases.

Imperforate anus manifests itself as an absence of intestinal enzymes. The isoform of alkaline phosphatase coming from kidney, liver, and bone, not the intestinal form, is observed (Figure 7.2C). The absence of disaccharidases will also confirm an intestinal anomaly.

Duodenal stenosis below the hepatic pancreatic duct results in a regurgitation of biliary enzymes into the amniotic fluid and an increase in the level of gammaglutamyl transpeptidase at a time when its level is minimal. Figure 7.2B shows a twin pregnancy where one of the twins had a duodenal stenosis. An unexpected finding of an echogenic abdominal mass in the right iliac fossa, producing meconium ileus, is a difficult situation. As this could represent a fetus affected with cystic fibrosis, the study of digestive enzymes in amniotic fluid can be done if the pregnancy is not beyond 20 weeks (by ultrasound).

Normal levels or levels evolving to normal within a period of a week do not favour the diagnosis of cystic fibrosis (Fig. 7.3B). Low levels of digestive enzymes (Fig. 7.3A), as observed in pregnancies affected by cystic fibrosis (see p. 145), confirm the intestinal obstruction and ileus. Is this a case of cystic fibrosis where the couple's genetic risk is unknown, realizing that there is 1 affected child in 2000 births? In these circumstances fetal DNA analysis should be done (from amniotic fluid cells or chorionic villi obtained transabdominally); if the fetus has one of the more common mutations or haplotypes associated with cystic fibrosis (KM-19 allele 2 in particular, see p. 144), one must consider this an affected fetus. In other circumstances the ileus must have another cause, trisomy 21 for example.

Urinary tract malformations   On bilateral obstructive uropathies it is possible to assess renal function not only indirectly by measuring volume of amniotic fluid or by the thickness of the renal cortex, but also by enzyme study of fetal urine. Several parameters make it possible to differentiate between renal dysplasia resulting in neonatal death by pulmonary hypoplasia, and other less severe obstructive uropathies. These parameters are sodium, chlorine, osmolarity, glucose, protein, calcium, and phosphorus. Figure 7.4 shows our experience

Fig. 7.2A Biliary
atresia. Digestive
enzyme levels in
amniotic fluid.
Amniotic fluid
drawn at 17 weeks
in one case and at
23 weeks in
another. GGTP,
gammaglutamyl
transpeptidase;
LAP, leucine
aminopeptidase;
PAL, total
alkaline
phosphatase,
intestinal PAL,
intestinal alkaline
phosphatase; ★,
fetus affected; ■,
fetus not affected.

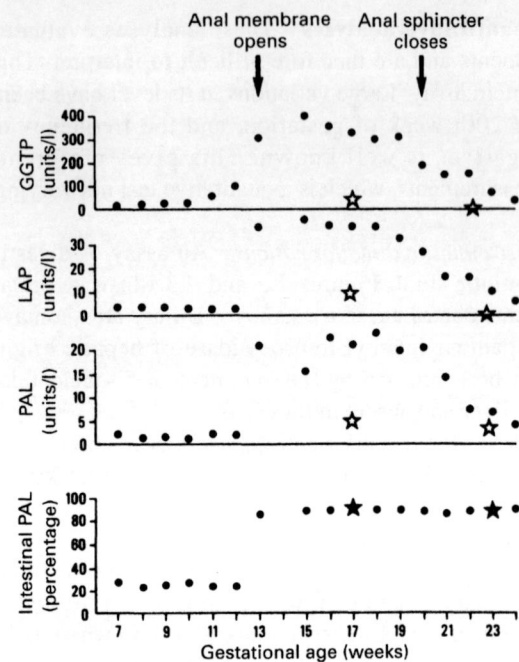

Fig. 7.2B
Duodenal atresia
below the
ampulla of Vater.
Amniotic fluid
drawn at 24
weeks from a twin
pregnancy. Only
one twin was
affected; the other
did not
present with
duodenal atresia.
Abbreviations as
in Fig. 7.2A.

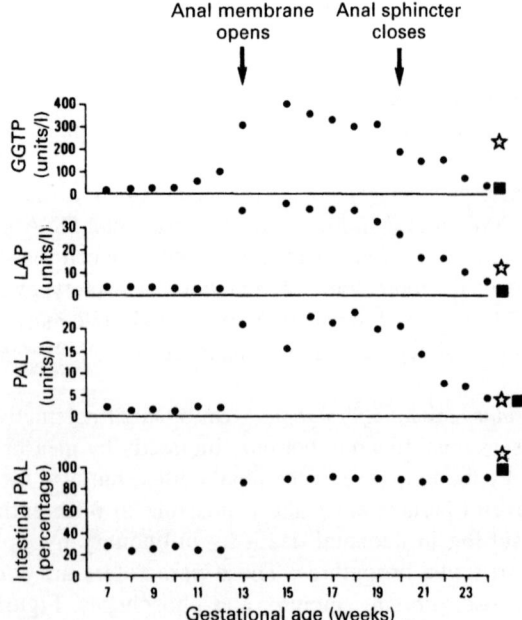

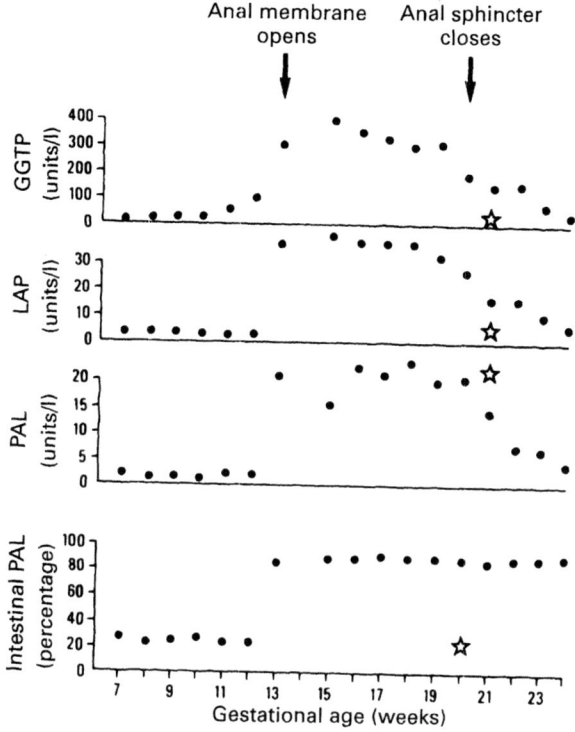

Fig. 7.2C Imperforate anus. Amniotic fluid drawn at 20 weeks. Levels of digestive enzymes in amniotic fluid. Abbreviations as in Fig. 7.2A.

with sodium values from 31 bilateral obstructive uropathies. Four parameters — urea, creatinine, ammonia, β2-microglobulin — allow the further differentiation of three groups of fetuses: those who will die at birth, those who at 1 year will have normal renal function (creatinine clearance < 50 μmol/L) and an intermediate group showing incomplete renal function (creatinine > 50 μmol/L). There is a correlation between the levels of β2-microglobulin and the degree of renal insufficiency at 1 year of age measured by creatininaemia (Fig. 7.5). Study of the biochemistry of fetal urine allows classification of the fetus into one of the three groups. It may be possible to confirm the poor prognosis illustrated by ultrasound finding of oligohydramnios and hyperechogenic kidneys, or reassure the parents if the prognosis is good. If the fetus is in the intermediary group, a second urine sample allows evaluation of the progress of the uropathy. A rise in calciuria may be the first sign of a tubular insufficiency in the fetus (Fig. 7.6) and an *in-utero* shunt can be decided upon on the basis of these criteria of function, although the benefits of intervention *in utero* have not yet been demonstrated.

Fig. 7.3A
Intrabdominal
echogenic mass.
Levels of
digestive
enzymes
in amniotic fluid
drawn after
ultrasound
finding of an
echogenic mass
in the right iliac.
Amniotic fluid
drawn at 18 and
20 weeks.
Enzyme levels
decrease during
that time, and the
fetus has
meconium ileus.

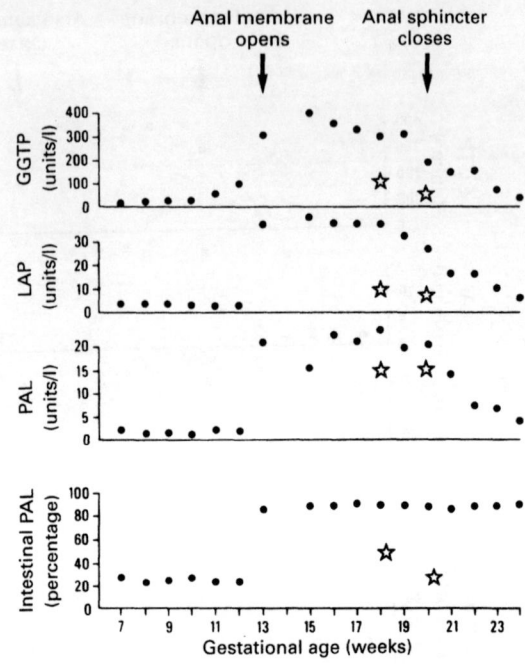

Fig.7.3B Normal
fetus. Amniotic
fluid taken at 18
and 20 weeks. At
18 weeks values
are below normal;
at 20 weeks they
are normal. The
child is normal at
birth.

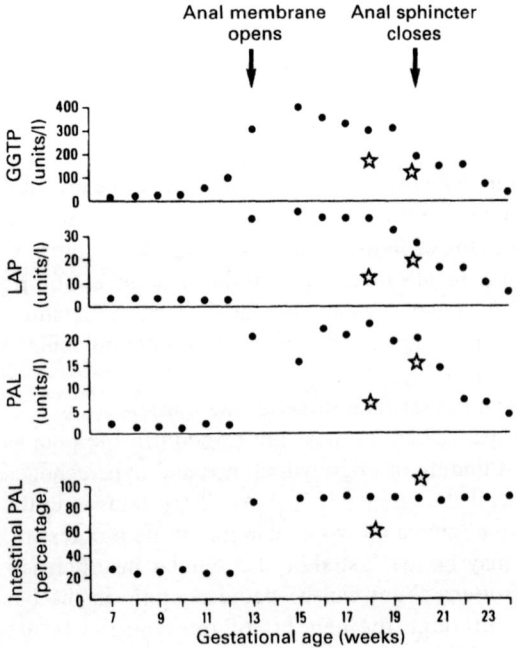

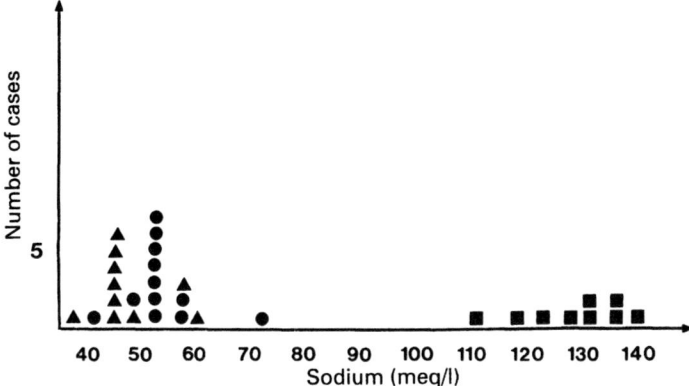

Fig. 7.4 Sodium levels in fetal urine sampled *in utero* for bilateral obstructive uropathy. ■, fetuses with renal dysplasia on histological examination, ▲, children presenting 1 year after birth with a serum creatinine of greater than 50 μmol/L; ●, children presenting 1 year after birth with normal renal function, a serum creatinine of less than 50 μmol/L.

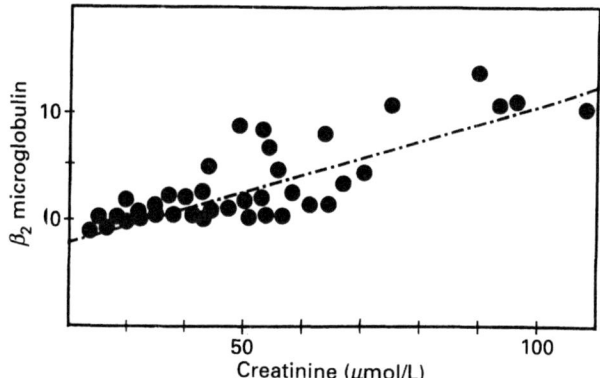

Fig. 7.5 β-2 microglobulin measured in fetal urine and serum creatinine in a child at 1 year of age. ($r = 0.78$, $p = 0.01$).

For other types of malformation, cardiac for example, there are no measurements which can help to confirm diagnosis or prognosis.

Sampling methods

Prior to sampling, the studies to be done must be determined with the laboratory, taking into consideration ultrasound findings, gestational age, and the likely time required for the analyses. For fetal karyotyping there are two possible sampling

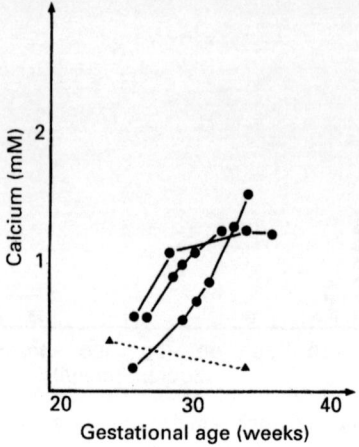

Fig. 7.6 Calcium levels in fetal urine during development. ▲, in the fetus who will have normal renal function at birth (clearance ≥ 50 ml/min/1.73 m²); ●, in the fetus who will have altered renal function at birth (clearance ≤ 50 ml/min/1.73 m².

methods. *Amniocentesis* imposes the smaller risk, and renders possible biochemical analysis of the supernatant. The time required for karyotyping varies from one laboratory to another: 2–3 weeks for some and a month for others. *Fetal blood sampling* requires a trained team in order to minimize risk to the fetus. It is the method of preference if a chromosomal anomaly is being specifically looked for, and if the sampling can be done immediately. However, if there is some delay in organizing an appointment in a specialized centre, then it is no longer a rapid karyotyping and it is best to do an amniocentesis immediately, particularly when the cytogenetics laboratory can give an early result and when biochemical analyses are required.

Discovery of an anomaly by ultrasound examination can be late. Table 7.7 gives results of chromosome anomalies in relation to gestational age. It can be

Table 7.7 Frequency and types of chromosomal anomalies detected after normal ultrasound findings at various gestational ages

Type of anomaly	Date of amniocentesis			
	≤ 22 weeks	22–27 weeks	28–31 weeks	≥ 32 weeks
Trisomy 21	4	17	16	11
Trisomy 18	11	25	19	12
Trisomy 13	–	10	1	5
45X	16	5	7	1
47XXY, 47XXX	–	2	1	1
Triploidy	–	7	2	1
Other anomalies	3	11	6	8

seen that results are often late. It is likely that in the future experience gained by ultrasonographers will allow an earlier diagnosis.

References and further reading

Benacerraf, B. R., Gelman, R., and Frigoletto, F. D. (1987). Sonographic identification of second-trimester fetuses with Down's syndrome. *New Engl. J. Med.*, **317**, 1371–6.

Benacerraf, B. R., Harlow, B., and Frigoletto, F. D. (1990). Are choroid plexus cysts an indication for second-trimester amniocentesis? *Am. J. Obstet. Gynecol.*, **162,** 1001–6.

Boué, A., Muller, F., Briard, M. L., Boué, J. (1988). Interest of biology in the management of pregnancies where a fetal malformation has been detected by ultrasonography. *Fetal. Ther.*, **3**, 14–23.

Boué, J., Vignal, P., Aubry, J. P., Aubry, M. C., Mac, A., Leese, J. (1982). Ultrasound movement patterns of fetuses with dimensional anomalies. *Prenatal. Diagn.*, **2**, 61–5.

Chitkara, U., Cogswell, C., Norton, K., *et al.* (1988). Choroid plexus cysts in the fetus: a benign anatomic variant or pathologic entity? Report of 41 cases and review of the literature. *Obstet. Gynecol.*, **72**, 185–9.

Filkins, K. and Russo, J. (1990). *Human prenatal diagnosis*, 2nd edn. Marcel Dekker, New York.

Harrison, M. R., Golbus, M., and Filly, R. A. (1990). *The unborn patient. Prenatal diagnosis and treatment*. W. B. Saunders, Toronto.

Hasan, S. and Hermansen, M. C. (1986). The prenatal diagnosis of ventral abdominal wall defects. *Am. J. Obstet. Gynecol.*, **155**, 842–5.

Herrmann, U. J. and Sidiropoulos, D. (1988). Single umbilical artery: prenatal findings. *Prenat. Diagn.*, **8**, 275–80.

Milunsky, A. (1988). *Genetic disorders and the fetus*, 2nd edn. Plenum, New York.

8   Maternal infection

Introduction

More than forty years after Gregg's description of the congenital rubella syndrome, microbiological, clinical immunological and epidemiological studies have provided much information on fetal and neonatal risks as a consequence of transmission of maternal infection. Despite these studies, much remains obscure, mainly because of methodological difficulties inherent in such investigations.

From a clinical point of view, infections with characteristic symptoms are not frequent in the mother because they are often childhood viral diseases (chickenpox, measles, mumps, etc.) Other infections have specific symptoms (respiratory, digestive and eruptive conditions) and many infections are asymptomatic (cytomegalovirus infection, for example).

The problem is even more complex when studies based on disease in neonates must be used. Other than a few malformative syndromes (congenital rubella, cytomegalovirus infection, congenital toxoplasmosis) many of the pathological manifestations, for example neurological and hepatic deficiencies, are common to various intrauterine or perinatal infections. As for long-term consequences (mental handicap, hearing loss) retrospective studies, even those amenable to laboratory testing, remain difficult to interpret.

In a single and immunologically mature person, child or adult, development of an infection and its symptoms are consistent and predictable. In embryos, fetuses, or neonates, affected as a consequence to a maternal infection, one is faced with two non-independent organisms, resulting in a complex transmission of the infection and a complex passive and active defence mechanism.

Various consequences of a particular infection

A particular infection may have various consequences resulting from the interaction of numerous parameters.

1. The type of infection: maternal infection may be due to primary infection, secondary infection, or recurring infection (herpes or cytomegalovirus for example) or the mother may be a carrier of the virus (hepatitis B, HIV).

2. The timing of maternal infection in relation to fetal development.

3. The mode of transmission to the fetus, either directly through the blood or first through infection of the placenta; by contamination at birth, either through

216

the membranes or by exposure to the maternal genital tract at the time of delivery.

4. The type and timing of maternal immunological response determines the time of transfer of antibodies to the fetus.

    (a) Pregnancy puts the mother in a particular immunological status, and the immunological response to a particular infection may be different to that occurring in the non-pregnant state.

    (b) Infection of embryo or fetal tissues may occur either before or after transmission of the mother's specific immunoglobulin; the consequence may be protection of the fetus and newborn, or a disease state caused by an antibody–antigen reaction occurring in the fetus.

5. The timing of the onset of mature immune response in the fetus. The development of the fetal immune system (see p.8), and evolution in its ability to respond to a foreign antigen, will moderate the disease consequences induced by infectious agents reaching the fetus.

Experimental data from animal studies show that viruses that are benign in the adult may be responsible for serious neurological damage in the embryo. An example is the attenuated virus, blue tongue, observed in sheep. Conversely, viruses pathogenic to the adult, may not have any disease consequence for the fetus: an example is lymphocytic choriomeningitis in mice.

Similar observations have been made in humans: triponema will result in congenital syphilis after a fetal age of 5 months, that is at the time when the fetus can have an inflammatory response which is the cause of the lesions.

In congenital rubella, non-inflammatory embryopathies and inflammatory fetopathies may result from chronic infection of tissues during development; in cytomegalovirus infection it is the formation of immune complexes resulting in tissue damage which interferes with defence mechanisms.

In the neonate, the same infection can have serious consequences in cases of transmission at the time of birth (as in neonatal herpes), or may be completely asymptomatic if the mother-to-child transmission occurs a few days later.

At times, a particular sensitivity to infection is observed in the newborn, as with the syncytial respiratory viral infection in the first months of life or the dengue virus where the more serious forms (dengue shock syndrome) are observed, when the mother is seropositive and the baby is less than one year old, and at a stage when transmitted maternal antibodies are still present.

Diagnosis of an infection

Only a few maternal viral, parasitic, or bacterial infections can result in disease in the embryo or fetus and in most of these infections (rubella, cytomegalovirus, toxoplasmosis) fetal disease would only be observed in the case of primary infection of the mother during pregnancy.

1. The *first goal* is testing to determine the presence of such a primary maternal infection. This requires:

(a) A knowledge of the mother's immune status prior to pregnancy. For some of these infections (rubella and toxoplasmosis) blood tests are performed systematically; different blood screening techniques have been developed, each capable of evaluating a large series, while conserving sensitivity.

(b) Availability of firm data from blood analysis confirming the presence of the primary infection, the best criteria being evidence of seroconversion.

Detection of specific IgM antibodies is imperative in diagnosis of rubella and toxoplasmosis; it is useful for other viral infections, in particular the herpes virus groups (cytomegalovirus, herpes simplex) where recurrence episodes may be accompanied by the presence of specific IgM antibodies.

Determination of specific IgM antibodies can be done by various techniques, but some result in a significant number of false positives and should be eliminated (in particular ELISA); even more so, now that recent techniques based on the immunocapture reaction provide reliable results. Paradoxically, the drawback of immunocapture reactions are due to their high sensitivity which reduces the threshold of antibody detection leading to a detection of a low level of IgM persisting more than 10 weeks after the primary infection. Interpretation of results should be correlated with the clinical picture and epidemiological data.

2. *The second phase is* to demonstrate fetal infection. There has been much progress in this area because of the possibility of fetal sampling (amniocentesis and particularly fetal blood sampling) which allows, depending on the case, isolation of the infectious agent (toxoplasmosis), determining a specific immune response based on the detection of specific IgM; since IgM does not cross the placenta, it can only be of fetal origin.

3. *The third phase of diagnosis is* evaluation of the disease risk in the presence of a fetal infection. In each situation, those factors which allow an appreciation of the risk will be considered; clinical, laboratory, and epidemiological.

Fetal infection can be observed with viruses which remain present in the maternal system even long after the primary infection. These infections may have serious consequences after birth: neonatal herpes, hepatitis B, and now HIV. These neonatal and infant disease states go beyond the aims of this book, and will be only briefly discussed for each type of infection.

Certain maternal bacterial infections such as listeriosis may have serious consequences for the fetus in the first two trimesters; in all these cases fetal sampling for microbiological analysis are contraindicated as there is a risk of infecting the fetus.

Rubella

The vaccination programme introduced in France in 1983 has aimed to eliminate the rubella virus, the best way of eliminating congenital rubella. Despite this vaccination campaign and the fact that less than 10 per cent of reproductive women are susceptible, congenital rubella has not disappeared. Although the number of cases has been reduced, 200–250 cases a year of maternofetal infections are still observed in France.

Primary rubella infection

Congenital rubella is always due to a primary infection occurring in the first 3 months of pregnancy. Maternal viraemia with or without eruption (in 50 per cent of rubella infections there is no eruption) leads to placental infection and a viremia in the embryo, resulting in the death and loss of the fetus or in the birth of a malformed child or, on occasion, the birth of a healthy child.

Documentation of the fetal consequences of rubella infection has progressed rapidly. During the first 12 weeks of pregnancy more than 80 per cent of infections are transmitted to the fetus, resulting in a 20 per cent risk of miscarriage and, importantly, when the pregnancy continues, leading to a greater than 90 per cent risk of congenital rubella. It is in this period of pregnancy that more serious malformations are observed. The risk of fetal transmission decreases in the 12–16 week period. At more than 16 weeks of pregnancy the risk of malformation is negligible, deafness appearing to be an exceptional consequence. Studies by Miller *et al.* (1982) (Table 8.1) and by Munro *et al.* (1987) and Grillner (Table 8.2) give comparable data on risks.

Recurring infection

This is characterized by a memory effect and a rise in IgG antibodies. There is no viremia and therefore no fetal risk. In some rare cases low levels of IgM specific antibodies have been observed. These were mostly in vaccinated women or women who had already had the disease. In renewed contact with the rubella virus they have had a subclinical infection. The important point in all these cases was that the children were born healthy. In other words, rubella re-infection in pregnant women, even if specific IgM antibodies are present, does not result in fetal infection.

Table 8.1 Malformations in children exposed to rubella virus at different stages of prenatal life. Prospective study by Miller *et al.* (1982)

	12 weeks	13–16 weeks	17–22 weeks
Frequency of congenital infection	90 per cent	53 per cent	36 per cent
Number of children seropositive at birth	9	26	
Cardiopathies and other malformations	5	0	0
Isolated hearing loss	4	9	0
Risk of malformation	90 per cent	18 per cent	0 per cent

Table 8.2 Malformations in children where rubella infection has been confirmed serologically. From Munro *et al.* (1987) and Grillner (1983)

	Time of maternal rubella infection				
	3–8 weeks	9–12 weeks	13–16 weeks	> 17 weeks	17–24 weeks
Multiple malformations (heart, CNS, eyes, hearing)	10	11	1[a]	–	–
Isolated hearing loss	8	14	20	1	1
No malformations	2	6	11	21	116
Total	20	31	32	22	117

[a] cerebral motor defect

Diagnosis of maternal rubella infection

Figure 8.1 shows the kinetics of antibody appearance during a primary rubella infection with eruption. An understanding of this schema is essential in analysing various situations involving pregnant women in contact with the rubella virus.

What are some of these situations and what factors should be considered in their interpretation?

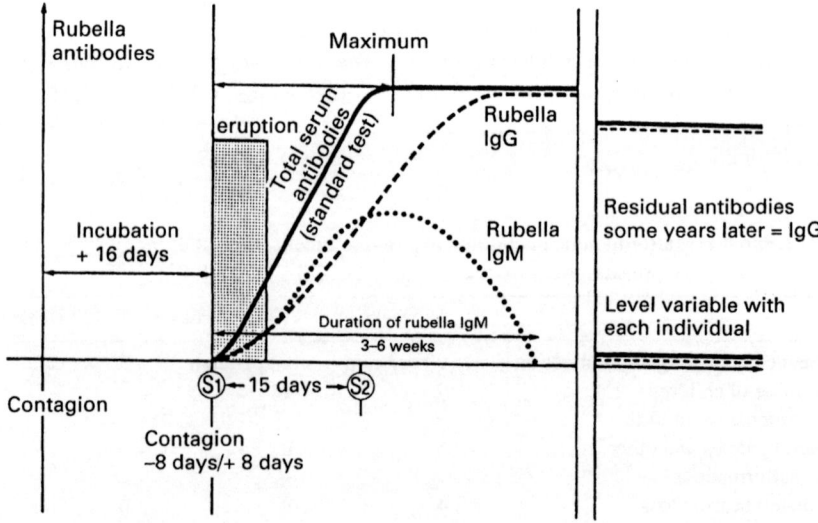

Fig. 8.1 Levels of antibodies at the time of primary rubella infection with eruption.

A case of suspected rubella eruption in early pregnancy
A woman seeks medical advice early (less than 10 days after an eruption) A blood sample, which we still call S1, should be taken and rubella antibodies should be looked for by the haemagglutination inhibition test (HAI).

1. If S1 is negative by HAI, the woman is not immunized and is therefore susceptible. A second sample (S2) must be drawn 15 days after S1 to demonstrate any rise in rubella antibodies. There are two possibilities:
  (a) S2 is negative by HAI. In this case there is no ongoing primary infection. The eruption has a different underlying cause. The woman should be followed serologically until the 4th month and minimize exposure to any source of infection (after 4 months there is no risk to the fetus). A vaccination after delivery should be proposed, with a blood follow-up to confirm immunization.
  (b) S2 is positive by HAI. There is seroconversion. This is probably a primary rubella infection which should be confirmed by looking for specific IgM in S2. If seroconversion occurs in the first 16 weeks of pregnancy there is a risk of fetal malformation.
2. S1 is positive by HAI. These women have rubella antibodies, and on this first sample a search for specific IgM will determine whether it is a primary infection, immunocapture techniques being very sensitive. There are two likely outcomes:
  (a) The presence of specific IgM is observed: therefore there is a primary rubella infection and a risk of malformation if occurring during the first 16 weeks of pregnancy.
  (b) The absence of specific IgM is observed: there is no primary infection and there is no risk for the fetus.

The second serum, S2, drawn 15 days after S1, may show a rise in antibodies, representing a recurring infection and of no risk to the fetus. It may show the same level of antibodies as S1 if the eruption is due to another type of infection.

A woman seeks medical advice late (more than 15 days after eruption) She has no known history of rubella, but it is well known that a history of eruption as a clinical sign of rubella is of little value. A sample S1 should be taken as above.

1. S1 is negative by HAI. This is not an ongoing primary rubella infection, but the woman is not immunized. She should be followed with blood work-up each month until 4 months' gestation, and avoid any source of infection.
2. S1 is positive by HAI. One must look for antirubella-specific IgM by immunocapture. There are two possibilities:
  (a) Presence of specific IgM. Primary infection with fetal risk of malformation if the eruption occurred in the first 16 weeks of pregnancy. In some cases, when the date of maternal and therefore fetal infection is difficult to pinpoint, fetal blood sampling may be an option.

(b) Absence of specific IgM. No primary infection. The eruption is associated with a cause other than a primary rubella infection.

Pregnant woman who may have been in contact with the rubella virus early in pregnancy

She seeks early consultation (within 1 week of contact) First, it is to be established whether she has had rubella and whether any antibody titres have been measured. If titration has been done appropriately and if it is positive, this woman can immediately be reassured. If she was susceptible at the time of contact she would not have any antibodies.

Otherwise, a first blood sample, S1, should be taken as above.

1. If S1 is HAI positive, this woman is immunized, and her antibodies were acquired before testing; either by herself contracting rubella or by vaccination. There is no risk to the ongoing pregnancy.

2. If S1 is HAI negative, this non-immunized woman is susceptible. She may have been contaminated during this recent contact. A second blood sample, S2, must be drawn 3 weeks after the first. This time is required to cover the incubation period (15 days), observe any eruption, and demonstrate any rise in antibodies. There are two possibilities:

(a) If S2 is HAI negative, this women does not have a primary rubella infection. She must be followed serologically on a monthly basis until the 4th month of pregnancy and she must avoid any source of infection.

(b) If S2 is HAI positive, specific antirubella IgM antibodies must be searched for. The presence of specific IgM indicates that there is primary rubella infection and risk of congenital malformation if present during the first 16 weeks of pregnancy. Absence of specific IgM indicates that there is re-infection, with a low residual level undetectable by present measuring techniques. There is no risk to the fetus.

Medical advice is sought a long time after contact (more than 3 weeks later) As previously, first it will be established whether the woman has had a rubella infection documented by antibody titres. A blood sample, S1, should then be drawn.

1. S1 is negative by HAI. This woman has not been infected; she does not have a rubella infection, but she is not immunized. She must be protected from any source of infection and be followed on a monthly basis for the first 4 months.

2. S1 is positive by HAI. Specific IgM should be looked for by immunocapture. The presence of specific IgM indicates a primary rubella infection, and there is a risk to the fetus. The absence of specific IgM indicates that there is no ongoing infection. There are antibodies present from a previous infection, and there is no risk to the fetus.

Serological assay of rubella as routine screen in pregnancy without knowledge of contact or eruption   If the serum is negative by HAI, the woman is susceptible. If the serum is positive by HAI, the woman is immunized. Our experience has shown that in the absence of known contact and eruption in the preceding weeks these antibodies are more often related to an old immunization.

One must emphasize that an antibody titre is proof of an antiviral immunity, but it does not tell us when immunity was established. A low antibody titre does not indicate an old immunization, neither does a high antibody titre indicate a recent immunization or an ongoing infection. Consequently, one must not concern the patient with an antibody titre observed during routine screening. Routine search for antirubella specific IgM in those blood tests indicating a raised level of antibody is not indicated. This search for IgM, which is technically difficult, has specific indications.

Fetal infection

How does one diagnose an affected fetus when a primary infection has been serologically demonstrated in the mother? This diagnosis cannot be done by isolation of the virus in a fetal sample (amniotic fluid or blood) as there is no good isolation technique for this virus. Diagnosis is, therefore, indirect. By fetal blood analysis, we can confirm a viral infection of the fetus with virus-specific techniques. The presence of antirubella-specific IgM is demonstrated by the immunocapture technique. It is only from the 22nd week of gestation that the study of these criteria has any value: this is quite late in pregnancy. Fetal blood analysis is done using non-specific criteria, which indicate an infectious process in the fetus:

- rise in total IgM (more than 10 mg/100 mL);
- erythroblastosis;
- moderate thrombocytopaenia;
- rise in gammaglutamyl transpeptidase confirming an infection in the liver.

The determining factor in diagnosis of fetal infection is the demonstration of antirubella-specific IgM.

From a practical point of view, two factors should be considered:

1. The risk of viral infection of the fetus. Roughly, until the 12th week of pregnancy the fetus is affected by the virus in 90 per cent of cases, between 12 and 16 weeks in 50 per cent of cases, and beyond 16 weeks in 35 per cent of cases.

2. The risk of disease due to this infection. Tables 8.1 and 8.2 show the frequency and severity of the viral infection.

When maternal rubella (dated by eruption or blood testing) has occurred earlier than 12 weeks of pregnancy, the high frequency of fetal infection and the frequency and severity of disease consequences do not necessitate confirmation on fetal blood, which would result in many anxious weeks of waiting for results.

When maternal rubella infection occurs after 16 weeks of pregnancy, it is known that even if there is fetal infection there is no disease consequence. Demonstration of viral infection by blood sampling is useless and may result unnecessarily in maternal anxiety.

It is only when a maternal rubella infection occurs between 11 and 16 weeks, or when the time of infection is not exactly known but is earlier than 16 weeks of pregnancy, that fetal blood sampling at 22 weeks is justified. Between 12 and 16 weeks of pregnancy viral infection of the fetus results in deafness in only 20 per cent of cases; one should be aware of this information if a termination of pregnancy is being considered.

Laboratory techniques

There are two techniques: those which permit appreciation of a woman's immune status with regard to rubella and those which permit demonstration of a primary infection in the mother or fetus.

Techniques evaluating immune status

Haemagluttination inhibition test (HAI)   This is the technique in use the longest, and the one still most frequently used (Fig. 8.2).

1. *Rationale.* It uses the haemagluttination property of the rubella virus. The reaction is a competitive one. Viral-specific antibodies prevent the absorption of rubella virus on red blood cells by coming between the viral haemagluttinin and the red blood cell receptor.

2. *Specificity.* There are non-specific inhibitors of haemagluttination in human serum, and these are essentially lipoproteins. Prior to titration for antirubella antibodies these inhibitors must be eliminated. The ideal method allows removal of all lipoproteins without losing immunoglobulins. Several techniques are suggested for handling the sera. It is difficult to confirm in some

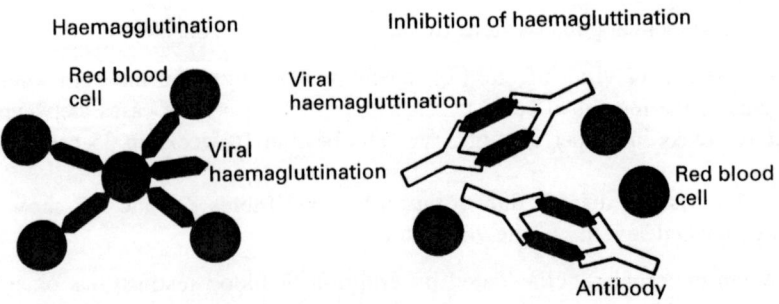

Fig. 8.2 Haemagluttination inhibition assay.

cases that there is no persistence of trace inhibitors associated with a risk of false positives. Inversely, there could be destruction of specific antibodies resulting in false negatives. Also, it is not unusual to have a difference in antibody titre, even after one or two dilutions, depending on what technique is used to eliminate the non-specific inhibitors. Use of a standard reference serum measured in international units, good control on reaction and measurement of results in international units allows a more homogeneous result.

3. *Sensitivity of methods.* A woman is considered immunized if her antibody titre is higher than 1/20 by HAI. Studies have shown that low levels of antibody undetectable by haemagluttinin inhibition could be sufficient to ensure immunity; this means that a serum diagnosis of rubella, negative by HAI, does not necessarily reflect non-immunization. When antibody titres are low, less than 1/20 by HAI, it is wise to consider rubella vaccination. Antibody titres obtained after vaccination are not very high; in our experience rarely higher than 1/40 by HAI. Moreover, after vaccination, no specific antibodies are detected even though the person has been immunized.

Other more recent techniques   These are very specific, as they do not interfere with non-specific inhibitors.

ELISA
1. *Rationale.* This is a solid-phase immunoenzymatic technique called an 'ELISA-sandwich'. The rubella antigen is fixed to a solid support (polystyrene plaque), and the maternal serum to be titred is applied. The rubella-specific IgG will then fix to the rubella antigen. IgG are revealed by addition of a human anti-IgG marked by an enzyme. An immune complex is formed: rubella antigen/antirubella IgG/conjugated to anti-IgG revealed by the enzyme's chromogenic substrate. After stopping the reaction, the optic density obtained is proportional to the level of antirubella IgG antibodies present in the serum (Fig. 8.3).

2. *Comments.* The advantage of this technique is that it is more sensitive than HAI, but the methodology as well as the interpretation of these results requires rigorous evaluation to determine whether the low levels of antibody detected are sufficient to confirm that a person is immunized. The threshold which determines immunization appears to be 15 IU.

Latex test
1. *Rationale.* This is an agglutination test done on slides. Latex particles sensitized by purified rubella haemagluttinin are agglutinized by the antibodies of the serum being tested. It is easily done; its advantage is the short time it requires to do.

2. *Comments.* The sensitivity of this technique seems better than that of HAI. None the less, it requires great care in the interpretation of results. Therefore, when working with pure sera, one must watch for the zone phenomenon (excess

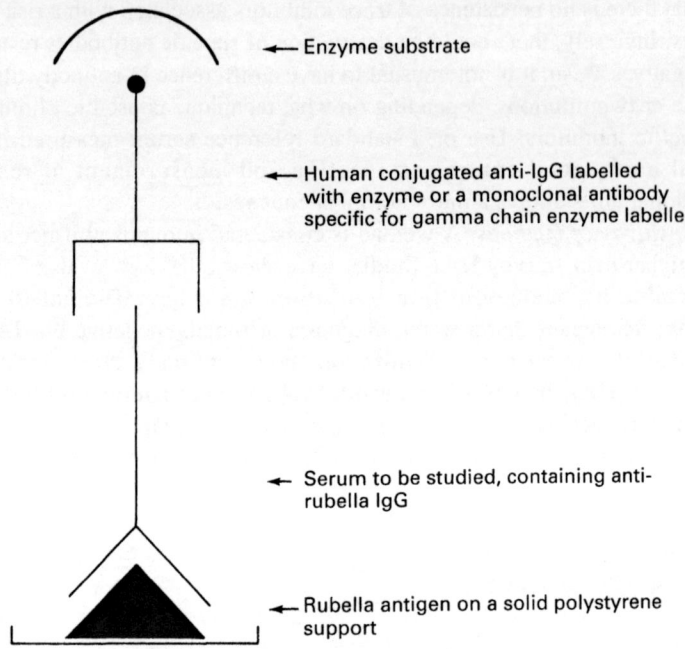

←— Enzyme substrate

←— Human conjugated anti-IgG labelled with enzyme or a monoclonal antibody specific for gamma chain enzyme labelled

←— Serum to be studied, containing anti-rubella IgG

←— Rubella antigen on a solid polystyrene support

Fig. 8.3 ELISA-IgG technique: reaction scheme.

of antibody), which will lead to false-negative results. It is also important to know whether the low levels of antibody are protective enough. There must be agreement on the threshold of sensitivity of this technique.

Techniques for the diagnosis of a primary rubella infection: serological tests

These tests must demonstrate rubella-specific IgM. This specific IgM appears only in the case of a primary infection (Fig. 8.1).

Ultracentrifugation   A classical technique, long considered the standard test, ultracentrifugation can separate serum IgM from IgG by molecular weight using centrifugation in a saccharose gradient. Antirubella antibody activity is then measured by HAI. This method is long and expensive, and for correct interpretation requires a strict control of reaction parameters. In particular, a good separation of IgM and IgG is required: any trace of IgG results in false positives. This can occur when the total amount of immunoglobulin is raised and aggregated IgG migrates with IgM. Similarly, it has been demonstrated that serum IgA polymers can also contaminate IgM.

Although this technique has been of great service, it presents many problems of sensitivity and specificity. In fact, due to its low sensitivity, specific IgM after primary rubella infection can be measured only within a short period of time,

2–3 weeks after an injection. Moreover, a relatively large amount of serum is required for ultracentrifugation. Other more sensitive and specific techniques have been proposed.

ELISA–IgM

1. *Rationale.* In the serum sample tested, this technique allows detection of IgM which becomes fixed to a rubella antigen (fixed to a solid structure) because of the presence of an enzyme-labelled anti-μ IgG.

2. *Comments.* This method of detection has many drawbacks and should not be used. It gives rise to false positives because of detection of IgM rheumatoid factors often found particularly in pregnant women; these factors react with the IgG fixed to the viral antigen. A number of ways of eliminating the rheumatoid factor have been proposed, but they have not given satisfactory results. This technique also gives rise to false negatives when the serum has high levels of antirubella IgG. There is then competition between IgG and IgM for the antigen, which reduces the sensitivity of the test.

Immunocapture   This is a reliable technique which has advantages over ultracentrifugation and ELISA IgM without the risk of false positive and false negative results.

1. *Rationale.* Animal IgG which are anti-human μ chain are fixed to a solid structure (polystyrene microplaque). If there is IgM present in serum it will attach to IgG anti-μ; this is known as immunocapture. The rubella antigen is added. If there is antirubella IgM, the rubella antigen will attach to this specific IgM, resulting in specific complexes on the solid structure (anti-μ/rubella IgM/rubella antigen). This complex can then be revealed in a number of ways:

- by HAI using red blood cells which use the agglutination properties of the rubella virus;
- by an ELISA reaction produced by the use of an anti-rubella IgG marked by an enzyme;
- most efficiently, by a labelled monoclonal antibody (Fig. 8.4).

2. Comments. This immunocapture technique has many advantages:

- sensitivity: absence of IgG/IgM competition, detection of low levels of IgM (useful in fetal blood testing);
- specificity: absence of interference with the rheumatoid factor, as the IgG cannot attach to anti-μ on the solid structure.
- the amount of serum required for testing is small, which is of particular interest when working on fetal blood.

Because of its sensitivity and specificity, this technique has allowed confirmation of an affected or unaffected fetus in clinical cases that were difficult to interpret.

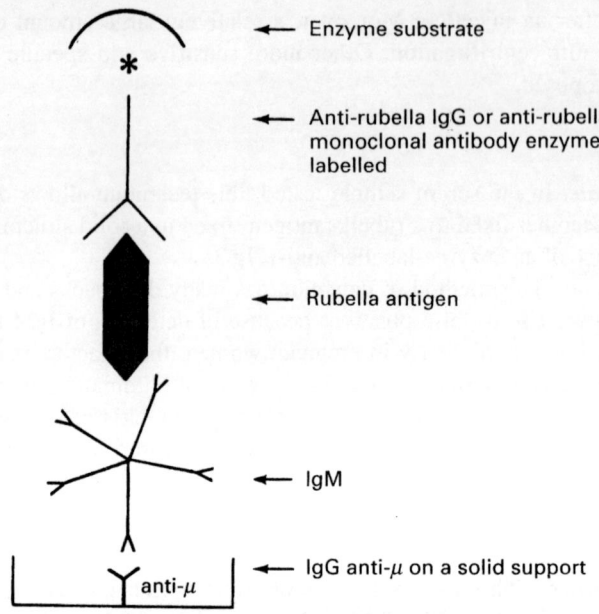

Enzyme substrate

Anti-rubella IgG or anti-rubella monoclonal antibody enzyme labelled

Rubella antigen

IgM

IgG anti-μ on a solid support

anti-μ

Fig. 8.4 Immunoabsorption reaction to detect rubella IgM.

This method is the most sensitive of those presently used, as it has been demonstrated that IgM can be observed 15 weeks after cutaneous eruption. This means that the infection could have occurred prior to conception.

Toxoplasmosis

In its acquired form, toxoplasmosis is either asymptomatic or presents with very mild clinical symptoms. Serious forms, at one time rare, have increased since the appearance of AIDS.

Toxoplasmosis contracted during pregnancy can result in serious damage to the fetus, resulting in congenital toxoplasmosis which in its most severe form is associated with hydrocephaly, intracranial calcifications, chorioretinitis, and neurological manifestations which progress to psychomotor sequelae. The multi-origin form combines encephalitis and multiple affected organs, and progress is the same as in the major form. These two forms are observed much less often today.

Subclinical forms are more common; untreated complications include eventual chorioretinitis in one-third of cases. This new situation is due to maternal screening for toxoplasmosis in pregnancy and good treatment during pregnancy.

In France, the prevalence of toxoplasmosis infection in young female adults has decreased substantially. The percentage of seropositive individuals in Paris, which corresponds to the national average, went from 83 per cent in

1970 to 54 per cent in 1983. Consequently, the number of women of reproductive age who are not immunized has gone up.

Risk assessment

The level of toxoplasmosis contamination in pregnant women is estimated at 6.4/1000 for the duration of pregnancy. This level has remained almost constant: in 1970 a 7.7/1000 frequency was established. For an infected pregnant woman the risk of having a clinically affected fetus is estimated to be 3 per cent.

The risk of a mother transmitting toxoplasmosis to her child increases steadily from the beginning to the end of pregnancy: transmission is rare when maternal infection is around the time of conception (less than 2 per cent), around 4 per cent if infection occurs between the 6th and 16th week, and 20 per cent between the 16th and 25th week. It is common (80 per cent) if infection occurs close to term.

Clinical expression of congenital toxoplasmosis varies with respect to three main criteria:

- date of maternal infection: in the first 3 months there is a predominantly florid form, but after 3 months subclinical forms are predominant;
- maternal treatment: severely affected children occur more frequently to mothers left untreated;
- placental infection: when the placenta is infected, fetal infection is certain.

Criteria for diagnosis of maternal toxoplasmosis infection in pregnancy
Serological methods   Diagnosis of infection is by blood work-up. In a primary *Toxoplasma gondii* infection, humoral immunity is initiated by formation of specific antibodies directed first to the parasite's membrane and then to its cytoplasmic constituents. The first immunoglobulin to appear is IgM, followed by IgG which remains throughout life.

The multiplicity of techniques used testifies to the difficulty of making such a diagnosis.

1. The *Dye test* or *Sabin and Feldman lysis test*. When live toxoplasmosis is put in contact with serum to be tested the presence of antitoxoplasmosis antibodies is revealed by lysis of parasites. The main drawback of this method is the necessity for live toxoplasmosis, which makes it a technique reserved for specialized laboratories. In addition, only IgG is measured. Nevertheless it is the standard method, having high sensitivity.

2. *Indirect haemagglutination reaction*. Agglutination of animal red blood cells sensitized by the toxoplasmosis antigen. Treatment of serum with dimercaptoethanol permits identification of IgM and IgG.

3. *Direct agglutination reaction method*.
  (a) Formol-treated antigen sensitized by enzymatic treatment (ADHS) is a reaction as sensitive as the Dye test and allows detection of IgG only. It is an excellent test for seronegative women.

(b) *Acetone-treated antigen*. The toxoplasmosis is treated with acetone which alters the parasite's antigenic structure.

These two reactions allow evaluation of the progress of acquired toxoplasmosis. In acute cases, the patient's serum agglutinates antigen HS as easily as antigen AC. In the case of a previous infection, only antigen HS is agglutinated.

4. *Indirect immunofluorescence* (IFI). This is the most commonly used test and, with the Dye test, is a standard method. It allows testing for IgG and IgM (Remington test).

Although IgG testing is reliable, sensitive, and specific, detection of IgM has many inconveniences which must be kept in mind to minimize false positives and false negatives. False negatives occur in the presence of raised levels of IgG because of competition for antigen sites. False positives are linked to the presence of rheumatoid factors or antinuclear antibodies. Initial treatment of the patients's serum by neutralization of IgG antibodies eliminates this cause of error. New techniques permit detection of IgM with very good sensitivity and specificity, making it possible to avoid the errors of previous methods. They are based on initial capture of serum IgM using IgM antibodies and then detection of specific IgM in various ways, such as agglutination and immunoenzymology.

5. *Immunosorbent agglutination assay* (ISAGA). Serum IgM is captured by an anti-IgM monoclonal antibody fixed to the bottom of the microtitration plaque and antitoxoplasmosis IgM is revealed by agglutination of formol-treated toxoplasmosis. This is a very sensitive method, the best technique for measuring IgM in fetal blood or in the newborn. Its main drawback is the persistence of a false positive reaction during a long period, as much as a year, well beyond the acute infectious period.

6. *Immunoenzymatic reaction* (ELISA): This is of value in detection of antitoxoplasmosis IgM in the same way as the immunosorbent agglutination assay: primary capture of serum IgM and detection of specific IgM by coupling of IgM antigen and antibody labelled with an enzyme (the specificity can be improved by using a monoclonal antibody). This method, known as 'reverse' of 'immunocapture double sandwich' can eliminate false positives (due to antirheumatoid factor and antinuclear antibody) and false negatives (due to raised levels of IgM). The use of parasite membrane antigenic extract also improves early detection of IgM.

7. *Enzyme-linked immunofiltration assay* (ELIFA). This is a precipitation technique permitting a comparison of the mother's blood with that of the newborn.

Interpretation of results   Interpretation of serological test results detecting toxoplasmosis infection must take into account a change in the kinetics of antibodies observed in new techniques (ELISA, ISAGA). Persistence of IgM for several months after infection means that the presence of IgM alone does not necessarily indicate an ongoing toxoplasmosis infection. In practice, two complementary serological techniques should be used together and correlation between clinical and laboratory results is essential to avoid errors of interpretation.

1. *First scenario.* The woman's immune state is known from a serological test carried out before the onset of pregnancy.

If serology is positive with an IgG titre stable after two tests done at 3–4 weeks' interval, then the woman is immunized with no risk of the fetus being infected with toxoplasmosis. If serology is negative, then the non-immunized woman is at risk for toxoplasmosis infection. A serologically negative woman should be tested every month to observe seroconversion, which would be an indication of infection with toxoplasmosis. To reduce the risk of infection, the seronegative mother must be rigid in her dietary hygiene.

- exclusion of raw or rare meat (freezing destroys the parasite) and handling of such products with bare hands;
- avoidance of all contact with cats;
- avoidance of all handling of soil;
- careful washing of fruits and vegetables eaten raw.

2. *Second scenario.* A woman with unknown immune status before pregnancy and serological testing during pregnancy is positive.

Infection is certain if seroconversion is demonstrated in pregnancy in a woman who was seronegative before pregnancy or in early pregnancy. Infection is probable when there is a significant rise in antibody titre on successive measurements, but this is a delicate interpretation. Infection is possible when peripheral adenopathies are associated with an elevated antibody titre. Gestational age at the time of maternal infection is difficult to assess. Once maternal infection is confirmed, treatment with spiramycin must be initiated and continued until the end of pregnancy at a dose of 3 g per day. One should be aware of the serological effect of spiramycin on toxoplasmosis. If treatment is initiated early, that is in the first days after detecting the antibody, the production of antibodies will slow down as the treatment affects proliferation of toxoplasmosis, therefore at the end of treatment there is a rise in antibody. In the child there is a significant synthesis of antibodies observed at birth.

When the mother has not been treated, the low level of specific IgG antibodies observed in the newborn results from the repressor effects of specific IgG transmitted passively to the fetus.

Assessing fetal infection   The main role of prenatal diagnosis is to recognize those cases of early transmission (before 20 weeks) where fetal risk is significant and where a termination of pregnancy is often justified. A serological and ultrasound monitoring protocol should be implemented.

Isolation of toxoplasmosis   This is the best criterion for diagnosis of fetal infection. Isolation can be done by withdrawal amniotic fluid or by cord blood sampling (in both cases, it is the cell pellet obtained after centrifuging which will be innoculated). The same methods used in determining infection in the newborn are used here, but on a mixture of trypsinized placenta.

Two methods allow for isolation: intraperitoneal innoculation of the mouse, a classical technique where results take 4–6 weeks; the second technique involves inoculation of human fibroblast cultures. The latter technique is trickier. It gives results equivalent to those obtained in mice, but more particularly the presence of the parasite can be demonstrated on cells by immunofluorescence with a labelled specific serum after 72 hours in culture.

In practice the method of isolation of the parasite will be determined by the time at which the patient is seen. Amniocentesis can be done at 16–17 weeks of pregnancy. It can be repeated if necessary, considering its low risk. Fetal blood sampling should not be done too early if one wants serological testing by isolation of the parasite, and the method of isolation should be determined by what serological methods are available, in particular by the availability of the fibroblast technique which allows for a quick result.

Fetal blood testing
1. *Specific serology.* This must be done systematically and in parallel with identification of toxoplasmosis.

As IgM is not transmitted from mother to fetus, detection of even low levels in the fetus is of great value in diagnosing fetal infection. A comparative study with maternal blood is possible by comparing immunological profiles, and allows certain identification of fetal IgM. IgM detection techniques should be of high sensitivity. ISAGA is the best procedure for this type of analysis.

IgG is measured by the Dye test, IFI, or ELISA. To distinguish between fetal antibodies and transmitted maternal antibodies it is important to measure the antibodies in maternal blood and fetal blood in parallel. The immunological status can then be measured:

Immunity status in IU/mg = specific IgG in IU/ml/total IgG in mg/ml.

When the antibodies are of fetal origin the level of antibody is four times that in maternal blood.

The more sensitive techniques are not entirely satisfactory because the synthesis of antibodies by the fetus may be too low to measure; only a true positive result is of any value, and the absence of specific IgM does not eliminate the diagnosis.

2. *Non-specific laboratory evidence for infection.* All the limitations mentioned above require one to turn to non-specific signs, which may nonetheless be decisive factors when they are clearly positive and associated.

The non-specific criteria to be considered are:

- a significant increase in the level of total IgM as proof of fetal response to antigenic stimulation;

• haematological factors of the particular parasitic infection, e.g. search for eosinophils or for thrombocytopaenia;
• signs of hepatic involvement, the best being a significant increase of gammaglutamyl transpeptidase.

Ultrasound surveillance as a complement to laboratory testing   Based on the interpretation of results from the four approaches — isolation of toxoplasmosis, specific fetal serology, non-specific evidence for infection in fetal blood, and ultrasound — the prenatal diagnosis of a toxoplasmosis infection can be obtained in a day or two.

Herpes

Cytomegalovirus (CMV), the herpes simplex virus (type I or II), varicella, and zoster can cause disease in the fetus and newborn in the case of maternal infection during pregnancy. On the other hand, primary infection by Epstein–Barr virus (infectious mononucleosis) does not impose a risk to the fetus.

These viral infections have common factors:

1. Primary infection is accompanied by viraemia, and the virus can reach the fetus and have disease consequences (for example cytomegaly inclusions). After primary infection, these viruses remain in the organism in a latent form; either in the peripheral nerve system (herpes, varicella) or in blood cells (CMV).

2. Pregnancy is one of a number of circumstances which provide an opportunity for the virus to recur. Briefly: for viruses found in the peripheral nervous system (herpes, varicella, and zoster), during periods of recurrence the virus travels through the nervous system and absence of viraemia prevents fetal infection. For those viruses latent in blood cells, the fetus may be infected through the bloodstream (CMV) but there are no known consequences associated with these episodes of recurrence.

Cytomegalovirus

Cytomegalovirus (CMV) is ubiquitous but, because of its fragility, its transmission requires intimate contact (transfer of saliva, sexual intercourse, maternal–fetal (transmission).

Primary infection usually occurs in the first year of life, with the mother playing an important role in its transmission (birth canal, saliva, milk). The lower the socioeconomic status, the greater the chance of the child being infected in its first year of life. A second peak of infection occurs in the teenage years and in young adulthood at the onset of sexual activity.

This primary infection is usually asymptomatic. It sometimes presents as a flu-like or mononucleosis-like syndrome (without tonsilitis and with a Paul–Bunnel–Davidson negative reaction). It is accompanied by uraemia, which can persist for several weeks. Viral excretion is by urine, sperm or saliva, and may last from several months to several years. The only way to make a diagnosis, if blood drawn at the right time is available, is to detect seroconversion with presence of specific IgM.

After primary infection CMV remains latent, and may be reactivated at different times, for example in pregnancy (10–28 per cent of pregnant mothers excrete virus at the cervix during the 3rd month of pregnancy). The reactivations are asymptomatic. There may be viraemia, and the level of antibody may be stable or may increase. Specific IgM can be detected in certain cases. Serological differences between a primary infection and re-infection are difficult to find unless there are test results testifying to a prior infection.

Cytomegalovirus infection during pregnancy   The problem is primarily the following:

- the infection which occurs during pregnancy is virtually always without obvious signs;
- the risk of disease in the fetus is low as, once the virus goes from mother to child, only 1/10 will have signs at birth and there is no prenatal test to predict it.

At birth, 0.3–2 per cent of neonates excrete virus, which is proof of intra-uterine infection; of them, only 5–10 per cent present with CMV inclusions characterized by hypotrophy, jaundice, hepatosplenomegaly, thrombocytopaenia detected by petechiae, anaemia, microcephaly, intracerebral calcifications, or chorioretinitis, and at times resulting in death or severe psychomotor retardation.

CMV inclusion disease affects 2/10 000 births. Amongst the 90–95 per cent who have no symptoms at birth, about 10 per cent may develop deafness later.

Fetal infection during pregnancy can occur during primary infection or after reactivation of latent virus.

Primary infection   This occurs on average in 1 per cent of pregnant, sero-negative women. The percentage of seronegative pregnant women depends mainly on the socioeconomic level: 30–40 per cent when the socioeconomic level is average or high, 1–2 per cent when it is low. The virus is transmitted to fetus in one out of two cases, with no association to the time in pregnancy that the maternal infection occurs.

Latent virus reactivation   Virus can be transmitted to the fetus, but the risk of fetal disease is lower and less severe. In fact, once a mother has given birth to a child with inclusion disease, a second affected child in the sibship has never been reported even though these children often carry the virus at birth. The usual absence of clinical signs in the mother and the fact that the fetus while infected rarely has symptoms, renders prevention of the birth of children born with CMV inclusion extremely difficult.

Some have proposed routine blood tests to detect seronegative women in order to follow them through pregnancy. There are a number of arguments against this:

1. There is no universally recognized serological test for the diagnosis of CMV infection. Complement fixation is not sensitive and a rise in antibodies during a recurrence episode can simulate seroconversion, because a low level of antibody is not detectable by this technique. Other very sensitive techniques have been suggested — passive haemagglutination, ELISA, indirect immuno-fluorescence, latex particle agglutination — but none of these techniques is accepted unanimously.

2. Detecting seroconversion in the mother will not prove that the fetus is infected, or that this infection will have disease consequences. Systematic blood testing would therefore give women false hope of prevention, when there is no way to solve the problem should seroconversion be observed.

In practice

1. A warning may be given by discovery of fetal anomalies on ultrasound examination (hypotrophy, intracranial calcifications, microcephaly). In the differential diagnoses of these anomalies, CMV is one possibility. The search for it implies — documentation of viraemia, viruria, and anti-CMV specific IgM in the mother, which will contribute to the diagnosis. A CMV-positive viraemia proves the presence of an active infection, but does not prove a primary infection. Presence of specific IgM may be due to a primary infection, reactivation, re-infection, or extended synthesis of IgM.

Confirmation of infection in the fetus can be done by:

(a) *Amniocentesis* to look for CMV by isolation from embryonic fibroblast cultures, the only cells receptive to CMV. Indirect immunofluorescence with monoclonal antibodies applied to cells (after 48 hours' infection) accelerates diagnosis, as the cytopathogenic effect appears in a variable time frame (between 3 days and 3 weeks); but CMV is a sensitive virus, and suitable transport conditions for the sample (on ice) are essential.

(b) *Fetal blood sampling*, which allows search for specific IgM anti-CMV by immunocapture. This technique eliminates interference with rheumatoid factors and is the preferred method because other techniques (ELISA, indirect immunofluorescence) may be influenced by cross-reaction with other herpes-type infections. Diagnosis of viraemia is theoretically possible, but the likelihood of isolating CMV on such a small sample is low. Analysis of fetal blood allows for observation of indirect signs: complete blood count, levels of interferon, levels of total IgM, levels of hepatic enzymes.

2. A maternal infection is clinically evident, (mononucleosis-like syndrome, extremely rare). It is important to confirm the underlying cause because mononucleosis caused by Epstein–Barr virus imposes no risk to the fetus.

Virological and serological tests (see above) will confirm a CMV infection. It is then important to look for signs of an affected fetus more than signs of CMV infection as such, as in more than 90 per cent of cases the fetus will not be affected. To do this, it is important to do a detailed ultrasound looking for specific anomalies. A problem is prevention of CMV in seronegative pregnant women who are in regular contact with children who can excrete CMV and be potential transmitters (in particular babies and small children in day nurseries, schools, etc.)

Identifying children who are CMV carriers is not recommended because excretion of virus is intermittent, blood sampling and transport pose a considerable practical problem and this screening policy is expensive.

Blood screening of seronegative women and their transfer into other work areas is not recommended either, as studies using genetic markers for the virus have shown that children are rarely the source of primary infection observed in the caregivers and, in addition, the reliability of these tests is not perfect. Only normal hygienic care is recommended (handwashing after each diaper change, or after contact with urine or other secretions).

Herpes simplex

There are two types of herpes simplex virus (HSV):

- type I (HSVI) which is responsible for infections 'above the belt' (muco-cutaneous and ocular infections) and occasionally genital herpes (15–20 per cent of genital herpes infections are HSV1), and neonatal herpes (25 per cent);
- type II (HSVII) which is responsible for infections 'below the belt' (genital herpes), neonatal herpes, and occasionally orolabial herpes (15–25 per cent of orolabial infections are HSVII).

The HSVI primary infection usually occurs in childhood and is asymptomatic in 90 per cent of cases. HSVII primary infection occurs at the beginning of sexual activity. Its frequency is on the increase.

Whatever the virus, HSVI or HSVII, the infection is marked by latency and recurrence. After the primary infection, the latent virus remains close to nerve ganglions and under favourable conditions there may be recurrence of infection at the same site as the primary infection. The frequency of recurrence of HSVII genital infection is 8–10 times more frequent than HSVI genital infection. HSVI orolabial infection has a recurrence frequency much higher than that of the HSVII type. The frequency of genital herpes is higher in the pregnant woman, but in about half of cases there are no signs of the infection.

Fetal risk
Orolabial herpes　Primary infection in the young adult is rare. With this in mind, the virus can only be transmitted from mother to child through viraemia which is not systematic. The consequences to the fetus depend on gestational age. Before

20 weeks of pregnancy there is a risk of fetal loss and, rarely, of congenital mal-formation. Later on in pregnancy there is no risk. In cases of recurrence, which occur most frequently, there is no risk to the fetus at any time in pregnancy.

Genital herpes   Risk to the fetus exists when the mother has a primary infection:

1. Prior to 20 weeks' gestation

- risk of fetal loss (frequency 25–30 per cent);
- rare risk of congenital malformations, like those observed with CMV.

2. After 20 weeks' gestation

- risk of premature delivery.

3. At term

- the virus can be transmitted from genitalia to uterus if membranes have been ruptured for more than 4–6 hours;
- more often, infection occurs at delivery by direct contact of fetus and infected birth canal.

4. In both cases there is risk of neonatal herpes; though still rare, the frequen-cy has been increasing over the years. In 75 per cent of cases it is due to HSVII and is more severe. Asymptomatic forms are the exception.

In cases of recurrence there is no risk to the fetus. Risk of infection of the newborn during delivery is much less likely as at the time of recurrence the number of lesions in the birth canal is less than at the time of a primary in-fection, the infection does not last as long (8–10 days versus 2–3 weeks in a primary infection), maternal antibodies partially protect the newborn, and the cervix is rarely involved. More than one child with neonatal herpes has not been observed in the same woman.

In practice   The mother presents with genital or orolabial herpes.

From the history it should be known whether these are the first clinical signs ever, or whether this is a recurrence. Diagnosis of a primary infection is not easy when signs of general infection are not observed. In some cases, one must confirm by maternal testing whether it is a herpetic infection. For this, the sensi-tivity of tests will be determined by the stage of the infection (virus is more likely to be isolated from a recent lesion), the quality of samples, and the speed of transport to the virology laboratory (HSV virus is very sensitive because of its coating). It is in one's interest to collaborate with the virology laboratory to find out the sample preparation required for transport.

1. *Isolation of virus taken sterily from cutaneous or mucous tissue, or from a vaginal swab.* The sample is inoculated into cells sensitive to herpes, and the cytopathogenicity appears after 1–4 days in the form of clusters of distended

cells which expand through the whole layer. To accelerate detection of cyto-pathogenic effects, one uses immunological techniques (immunofluorescence, immunoenzymology) which also permit typing.

2. *A rapid diagnosis permitting detection of the virus or its antigen either in effusions or in the cells sampled at the site of the lesion.* This strategy is of inter-est when rapid preventative or therapeutic measures are required.

Different diagnostic techniques are possible: on effusions, electron micro-scopy can be used (if the equipment is available) to give a result in less than one hour. One can also use immunoenzymology with monoclonal antibodies. On cells, Tzanck's cytodiagnostic method can be used; this allows demonstration of inclusions, testifying to a viral infection. This rapid low-cost technique is not highly sensitive, it is non-specific, and it requires an experienced staff. This last technique should be replaced by immunological methods which allow detection of viral antigens in cells using fluorescence (IF) or enzyme (IE) labelled antibod-ies. These methods are rapid and sensitive, but less sensitive than isolating the virus for asymptomatic infections.

What are the advantages of maternal serological tests?

With few exceptions, blood testing for herpes is of little interest for a mucocutaneous infection, either for total antigen or for specific IgM.

It must be remembered that the presence of antiherpes antibodies does not protect against recurrence or against maternal fetal transmission. It is only an indicator that the patient has been in contact with the virus.

The only serological sign of a primary infection is the seroconversion between two serum samples, one taken as early as possible after appearance of the lesions and the other 10–15 days later. Presence of antibody in the first sample, if taken at the onset of signs of infection, speaks in favour of recurrence, particularly if the level remains stable in the second sample. The search for IgM does not allow differentiating between primary infection and recurrence. The presence of specific IgM may signify either a primary infection (presence of IgM in 90 per cent of cases), a recurrence (presence of IgM in 40–50 per cent of cases), a persistence of IgM (which may be seen in some cases a long time after the primary infection), or a polyclonal reactivation with synthesis of IgM by another virus at the time of infection.

Fetal risk assessment

When there is a primary oral or genital herpes infection occurring before 20 weeks gestation, termination of pregnancy is not justified because congenital malformations are rare. Nonetheless it is important to know whether the fetus has been infected and if there are malformations. Ultrasound should be done to assess fetal development, looking for detectable cerebral malformations (micro-cephaly, hydrocephaly) and fetal blood should be drawn at 22 weeks when a response to the infection has had the time to occur. Because viraemia is so brief, a search for it is pointless. Serological tests sensitive enough to detect anti-HSV IgM are not available for the fetus, and total antibody count is useless because maternal antibodies are also present. None the less, indirect signs of fetal infection may be looked for: CBC, hepatic enzyme levels (e.g. gammaglutamyl transpeptidase, indicating liver involvement and proof of a general infection), interferon measurements (indicating a viral infection), total IgM (low when the fetus has not been in contact with antigen). There is no experience of looking for the virus in amniotic fluid.

Varicella and zoster

Primary infection, which is observed clinically as chickenpox, is followed by a period of latency in the sensory nerve ganglions with possibility of recurrence in the dermatomic area as zoster (shingles). Given the highly contagious nature of varicella and its high frequency in childhood, few adults are susceptible and it is rarely observed in a pregnant woman (0.1–0.7/1000 pregnancies).

Fetal risk

Varicella   Maternal varicella can be a risk to the fetus, when it occurs early in pregnancy and a risk to the newborn, when it occurs in the few days following delivery.

1. *First trimester.* The virus can be transmitted by a viremia, but this is no indication that the fetus will develop disease. Prospective studies indicate that the risk of congenital malformation is small, and there are about 15 cases reported in the literature. The clinical picture is of low birth weight, much scarring as a consequence of lesions, many aspects similar to amniotic bands, muscular atrophy, hypotrophy (including atrophy and limb paralysis), rudimentary fingers, microcephaly, epilepsy, chorioretinitis, cataracts, and psychomotor retardation. It is fatal in half of the cases.

2. *End of pregnancy.* There is a risk of neonatal varicella. The risks and consequences of infection are variable and depend largely on the time of maternal infection with respect to time of delivery; if maternal infection occurs more than 5 days before delivery, the baby will have received some protection from transmitted maternal antibodies and will theoretically present with a milder form. When the maternal infection occurs within 5 days of delivery the baby is not protected and is at risk of having severe varicella (disseminated skin lesions, multiple visceral organs affected) possibly leading to death in 15–30 per cent of cases.

Zoster   Zoster is a recurrence of infection by the varicella virus in an immune person having circulating antibodies. The virus is restricted to a single dermatomic area, there is no viremia and therefore no risk to the fetus, as confirmed by prospective studies.

Strategies

A pregnant woman acquires varicella during pregnancy   Usually clinical signs are characteristic, and further testing is unnecessary. When in doubt, a sample of the vesicles can confirm the diagnosis rapidly by immunofluorescence or immuno-enzymology. Sometimes two blood tests can be done at a 15-day interval to look for seroconversion. Once the diagnosis is made, there are two possibilities.

1. Eruption occurs in the first trimester: there is a theoretical risk of congenital malformation, but it is so low that a termination of pregnancy based solely on maternal expression of disease is not indicated. However, ultrasound surveillance should be done looking for abnormalities of head and limbs, intrauterine growth retardation and microcephaly. Tests on fetal blood samples drawn at 22 weeks of gestation can complement this by demonstrating specific or non-specific signs of viral infection.

There is not yet sufficient experience to decide on the value of these tests versus detailed ultrasound surveillance.

In our own experience, and that of other European centres adopting the same guidelines, ultrasound surveillance has demonstrated presence of a normal fetus which was then confirmed at birth. So far, no positive ultrasound diagnosis of an affected fetus has been reported, which shows the rarity of fetal disease in the presence of maternal varicella.

2. Eruption occurs in the days prior to delivery: labour should be postponed as long as possible. In this way, the fetus can acquire maternal antibodies and be partially protected. Nevertheless, it is recommended that the child be injected at birth with specific gammaglobulins (0.3–0.6 ml/kg) in order to prevent the onset of infection or to minimize the effects, and that the newborn be isolated.

Viral hepatitis

There are several forms of viral hepatitis: viral hepatitis A, viral hepatitis B, non A-non-B hepatitis and delta-virus hepatitis. Viral hepatitis A, which infects by orofaecal passages, is rarely severe; the A virus does not result in chronic disease. Viral hepatitis B, which infects by oral and salivary pathways, may be severe and results in a chronic carrier status.

The following antigen–antibody systems are associated with hepatitis B:

1. The HBs surface antigen and its antibody:

- the antigen is transient in patients with acute disease and is present for longer periods in a person chronically affected;
- the anti-HBs antibody is detectable after disappearance of the HBs antigen and protects against re-infection by virus B.

2. HBc antigen and its antibody:

- the HBc antigen corresponds to the viral core found in the hepatocyte nucleus during a virus B infection;

- the anti-HBc antibody may be present during acute disease, and is almost always present in those individuals chronically infected.

3. HBe antigen and its antibody:

- unlike Hbs and HBc, which are associated with the viral particle, HBe is a soluble compound found in the serum of some chronically-affected patients (HBs+). It testifies to active viral replication and to potential high contagiousness;
- the appearance of anti-Hbe antibodies corresponds to the end of the replication state and the likelihood for being contagious.

Non-A-non-B hepatitis is still an exclusion diagnosis, because the infectious agents have not been isolated.

Delta-virus hepatitis has recently been identified. This defective virus can replicate only in the presence of virus B. It may cause chronic hepatitis lesions.

Fetal risk

Maternal–fetal transmission of the hepatitis virus depends on the particular virus and on the time in pregnancy at which maternal infection occurs. A number of possibilities can be anticipated, such as when the mother has acute hepatitis in pregnancy or is a chronic asymptomatic carrier of HBs antigens (i.e. she synthesizes HBs antigen at a consistent rate without clinical or even subclinical liver disease).

Hepatitis A   There is hardly any risk of transmission because of the short duration of viraemia and absence of faecal contamination at delivery.

Hepatitis B
1. The mother has acute hepatitis in pregnancy:

- in the first trimester, there is no risk of transmission;
- in the second trimester, risk is low (7–25 per cent).

In both cases, if the mother is still a carrier of HBs at the time of delivery, there will be a risk for neonatal hepatitis.

- in the third trimester or in the first month of the post-partum period, the risk of transmitting the virus is high, of the order of 60–80 per cent.

2. The mother is a chronic asymptomatic carrier of HBs antigen: the risk of transmission is primarily dependent on the presence of HBe in maternal serum. The frequency of asymptomatic HBs carriers varies from one area of the world to another:

- 0.1–1 per cent in western Europe, North America, and Australia;
- 2–7 per cent in eastern Europe, the Mediterranean, the Middle East, and South America;
- 8–20 per cent in south-east Asia, China, subsaharan Africa, and Oceania.

Maternal–fetal transmission is much more common in these last areas of the world because of the high frequency of carriers and because of the high frequency of HBe-positive women carriers of HBs antigen. There are three possible cases:

- HBs+ and HBe+: the risk of transmission of virus to the child and therefore of neonatal hepatitis is about 80–90 per cent with an 80–85 per cent risk of the child becoming a chronic carrier;
- HB+, HBe–, anti HBe+: the risk of transmission drops to 20 per cent or even less. In cases of infection, progress to chronic carrier status is more rare;
- HBs+, HBe–, anti HBe–: the risk of transmission is about 12 per cent.

In addition to the presence of HBe, risk of transmission also depends on the level of HBs antigen in maternal serum and on the activity of serum DNA polymerase, which is a sensitive marker because it is positive in HBe+ women and in women who are anti HBe+ who transmit the virus. Fetal transplacental infection is possible, though rare, and the child usually becomes infected during delivery.

Viral hepatitis or the mother's chronic carrier status brings no increased risk of congenital malformation, spontaneous abortion, fetal death, or intrauterine growth retardation. The only risk is of neonatal hepatitis or of becoming a chronic carrier of the virus.

Non A-non-B Hepatitis   The risk of transmission has not been well evaluated, but appears to be greater in cases of acute hepatitis in the third trimester.

Delta hepatitis   Maternal–fetal transmission has recently been shown. Considering the dependence of this virus on hepatitis B, its transmission must follow the same rules.

AIDS

AIDS, acquired immune deficiency syndrome, is caused by a virus known as HIV (human immunodeficiency virus). Transmission is by blood and genital secretions. After a primary infection the viral genome will integrate into the T4 lymphocyte genome. This selective tropism is determined by a cell-surface receptor known as CD4. The virus may be found in other blood cells, in particular macrophages, and may be produced by them. Antibodies formed by the patient after primary infection testify to the presence of the virus in the body. This patient is likely to present with clinical signs and is potentially contagious.

Apart from the HIV-I responsible for virtually all cases of AIDS, a HIV-II virus has been isolated in western Africa. It is not as widespread, and its pathogenesis less understood.

One distinguishes two epidemiological types of HIV infection. The occidental type is made up of two large groups of at-risk cases: male homosexuals and drug addicts, though the number of affected heterosexuals is increasing. The African type is of mostly heterosexual transmission.

In Africa, and in more and more other countries, the number of seropositive pregnant women is on the increase and represents a great public health hazard.

Risk to the pregnant woman

Consequences for an HIV seropositive woman   Is pregnancy an aggravating factor? Is there a greater risk of a clinical form in asymptomatic women? Is there a poorer prognosis for symptomatic women?

There are not yet enough studies to evaluate these risks. There are theoretical arguments which support the likelihood of pregnancy aggravating the situation:

- the decrease in T4 lymphocytes observed during pregnancy, although this is moderate and of no prognostic value;
- the level of serum antigens, which increases during the last trimester but returns to normal levels after pregnancy;
- the fact that pregnancy provides a particular immune status with allogenic stimulation, and the fact that other infections are present.

Consequences to the child   Transmission of virus from the seropositive mother to the newborn represents a high risk, when one considers the poor prognosis for HIV children. Estimates of the rates of viral transmission from mother to newborn are variable, between 20 per cent and 60 per cent depending on the study. It must be remembered that the risk is greatly diminished when the mother is asymptomatic and that this risk increases with the length of time that the mother is seropositive. In general, the risk is higher in Africa.

Three criteria can serve as indicators of the risk of transmission from mother to child (Table 8.3):

- level CD4 in the first trimester;
- presence of serum antigens during pregnancy;
- rate of viral replication.

In combining these criteria, one can evaluate the risk of transmission to the fetus (Table 8.4).

The mechanism of transmission is less well known. Possibly there is a prenatal pathway between 13 and 16 weeks of gestation, as shown by the presence of virus in the placenta observed at the time of pregnancy termination. It is suggested that more often, transmission is late, i.e. late in pregnancy or at the time of delivery (presence of virus on the cervical plug).

There are indirect arguments which favour late transmission: absence of embryo-fetopathology, as in other viral infections of the embryo, and absence of immunological deficiency in the affected neonates. It is also thought that post-

Table 8.3 Criteria for risk of transmission of maternal HIV to the newborn

Criterion		Risk of transmission (per cent)
CD4	$< 200/mm^3$	60
	$> 200/mm^3$	15
Agp 24	+	50
	–	23
Replication rate	rapid	58
	slow	21

Table 8.4 Combination of risk factors

Number of factors	Risk of transmission Percentage
0	22.5
1	55
2	65
3	71

natal transmission is an exception and the role of potentially infected maternal milk is disputable.

Laboratory tests

Two types of analyses may be used: serological tests which demonstrate different types of antibodies, and virology tests which demonstrate the presence of virus.

Serological tests   The ELISA test is the one most commonly used. The antigen is made up from the virus. It is sensitive with occasional false positives, which means any positive or questionable results should be tested again by ELISA and Western blot. Antibodies detected by ELISA are at a detectable level usually at 4–12 weeks after infection, but there may be a prolonged seronegative status. The Western blot technique uses purified viral antigen separated by electrophoresis and studied serologically. It detects antibodies for each antigen, protein or glycoprotein, specific to the virus. Certain bands are important and correspond to antibodies directed against surface proteins, gp 120 and gp 160.

In the newborn, transmitted maternal antibodies take a long time to disappear: antibody gp 160 can persist up to 10 months and antibody p25 up to 12 months. In HIV-infected neonates there is a more rapid decrease in maternal antibodies, and at 2 months only the antibody gp 160 persists. No method based on measurement of IgM-type antibody specific to the virus has been developed.

Virology   Virological testing uses various methods and will evolve in the near future by developments in molecular biology techniques.

Isolation of virus from cell cultures remains in the area of research. Demonstration of a viral constituent, p25, is a simple technique but unfortunately of low sensitivity. The p25 antigen appears at the onset of infection, and its presence in the blood is an expression of viral replication. This technique is not sensitive enough to be used at birth in cord blood. A promising method is identifying the presence of virus by molecular biology using the PCR technique (see p. 74), which allows considerable amplification of DNA fragment (here, that DNA segment corresponding to the virus) once a specific primer is available to initiate the reaction. Its great sensitivity should allow its use at birth, in cord blood. It is too soon to appreciate the real value of diagnosing HIV infections by PCR, and certainly too soon to know the frequency of false positive results.

Amongst other tests developed for study of HIV infection, one in particular can demonstrate the CD4 molecule, the cell receptor specific to the virus.

Examples and strategies

In practice, one finds oneself at a loss, as there are few certainties and those we do have are pessimistic. A seropositive woman has a 20–70 per cent chance of having an affected child with a poor prognosis. Antenatal diagnosis cannot be considered. In fact, there is potential risk of infecting the fetus during diagnostic testing (cord blood sampling) as the time of viral transmission from mother to fetus is not known; it may occur at the beginning or the end of pregnancy and/or at delivery.

A seropositive woman who is not pregnant   It is important to explain the risks of pregnancy, for the woman and for the future child. The tendency is to discourage pregnancy but, confronted with the profound wish of some women to have a child, as is often the case for previous drug addicts, one should attempt to evaluate the risks. If infection is recent the woman should be advised that the risk to the child will increase with time, and in the eventuality that this woman does want a child it seems preferable not to delay pregnancy.

A seropositive pregnant woman   The woman should know the risks to her and the child to be born. Laboratory tests may give some prognostic information regarding maternal infection.

In the first trimester, after evaluation of the risks, a request for termination of pregnancy seems acceptable. When the woman seeks consultation too late in pregnancy for termination, or if she wishes to carry on with the pregnancy, it is essential to monitor the pregnancy (risk of premature delivery, premature rupture of membranes) and to look regularly for signs of AIDS-related-complex ARC or AIDS. This monitoring should continue after birth.

Systematic blood testing at premarital sessions or for all pregnant women   One must first clearly understand the significance of blood test results, which are very different from that of other systematic blood tests (rubella, toxoplasmosis) where the positiveness implies a definite protection. For AIDS, a positive result means a viral infection with risk of disease and its transmission. A negative result generally means that at the time of blood testing there was no viral infection (in some rare cases, the sampling may have been in the early period of infection when antibodies had not yet appeared), and that the woman is susceptible to the virus.

A systematic blood test, be it premarital or prepregnancy, has a number of problems. First, the incidence of infection in the population, which shows particularly large variation between urban and rural areas. For example, a study in Massachusetts showed an incidence of 8/1000 pregnant women in Boston and 0.9/1000 in rural areas. Another important point is recognition of high-risk groups, which was shown by a study of maternity wards in Paris where an incidence of 4/1000 was observed. In 97 per cent of these HIV-positive women, the most probable route of infection could be determined by questioning. Drug addicts represented 56.5 per cent, women whose partner originated from a region where infection is endemic (black Africa in particular) 19.8 per cent, heterosexual infection by a partner belonging to a high-risk group (drug addict, bisexual, or known HIV positive) 16.8 per cent, previous transfusions 4.6 per cent.

In France, the National Ethics Committee has requested that information on the availability of serological diagnosis be systematically given to all pregnant women who are free to ask for blood testing.

Vaccinations

A frequent source of anxiety for the pregnant woman is vaccination, particularly with viral vaccines, which are often like an infection that can impose risks on the fetus. Knowing the nature of the vaccine is important in assessing the potential risk it represents. There are two types of vaccine.

Vaccines which can be used by pregnant women at any time in pregnancy

These are vaccines made of killed or inactivated viruses. The term 'killed' means that the viral preparation has lost its ability to infect or to be pathogenic but has retained its antigenic component or immunogenic ability. Examples are:

1. Inactivated poliomyelitis vaccine;
2. Flu vaccine: the potential risk of flu in pregnant women (miscarriage) and its possible teratogenicity are arguments for advising vaccination, and protecting the mother ensures passive immunity of the newborn for at least the first 4 months of life.
3. Hepatitis B vaccine: the antigen used for vaccination is the purified viral envelope carrying the HBs antigen. This antigen has no ability to infect, but retains immunogenic abilities.
4. Diphtheria and tetanus toxoids.

Vaccines to be avoided by pregnant women

Live or attenuated viruses must be avoided. Viral strains used for vaccine retain an antigenic component, that is, the immunogenic ability of the wild virus as well as the ability to replicate in humans. Their ability to cause disease has been removed, and they cause an infection with few clinical signs or without any signs at all. Pregnancy is a contraindication to these vaccines because of a theoretical sensitivity of embryonic tissue to the viral infection. They are legally forbidden during pregnancy mostly as a precaution, as one might associate the vaccine to a congenital malformation, which is of a completely different origin. Examples are:

1. Oral polio vaccine: Of the millions vaccinated around the world, epidemiological and clinical studies have demonstrated the absence of fetal pathogenesis of the oral vaccine.

2. Rubella vaccine: Prospective studies on pregnant women having received a rubella vaccine 3 months before or after the presumed time of conception, have shown that all susceptible (non-immunized) mothers, who have decided to carry their pregnancies to term, have given birth to babies without any sign of abnormality known to be associated with congenital rubella. Some children had shown signs of intrauterine infection, but their growth and development progressed normally. Amongst these women, some were vaccinated at a time considered of most risk for viraemia and congenital malformations (in the week before conception or 4 weeks after). Pregnancy remains a contraindication to rubella vaccine, and precautions must be taken to avoid vaccination of pregnant women. In cases of inadvertent vaccination in the month preceding, or in the 3 months following conception, the risk of congenital rubella does not constitute a reason for termination of pregnancy. It is useless to do fetal blood analysis to demonstrate possible fetal infection because, even when infection can be demonstrated, it does not have any disease effects on the fetus.

3. Yellow fever vaccine: Studies done around the world demonstrate that this vaccine is innocuous at any time in pregnancy. However, this vaccine is not advised for pregnant women, except when epidemiological circumstances impose the need for vaccination.

4. BCG is the only live attenuated bacterial vaccine. Though without any teratogenic effect, BCG is not recommended in pregnancy. In case of infection, antitubercular chemotherapy can be used.

References and further reading

Alagille, D. (1985). Vertical transmission of HBV hepatitis to fetuses and infants: current advances in prevention. *J. Pediatr. Gastroenterol. Nutr.*, **4**, 515–16.

Arvin, A. M., Hensleigh, P. A., Prober, C. G., *et al.* (1986). Failure of antepartum maternal cultures to predict the infant's risk of exposure to herpes simplex virus at delivery. *New Engl. J. Med.*, **315**, 796–800.

Blanche, S., Rouzioux, C., Guihard, M. L., *et al.* (1989). A prospective study of infants born to women seropositive for human immunodeficiency virus type 1. *New Engl. J. Med.*, **320**, 1643–8.

Boué, A. and Malbrunot, C. (1985). Infections virales du foetus et du nouveau né. In *Médecine néo-natale* (ed. P. Vert and L. Stern), Masson, Paris.

Brown, Z. A., Vontver, L. A., Benedetti, J., *et al.* (1987). Effects on infants of a first episode of genital herpes during pregnancy. *New Engl. J. Med.*, **316**, 240–4.

Buffet, C. (1985). Hepatites virales en cours de grossesse et transmission materno-foetale du virus B. *Presse Med.*, **14**, 419–22.

Coulaud, J. P. (1988). L'infection VIH et le Sida, les manifestations maternelles et infantiles. *L'enfant en milieu tropical.*, **172**, 7–52

Daffos, F., Forestier, F., Capella-Pavlovsky, M., *et al.* (1988). Prenatal management of 746 pregnancies at risk for congenital toxoplasmosis. *New Engl. J. Med.*, **318**, 271–5.

Derouin, F., Thulliez, P., Candolfi, E., *et al.* (1988). Early prenatal diagnosis of congenital toxoplasmosis using amniotic fluid samples and tissue culture. *Eur. J. Clin. Microbiol. Infect. Dis.*, **7**, 423–5.

Enders, G., Nickerl-Pacher, U., Miller, E., *et al.* (1988). Outcome of confirmed periconceptional maternal rubella. *Lancet*, **i**, 1445–6.

Grangeot-Keros, L. and Pillot, J. (1985). Étude critique du sérodiagnostic de la rubéole. *Bull. Inst. Pasteur*, **83**, 375–88.

Hoff, R., Berardi, V. P., Weiblen, B. J., *et al.* (1988). Seroprevalence of HIV among childbearing women. *New Engl. J. Med.*, **318**, 525–30.

Huraux, J. M. and Nicolas, J. C. (1985) *Virologie*, pp. 216–22. Flammarion, Paris.

Katz, S. L. and Wilfert, C. M. (1989). Human immunodeficiency virus infection of newborns. *New Engl. J. Med.*, **320**, 1687–9.

Miller, E., Cradock-Watson, J. E., and Pollock, T. M. (1982). Consequences of confirmed maternal rubella at successive stages of pregnancy. *Lancet*, **ii**, 781–4.

Minkoff, H., Nanda, D., Menez, R., *et al.* (1987). Pregnancies resulting in infants with AIDS or AIDS related complex. *Gyn. Obstet.*, **69**, 285–91.

Munro, N. D., Sheppard, S., Smithells, R. W., *et al.* (1987). Temporal relations between maternal rubella and congenital defects. *Lancet*, **ii**, 201–4.

Paryani, S. G. and Arvin, A. M. (1986). Intrauterine infection with varicella zoster virus after maternal varicella. *New Engl. J. Med.*, **314**, 1542–6.

Pinon, J., Poirriez, J., Leroux, B., *et al.* (1987). Diagnostic précoce et surveillance de la toxoplasmose congénitale. *Presse Med.*, **16**, 471–4.

Prober, C. G., Sullender, W. M., Yasukawa, L. L., *et al.* (1987). Low risk of herpes simplex virus infections in neonates exposed to the virus at the time of vaginal delivery to mothers with recurrent genital herpes simplex virus infections. *New Engl. J. Med.*, **316**, 240–4.

Snydman, D. R. (1985). Hepatitis in pregnancy. *New Engl. J. Med.*, **313**, 1398–1401.

Stagno, S., Pass, R. F., Dworsky, M. E., *et al.* (1982). Congenital cytomegalovirus infection. *New Engl. J. Med.*, **306**, 945–9.

Stagno, S. and Whitley, R. J. (1985). Herpes virus infections of pregnancy. Part II: Herpes simplex virus and varicella-zoster virus infection. *New Engl. J. Med.*, **313**, 1327–30.

Weber, D. J., Redfield, R. R., and Lemon, S. M. (1986). Acquired immunodeficiency syndrome: epidemiology and significance for the obstetrician and gynecologist. *Am. J. Obst. Gyn.*, **155**, 235–40.

IV   PRACTICAL APPLICATIONS AND THEIR CONSEQUENCES

9 Prenatal diagnosis and its applications

If one knows the indications for prenatal diagnosis, the techniques available and how to use them, it is appropriate to apply these techniques in all at-risk pregnancies and to evaluate their effects on the incidence of malformations at birth.

Data

Genetic epidemiology

One must first define the anomalies for which prenatal diagnosis is applicable. For this evaluation one must consider three points:

1. *Severity of the malformation*: lifespan, the extent of handicap, the effect on mental development, absence of treatment. All these factors led to the selection of chromosome and single-gene anomalies for which testing is currently suggested and which have been the subject of previous chapters.

2. *The mode of ascertainment of the anomaly*: well-defined hereditary transmission, structural chromosome anomaly, autosomal recessive anomaly, or X-linked recessive. The approach will be more complex when it is a *de novo* anomaly such as, for example, an abnormality of chromosome number, or a neural tube defect, where epidemiological data will identify at-risk groups which are sometimes difficult to define.

3. *Incidence of the anomaly in the population*: this element is important, to establish priorities in determining the number and specialization of the laboratories needed to implement a programme; for example a large number of local cytogenetic laboratories and a small number of centralized laboratories specializing in biochemistry and molecular biology.

There are some geographical locations where a high frequency of a particular anomaly will direct programmes to a certain area of expertise; this was the case with testing for neural tube defects in Scotland, Wales, and Ireland; haemoglobinopathies and sickle cell anaemia in black populations; and thalassaemia in Mediterranean countries.

Technical limitations

The application of prenatal testing will depend on the equipment available and on the availability of competent technical staff. Other than problems of funding, local circumstances may complicate matters when, for example, certain indispensable reagents are perishable or must be imported. This is the case for cell culture media and for radioactive materials required for molecular techniques. Therefore, in those regions where it is difficult to provide a good supply of carbon dioxide and quality media, direct chromosome analysis on chorionic villi would be better than analyses requiring cell cultures.

Acceptability of prenatal diagnosis

In industrialized countries, the large decrease in perinatal mortality and infectious disease in the first year of life has made genetic disease and congenital malformation a primary concern for parents. This awareness is concentrated around more common anomalies with characteristic phenotypic features, such as trisomy 21 and muscular dystrophy. In some regions, the particular prevalence of a disease (thalassaemia in Mediterranean areas, spina bifida in the Celtic population) renders the population receptive to prenatal screening techniques.

Education in this area consists of a balance between dramatizing the risk, thus creating excessive anxiety, and minimizing the risk, which leads to negligence. The availability of genetic counselling should reduce this problem.

What remains are the cultural, philosophical, and religious attitudes towards termination of pregnancy. Even more than profound personal conviction, the social attitude where a woman lives plays an important part with regard to this issue. In some regions where social pressures are important, early prenatal testing on chorionic villi, at a time when the pregnancy can go unnoticed, has made prenatal testing possible.

Recent experience

The basic question in providing a prenatal diagnosis programme is how to determine which pregnancies are at risk.

Prenatal diagnosis of chromosome anomalies

Tables 9.1 and 9.2 show the increase in number of prenatal tests done for chromosome anomalies from 1980 to 1987 in France by all the prenatal diagnosis laboratories grouped under the French Association for the Screening and Prevention of Handicaps.

Among the three main indications considered as priorities, the number of diagnoses for parental chromosomal anomaly or for a previous child with a numerical chromosomal anomaly have increased slowly and have remained stable. Diagnoses for maternal age of 38 or more have increased in number (2020 in 1980 to 12 114 in 1987) and in proportion (from 74.7 per cent of all chromosomal analyses in 1980 to 87.9 per cent in 1987). It must be noted that though the number of diagnoses done for advanced maternal age has increased sixfold during this time period, the number of women reached, who are eligible (38 years old and over), has increased only by 3.7 per cent. In fact, during the same period, even though the birth rate has varied only slightly, the number of at-risk

Table 9.1 Number of prenatal chromosome diagnoses by indication done in France from 1980 to 1987. Collaborative study by prenatal diagnosis centres collected for the Association Francaise pour dépistage et la prévention des handicaps (M. L. Briard, personal communication). Figures in brackets indicate the percentage diagnoses for these indications in one year

Year	Total number of diagnoses	Maternal age		Previous affected child		Parental chromosomal rearrangement	
1980	2759	2060	(74.7)	462	(16.7)	237	(8.6)
1981	3912	2968	(76.3)	625	(16.0)	301	(7.7)
1982	4440	3530	(79.5)	612	(13.8)	298	(6.7)
1983	5454	4400	(80.7)	761	(14.0)	293	(5.3)
1984	7124	5885	(82.6)	863	(12.1)	358	(5.0)
1985	9301	7880	(84.7)	1021	(10.9)	400	(4.3)
1986	11 665	10 126	(86.8)	1070	(9.2)	469	(4.0)
1987	13 783	12 114	(87.9)	1181	(8.6)	488	(3.5)

Table 9.2 Prenatal diagnosis in women over 38 years of age. Figures in brackets are percentages

Year	Number of diagnoses	Population at risk		Participation rate
1980	2060	14 964	(1.97)	(13.9)
1981	2986	15 686	(1.95)	(19.0)
1982	3530	16 296	(2.04)	(21.7)
1983	4400	15 651	(2.09)	(28.7)
1984	5885	17 207	(2.27)	(34.2)
1985	7880	19 754	(2.57)	(39.9)
1986	10 126	22 384	(2.38)	(45.2)
1987	12 114	23 500[a]	(3.06)	(51.6)

[a] estimated

pregnancies has increased considerably, from 15 000 to 23 500 (1.87 per cent to 3.06 per cent of total pregnancies). This clearly demonstrates the difficulty of predictions in this area and the difficulty in determining the cut-off point for eligibility, which itself is linked to financial constraints which then determines the number of laboratories. In recent years, chromosomal analysis as a result of ultrasound findings has substantially increased the number of chromosome anomalies detected (see p. 204).

Is it appropriate to do a chromosomal analysis when amniotic fluid is drawn for other reasons, considering the low risk of a chromosomal anomaly, the-laboratory overload, and the cost incurred by cytogenetic laboratories?

Table 9.3 Gammaglutamyl transpeptidase activity in amniotic fluid from a pregnancy carrying a trisomy 21 fetus

Study area	Number of fluids studied	Percentage with gammaglutamyl transpeptidase levels	
		Below median	Below 5th percentile
Copenhagen	16	94	56
Edinburgh	54	85	52
Paris	54	95	59

This is an issue that must be faced when amniocentesis is performed because of a risk of neural tube defect, determined by levels of maternal serum alphafetoprotein. The cytogenetic laboratory load may be reduced by measure of gammaglutamyl transpeptidase in amniotic fluid. A number of studies (Table 9.3) have shown that in the presence of a trisomic fetus, values are always below the median.

Applications to single-gene disorders, first determined by mode of transmission

For the larger number of autosomal recessive disorders, an at-risk couple can be recognized only after the birth of an affected child. Therefore, prenatal diagnosis can be considered only in a subsequent pregnancy. In general, the efficiency of such testing will be limited because only 23 per cent of children affected with an autosomal recessive disease are born into a family already recognized as being at risk (Table 9.4).

In some autosomal diseases, it is possible to recognize at-risk couples because of screening for heterozygotes. There are two points to consider:

- that the disease (and therefore the frequency of heterozygotes) be frequent enough; it has been already noted that most metabolic diseases are in fact rare;
- that heterozygote testing be reliable and relatively simple; but testing often involves a quantitative measure of an enzyme and, although median values in heterozygotes are usually around 50 per cent of normal values, there is great individual variation which leads to much overlap, rendering the test useless in practice.

At present, testing for heterozygosity has been proposed only for two populations at risk: for haemoglobinopathies where a precise qualitative test is available, and for Tay–Sachs disease in Ashkenazi Jews.

For X-linked recessive disease, it is theoretically easier to identify potentially at-risk mothers, sisters, maternal nieces and aunts of an affected child. In the more frequent diseases, such as muscular

Table 9.4 Impact of prenatal diagnoses on the prevention of inborn errors of metabolism. From Saudubray and Poenaru (198x). The table shows the effect of autosomal recessive disease in a family of three children. It is clear that once the diagnosis is made on the first affected child the number of fetuses affected and detected prenatally is 11/48 (23 per cent)

Type of family	Frequency of families	Number of affected	Number of children avoided by prenatal diagnosis
1 affected child	9^a	9	0
	9	9	0
	9	9	0
2 affected children	3^b	6	3
	3	6	3
	3	6	3
3 affected children	1^c	3	2
No affected child	27^d	0	0
Total	64	48	11

^{a} $1/4 \times 3/4 \times 3/4$
^{b} $1/4 \times 1/4 \times 3/4$
^{c} $1/4 \times 1/4 \times 1/4$
^{d} $3/4 \times 3/4 \times 3/4$

dystrophy (creatine phosphokinase assay), haemophilia (coagulation factor assay), X-linked mental retardation (evaluation of X-fragile sites), it is only when these test results are clearly positive that one can confirm that the mother is a carrier. An apparently normal result does not exclude the possibility that the mother is still a carrier. Variation in expression of these criteria is a result of lyonization. With the discovery of the gene mutation in fragile X syndrome, however, molecular analysis has clarified the uncertain cytogenetic results found in many families.

With DNA polymorphic markers, the segregation of the X chromosome, whether normal or mutant, can be followed in any one family to determine which women are carriers. The application of this method is expensive and depends on the availability of good laboratories.

Improvement and extension of prenatal diagnosis services

Improvement with available techniques
The issue that must be addressed is how to recognize at-risk pregnancies.

Main objective: diagnosis of chromosomal anomalies   What strategies can be used to extend prenatal diagnosis to all pregnancies? Figure 9.1 shows the

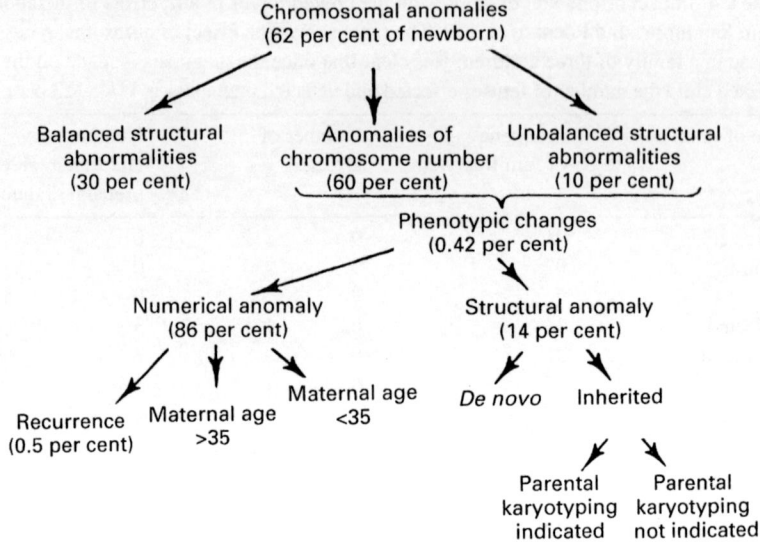

Fig. 9.1 Distribution of chromosomal anomalies. From Aymé *et al.* (1980).

chromosome anomalies leading to physical malformations and mental handicap at birth. Recently, the first step in implementing prenatal diagnostic techniques for chromosomal anomalies has been to classify women in to groups
that are easy to define: carriers of balanced chromosome rearrangement, mothers 38 years old or more, women with a previous child with a chromosomal
anomaly. Tables 9.1 and 9.2 demonstrate the outcome of such a scheme and
the effort still required to improve on the percentage of pregnancies benefitting
from prenatal diagnosis.

Assuming that such a programme is properly implemented, about two-thirds of
births with chromosomal anomalies would not be detected, because most births
occur to younger mothers and, despite a low incidence, three quarters of the cases
of trisomy 21 are born to this population of young mothers.

Lowering the maternal age in order to enlarge the at-risk group is unreasonable
and not very effective, because the number of invasive procedures would increase
rapidly while the proportion of cases detected in each age group would decrease.

The only viable proposal is to select, among young pregnant women, a group
where the risk of having a fetus affected with a chromosomal anomaly is equivalent to that of a woman of 40 or over. The efficiency of this proposal depends on
the ability to pick out at-risk women in a simple manner, as early as possible, and
to do so for all pregnancies. A number of directions have been taken in an attempt
to tap those at-risk groups.

Ultrasound indications Since 1980, ultrasound examinations done on fetuses with chromosomal anomalies detected by amniocentesis have been able to

show characteristic physical anomalies, for example finger position associated with trisomy 18, or signs linked to physical growth and development, such as a delay in overall fetal movement in trisomy 21. None the less, these analyses were too subjective to form the basis of screening

In recent years, amniocenteses done after an abnormal ultrasound have demonstrated the significant number of chromosomal anomalies (see p. 204). These amniocenteses can only permit detection of chromosomal anomalies which also result in major physical malformations, as in some cases of trisomy 18 and 21. In addition, the ultrasound finding is often late and presents a problem in terminating the pregnancy. One must therefore look for early and more subtle signs, allowing in particular the detection of trisomy 21. Different criteria have been looked at: femur length, dilatation of renal pelvis, etc. One of the most interesting signs is an increase in the nuchal thickness of the fetus; the characteristic nape of children with trisomy 21 is well known. Work by Benacerraf has shown that ultrasound detection of thickening of the nape or absence of nuccal folds (Fig. 9.2) associated with measurement of femur length (smaller than the 90th percentile) can be a useful sign, and may allow detection of 76 per cent of trisomy 21 fetuses.

Laboratory tests   With testing of all pregnancies in mind, only analyses of maternal blood can be considered, as has been done for neural tube defects.

Unless there is passage of a particular chromosomal constituent into maternal serum, one must direct testing towards quantitative measures of substances present in maternal blood during pregnancy which become abnormal in the presence of a fetus with a chromosomal anomaly. The substance must cross the placental barrier, and variations from the norm must be easily detectable.

Merkatz *et al.* (1984) demonstrated by retrospective study a relationship between trisomy 21 in the fetus and low alphafetoprotein in maternal serum which had been drawn at 17 weeks of gestation to rule out neural tube defects. These results have been confirmed by a number of studies.

In the last 20 years, various studies have shown that chromosomal anomalies are associated with growth retardation. At the cellular level this was shown by a slowing of the cell cycle of trisomic cells, in the embryo/fetal growth curve, and at birth where Naeye (1967) showed a reduction in cell density in trisomic neonates. Analyses done on amniotic fluid for a pregnancy with a trisomic fetus showed that levels of alphafetoprotein were almost always lower than the median, which itself was calculated for normal pregnancies. In the same way, studies showed that levels of gammaglutamyl transpeptidase in amniotic fluid were also lower in the presence of a trisomy 21 fetus (Table 9.3).

These two proteins originate from the liver and one may assume that low levels are a reflection of a reduction in number of hepatic cells because of growth retardation in trisomic fetuses. As a consequence, the level of alphafetoprotein in maternal serum is lower. The fact that alphafetoprotein is exclusively

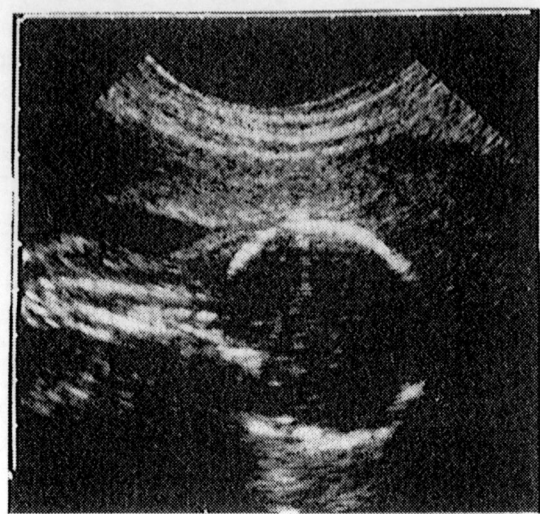

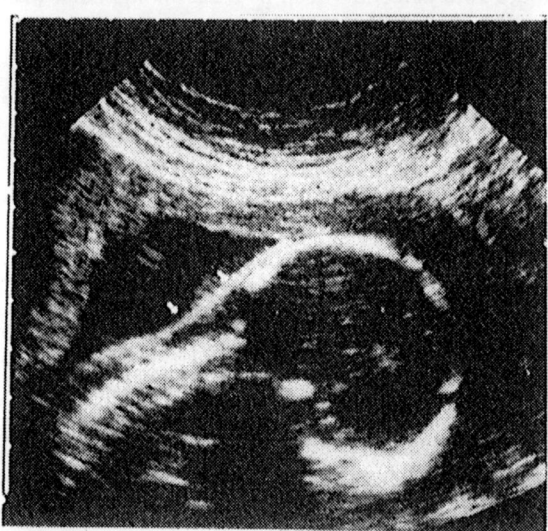

Fig. 9.2 Ultrasound picture of the nape of the neck of a trisomy 21 fetus. From M. C. Aubry and J. Boué.

of embryonic origin gives great value to this test. Figure 9.3 shows results obtained in our laboratory, which are similar to results obtained by other teams.

Applying screening tests to all pregnancies is not without problems. One must distinguish between inadvertent diagnosis of trisomy 21 in systems where screening is routinely done for neural tube defects, as in the United Kingdom, and systematic screening for trisomy 21, where blood is drawn with this goal in

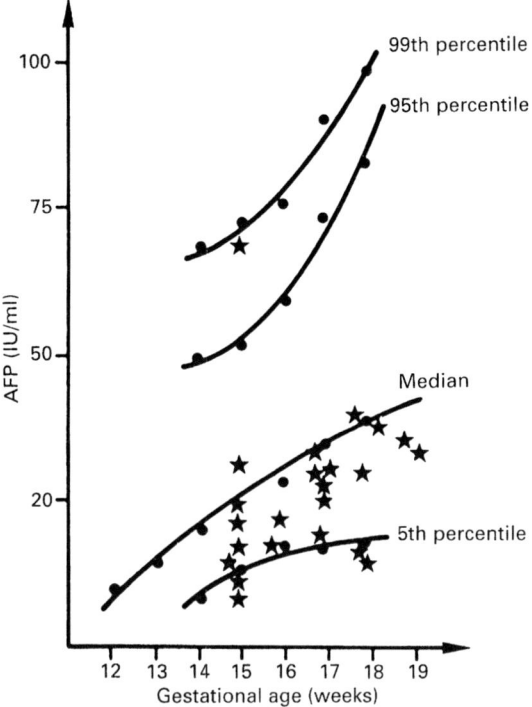

Fig. 9.3 Maternal serum alphafetoprotein value. ⋆, level in trisomy 21 pregnancies.

mind. In fact, as in the association between maternal age and trisomy 21, the correlation between low alphafetoprotein in maternal serum and trisomy 21 is merely an indication, not a diagnosis. In choosing the median as cut-off, half the women will have a serum level below this point. All of these are therefore in the group of women at risk for trisomy 21 and amniocentesis should be proposed. Such an approach will subject many normal pregnancies to amniocentesis. In choosing the fifth percentile as the cut-off limit, only 5/100 amniocenteses will be done, but also only 27 per cent of trisomy 21 will be detected. This relationship — 5 per cent of amniocenteses and karyotypes done, for 25–30 per cent of trisomy 21 detected — is appealing. In practice, however, a screening test for trisomy 21 will be done on all women. For 95 per cent of them the serum alphafetoprotein level will be 'normal', i.e. above the chosen cut-off, which serves to remove these women from the at-risk group, when the majority of trisomy 21 babies (70–75 per cent) will in fact be born to this group. The birth of a baby with trisomy 21 then becomes a 'medical error', unlike the birth of a trisomy 21 baby in a younger woman when maternal age criteria are used.

To increase the sensitivity of maternal screening methods, other biochemical markers have since been studied: human chorionic gonadotropin (hCG)

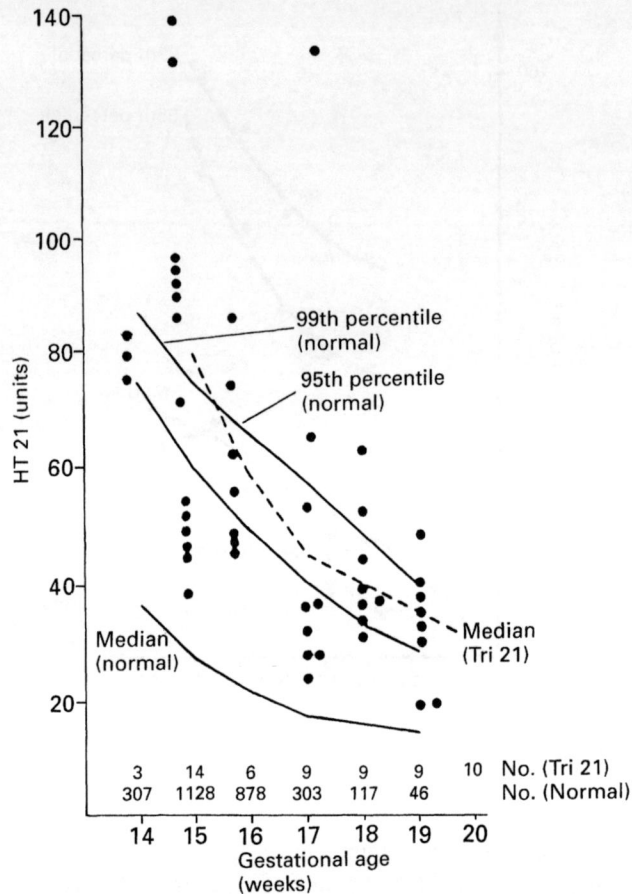

Fig. 9.4 Human chorionic gonadotroplin (hCG) values in maternal serum in 2779 unaffected pregnancies and 50 trisomy 21 pregnancies. From Muller and Boué (1990).

unconjugated oestriol, pregnancy-specific beta-glycoprotein. Several retrospective studies have been performed using hCG alone, or hCG combined with other serological markers and maternal age (Fig. 9.4). These retrospective studies indicated that hCG was a promising discriminant serum marker for screening pregnancies with an increased risk of trisomy 21. On the other hand the results obtained with unconjugated oestriol and pregnancy-specific beta-glycoprotein were controversial. To confirm the results of the retrospective studies, further prospective studies have been carried out (Table 9.5). The findings of the prospective studies largely confirmed the results predicted by the retrospective studies based on retrieved maternal serum specimens. Maternal serum hCG values combined with maternal age represented a discriminant test

Table 9.5 Prospective studies (below maternal age indication) ICHG Washington, October 1991. Figures in brackets are percentages. Abbreviations: M, maternal age; H, human chorionic gonadotrophin; A, alphafetoprotein; O, oestrogen

Centre	Reference	Techniques	Trisomy 21 detected Number	Proportion
London	Wald	M H A O	14 700	11/20 (64)
Maine–Rhode Island	Haddow	M H A O	25 000	30/35[a] (57)
Finland	Salonen	M H A O	6 800	5/8 (62)
Scotland	Crossley	M H A O	7 800	9/15 (60)
New York	Macri	M H A	24 000	17/25 (68)
Paris	Muller	M H	21 000	31/49 (63)

[a] expected number (pregnancies still in progress)

and allowed the selection of a group of women with an increased risk of chromosomal anomalies. The detection rate for trisomy 21 was 60 per cent. An interesting finding was that other severe chromosomal abnormalities have also been detected in this selected group of women (trisomy 13, trisomy 18). This detection rate has been improved by combination with ultrasonography performed when hCG values were very low.

These results supported the hypothesis that high levels of hCG reflected a high placental activity, allowing the survival of trisomic conceptuses. It is well known that trisomic fetuses reaching term represent only a small proportion of the trisomies conceived; it is estimated that, for one newborn trisomy 21, there are 5–8 trisomy 21 abortuses. In these latter cases low values of hCG have been observed (Table 9.6).

In trisomy 13 and trisomy 18 pregnancies reaching term, Kalousek *et al.* (1989) observed confined placental mosaicism, the diploid cytotrophoblast providing a functional compensation. No placental mosaicism has been observed in trisomy 21 at term. The elevated hCG levels in trisomy 21 pregnancies are not due to synthesis of abnormal hCG molecules, but may reflect some abnormalities in placental development. Pathologic examination of viable trisomy 21 placentas has shown a marked retardation of villus maturation with frequent persistence of the embryonic form of the villi. In normal pregnancies, the study of placenta histology in relation to hCG has shown that the cytotrophoblast regulates hCG production by maintaining a pool of transient intermediate cells whose numbers peaked at 8–10 weeks of gestation and declined thereafter. Thus, the fact that there is persistence of the embryonic cytotrophoblast structure in trisomy 21 placentas affords an explanation for the production of a high hCG level.

Table 9.6 Chromosomal anomalies detected after hCG maternal serum screening

| Maternal age (years) | Number of women tested | Trisomy 21 | | |
| | | Observed | Expected | |
			At birth	At 18 weeks[a]
30–34	2757	6	3.6	4.6
35–36	1085	4 + 1 born	3.9	5
37	503	4 + 2 born	2.6	3.4
38–39	572	1	4	5.2
> 40	251	5	3.5	4.5
Total	5168	23	17.6	22.7

[a] Evaluation based on INSERM figures corrected for the proportion of fetal deaths of trisomy between 18 weeks and birth, from Hook (1989).

The screening strategy depends on public health policies developed for prenatal diagnosis:

1. The age limit for maternal age indication for amniocentesis varies from one country to the other. Some pregnant women with maternal age indication are reluctant to have an amniocentesis; hCG values may represent an argument in counselling these patients, as practically all hCG values in pregnancies with fetal trisomy 21 are above median values.

2. The maternal serum alphafetoprotein screening programme. Most of the studies have been performed in countries where alphafetoprotein screening was routinely done because of the frequency of neural tube defects, even if alphafetoprotein levels did not represent a discriminant test for trisomy 21. When the epidemiological status of neural tube defects and the possibility of routine ultrasonography do not support a MSAFP screening programme, hCG alone is a reasonable choice.

The prospective studies have shown some practical problems linked to the application of this screening. The maternal parameters influencing the determination of the cut-off must be carefully checked for each case: the decreasing slope of the normal hCG values may be an important cause of false results if there is an error in dating pregnancy. Growth retardation is one of the characteristics of trisomy 21 conceptuses.

Multiple pregnancies give higher hCG levels than singleton pregnancies. Some racial factors may complicate evaluation; it has been shown that in black women normal hCG values are significantly higher.

Among the possible adverse effects, the fetal risk associated with amniocentesis must be balanced with the detection rate of trisomy 21. Also, an important point is the information given to the women at the time of blood sampling. This necessitates a co-ordinated strategy for the screening programme with a need not only for technical resources but also for genetic and supportive counselling, especially for women under 35, who had not been previously thought to be at increased risk of trisomy 21. It should be explained that the maternal serum screening is not a direct diagnosis of trisomy 21, but the evaluation of a change in the statistical risk in relation to their age. The last important adverse effect is that, with a reliable assay and good application, about 30 per cent of trisomy 21 fetuses remain undetected during pregnancy, and in these unfortunate cases, this represents a failure of the screening.

Clinical criteria based on previous obstetric history and clinical findings in early pregnancy. A high frequency of early spontaneous abortions in previous pregnancies, particularly in the pregnancy just prior to that of the current one, was observed in pregnancy histories of women where a chromosomal anomaly was detected by prenatal diagnosis. These were essentially women of advanced maternal age. A high level of metrorrhagia was also observed, particularly small and persistent metrorrhagias.

A strategy, based on the above criteria, ultrasonography, laboratory tests, and clinical findings, should be developed in order to gauge indications for fetal karyotyping.

Single-gene disorders

Improving the ability to recognize at-risk couples before the birth of an affected child is a difficult goal to attain. For autosomal recessive conditions where simple testing for heterozygotes is not available one can conceive a test of exclusion of heterozygosity for the mutant gene in some favourable situations. Cystic fibrosis is an example. In the affected child's sibship, for which the parental mutations or haplotypes associated to the mutant gene have been determined by molecular biological methods, it is possible to determine the normal homozygotes (for whom the risk is excluded) and the heterozygotes (in the sibship of the affected, two-thirds are heterozygotes). We have already seen (see p. 149) how a couple's risk can be adjusted when one member of the couple is known to be heterozygous and, if necessary, gauge the need for prenatal enzymatic testing of amniotic fluid.

In other autosomal recessive diseases such a strategy is difficult to conceive because disease incidence is small and so for a known heterozygous the chances that his/her partner is also heterozygous is low. Prenatal diagnosis is therefore limited to determining an unaffected fetus by exclusion (the fetus having received the haplotype of the normal chromosome), which is not satisfactory.

In X-linked disease, particularly in Duchenne muscular dystrophy, one must bear in mind that in one in three cases, the mutation is new and cannot be anticipated.

Extension of prenatal diagnosis

Prenatal diagnosis can be extended in terms of indications or in terms of available techniques.

New indications First, there is the problem of prenatal diagnosis in dominant conditions. Prenatal diagnosis of a dominant condition can be considered when the disease is of late onset (Huntington's disease), or when the disease is debilitating, but compatible with life (Steinert's myotonia); in these contexts there are serious ethical issues. Until recently, prenatal diagnosis for these particular conditions had limitations because the specific gene mutations were not known and only linkage analysis could be used. In other dominant conditions, such as tuberous sclerosis, even with the knowledge of informative polymorphic markers linked to the gene with a small risk of recombination, the family structure limits the possibility of diagnosis. For identifying a dominant disease gene, ideally one needs large families with live members in several generations, but in practice, families requesting testing are small and many ancestors are often deceased. Harper has clearly shown the limits in these kind of diagnoses:

1. First, in identifying those who have inherited the mutant gene but are asymptomatic, family structure means that only 15 per cent of cases will be provided with a diagnosis (Fig. 9.5a).

2. Also, in a possible request for prenatal diagnosis in families where markers linked to mutant genes are known, diagnosis is possible. When molecular biology cannot determine whether the parent has inherited from his/her affected parent the normal or the affected chromosome, then prenatal diagnosis may in some cases exclude risk to the fetus; in other cases the fetus may have the same theoretical risk as the parent, about 50 per cent (Fig. 9.5b). This diagnosis of

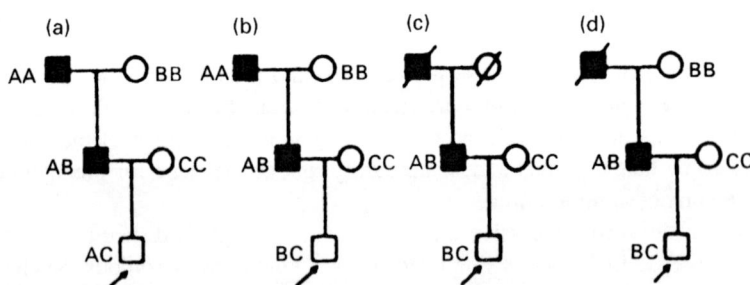

Fig. 9.5a An example of families where the risk of an autosomal dominant condition in an asymptomatic member must be determined. (a) The proband's grandparents are still living. The affected parent has markers A and B. Marker A, inherited from the affected grandparent, is linked to the gene and is transmitted to the proband who is therefore carrying the mutant gene (within the limits of possible recombinations). (b) In the same pedigree, the proband has inherited marker B and therefore the normal gene. (c) The grandparents are deceased and it is impossible to determine which marker, A or B, is linked to the mutant gene. (d) The affected grandparent is deceased, but one can deduce that the mutant gene is linked to marker A and that the proband has inherited the normal gene.

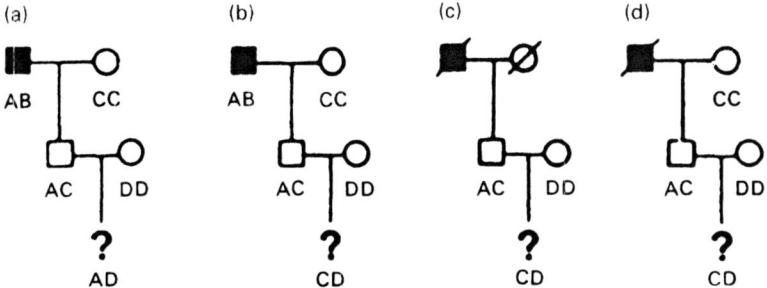

Fig. 9.5b Prenatal diagnosis for an autosomal dominant condition is requested when a risk cannot be assessed in the asymptomatic parent. (*a*) The fetus has inherited marker A from the affected grandparent and therefore has the same risk as his at-risk parent (i.e. 50 per cent). (*b*) The fetus has inherited marker C from the healthy grandparent and there- fore, within the limits of recombination, one can exclude the risk of his being affected. (*c*) both grandparents are deceased: diagnosis is not possible. (*d*) The affected grandparent is deceased: the at-risk parent has inherited the chromosome carrying the mutant gene but has transmitted the chromosome carrying the normal gene.

non-exclusion of risk is not satisfactory. Prenatal diagnosis of other dominant diseases such as polycystic kidney disease using this same strategy has been proposed.

New techniques In recent years, we have become accustomed to the develop- ment of new techniques completely overhauling methods of diagnosis. It is impossible to try to anticipate what will happen in the years to come.

The refinement of methods for determining heterozygosity for cystic fibrosis, as well as establishing automatic karyotyping, represent significant advances.

In this area, certain concepts must be looked at with care, for example pre- implantation diagnosis. Diagnostic techniques used in chorionic villi or amniotic fluid cells can be used on cells sampled from an embryo *in vitro* prior to implan- tation. For some techniques, cytogenetic or biochemical, the first obstacle is the necessity of a quantity of embryonic cells, ensuring a diagnosis as extensive and accurate as that obtained *in utero*. Direct analyses done on cells from embryos *in vitro* are difficult because implantation of embryos happens only 2–3 days after conception and at a time when the embryo consists of only eight cells. Indirect analyses may be done after culturing for a sufficient number of cells. For bio- chemical analyses (metabolic disorders) one must ensure that expression of the protein in cells at that stage is normal. It is known that the embryo's genome is only expressed after the 4–8 cell stage; proteins expressed before this may be oocyte proteins coded by the maternal genome. DNA amplification techniques are certainly useful as they allow amplification of DNA from one or two cells.

Even if solutions to the various problems are found, one must consider the medical implications of their application: these include *in vitro* fertilization, embryo freezing during analysis of cells, and re-implantation after results are available.

Couples at risk of having a child with a genetic disease are fertile. With *in utero* prenatal diagnosis, as presently practiced, pregnancy is on-going, the diagnosis is made and there is termination of pregnancy only in cases where the fetus is affected. In X-linked or autosomal recessive diseases, 75 per cent of fetuses are normal and pregnancy goes to term with subsequent delivery of a normal baby. In a dominant disease, 50 per cent of pregnancies result in the birth of a normal child. In *in vitro* embryo diagnosis, *in vitro* fertilization with re-implantation is required. Only about 15 per cent of pregnancies go to term, even though the embryo is normal (this is the highest success rate for *in vitro* fertilization), resulting therefore in the need to analyse many embryos which can be stored frozen, with a view to using them for another implantation if there is failure, or if there is a request for a second child. The result is that we replace the physical and psychological trauma of pregnancy termination by the physical and psychological trauma of *in vitro* fertilization in a fertile couple, a couple who will not cope well with repeated failures. Additionally, *in utero* prenatal diagnosis should be done to confirm *in vitro* diagnosis and possibly to detect a natural conception, which may have occurred in a fertile couple.

Finally, the deleterious effects on the fetus of pre-implantation cell sampling are not known. As this technology continues to evolve, it is also important to consider the cost which will be added to *in utero* prenatal diagnosis (already substantial), cost of handling, and cost of conservation of embryos, which then must be multiplied by the number of attempts (Davies, 1994).

References and further reading

Ayme, S., Mattei, J. F., Mattei, M. G., Giraud, F. (1980). Anomalies chromosomiques: facteurs de risque actuellement connus. *J. Genet. Hum.*, **28**, 155–78.

Benacerraf, B. R., Gelman, R., and Frigoletto, F. D. (1987). Sonographic identification of second-trimeter fetuses with Down's syndrome. *New Engl. J. Med.*, **317**, 1371–409.

Bogart, M. H., Pandian, M. R., and Jones, O. W. (1987). Abnormal maternal serum chorionic gonadotropin levels in pregnancies with fetal chromosome abnormalities. *Prenat. Diagn.*, **7**, 623–30.

Boué, J., Morer, I., and Vignal, P. (1980). Essai de définition d'un coefficient de risque d'anomalie chromosomique en début de grossesse. *J. Genet Hum.*, **28**, 149–53.

Boué, J., Vignal, P., Aubry, J. P., *et al.* (1982). Ultrasound movement patterns of fetuses with chromosome anomalies. *Prenat. Diagn.*, **2**, 61–5.

Canick, J. A., Knight, G. J., Palomaki, G. E., *et al.* (1988). Low second trimester maternal serum unconjugated oestriol in pregnancies with Down's syndrome. *Br. J. Obstet. Gynecol.*, **95**, 330–3.

Cuckle, H. S. and Wald, N. J. (1987). Vaginal bleeding in pregnancies associated with fetal Down syndrome. *Prenat. Diagn.*, **7**, 619–22.

Davies, K. (1994). PEPing up preimplantation testing. *Nat. Genet.*, **6**(1), 1–2.

Di Maio, M. S., Baumgarten, A., Greenstein, R. M., *et al.* Screening for fetal Down's syndrome in pregnancy by measuring maternal serum alpha-fetoprotein levels. *New Engl. J. Med.*, **317**, 342–6.

Garver, K. L. (1989). Update on MSAFP policy statement from the American Society of Human Genetics. *Am. J. Hum. Genet.*, **44**, 338–43.

Harper, P. S. and Sarfarazi, M. (1985). Genetic prediction and family structure in Huntington's chorea. *Br. Med. J.*, **290**, 1929–31.

Hook, E. B., Topol, N. N., and Cross, P. K. (1989). The natural history of cytogenetically abnormal fetuses detected at midtrimester amniocentesis which are not terminated electively: new data and estimates of the excess and relative risk of late fetal death associated with 47, +21 and some other abnormal karyotypes. *Am. J. Hum., Genet.*, **45**, 855–61.

Kalousek, D. K., Barret, I. J., and McGillivray, B. C. (1989). Placental mosaicism and intrauterine survival of trisomies 13 and 18. *Am. J. Hum. Genet.*, **44**, 338–43.

Merkatz, I. R., Nitowsky, H. M., Macri, J. N., and Johnson, W. E. (1984). An association between low maternal serum alpha-fetoprotein and fetal chromosome anomalies. *Am. J. Obstet. Gynecol.*, **148**, 886–94.

Muller, F. and Boué, A. (1990). A single chorionic gonadotrophin assay for maternal serum screening for Down's syndrome. *Prenat. Diagn*, **10**, 389–98.

Muller, F., Rebiffe, M., Der Sarkissian, H., *et al.* (1986). Diminution de certaines activités enzymatiques dans le liquide amniotique de foetus porteurs d'anomalies chromosomiques. *Ann. Genet.*, **29**, 27–31.

Muller, F., Aegerter, P., and Boué, A. (1993). Prospective maternal serum human chorionic gonadotropin screening for the risk of fetal chromosome anomalies and of subsequent fetal and neonatal deaths. *Prenat. Diagn.*, **11**, 29–43.

Naeye, R. L. (1967). Prenatal organ and cellular growth with various chromosomal disorders *Biol. Neonat.*, **11**, 248–53.

Nicolaides, K. H., Rodeck, C. H., and Gosden, C. M. (1986). Rapid karyotyping in non lethal fetal malformations. *Lancet*, **i**, 283–6.

Norgaard-Pedersen, B., Larsen, S. E., Arends, J., *et al.* (1990). Maternal serum markers in screening for Down syndrome. *Clin. Genet.*, **37**, 35–43.

Petrocik, E., Wassman, E. R., and Kelly, J. C. (1989). Prenatal screening for Down syndrome with maternal serum human gonadotrophin levels. *Am. J. Obstet. Gynecol.*, **161**, 1168–73.

Saudubray, J. M. and Poenaru, L. (1986). Diagnostic prénatal des maladies héréditaires du métabolisme. In *Le diagnostic prénatal* (ed. J. F. Mattei and Y. Dumez), pp. 55–73, Doin, Paris.

10 Fetal therapy

In utero transfusion for fetal–maternal incompatibility, first developed by Liley in 1963, has recently been improved by direct transfusion through umbilical vessels using ultrasound guidance. This same method has allowed treatment of severe thrombocytopaenia in the fetus at the end of the pregnancy.

In the present context, we discuss only possible approaches to be used in the treatment of abnormalities detected by prenatal diagnosis. Absence of a real possibility of therapy for most genetic anomalies of the fetus leads one to consider termination of pregnancy for those found to be affected at prenatal diagnosis. Fortuitous discovery of fetal anomalies by ultrasonography will lead to a decision regarding fetal therapy or termination of pregnancy. What role do laboratory tests have in this decision? Two types of therapy may be considered.

Surgical methods

Malformations observed only at birth could previously be corrected only by neonatal surgery, with variable results. Now, prenatal ultrasound detection of anomalies allows better-planned neonatal surgery with a greater success rate.

Open fetal surgery, experimented with in animals, has not been seriously considered for application in humans. Present work is directed to providing support intervention, with the aim of minimizing serious complications as development progresses and better preparation for neonatal surgery at birth.

These support procedures include puncture guided by ultrasound to release pressure in a particular cavity (hydrothorax for example), or the placing of a catheter to allow a shunt from the cavity containing liquid to the amniotic sac. The value of such interventions is still questionable. Some have been abandoned completely after catastrophic outcomes (in cases of hydrocephaly for example) and others, are trying by prospective study, to get a handle on which of these cases have appropriate indications.

Laboratory tests provide information which may provide a clearer diagnosis and prognosis. In fact, there are two questions to consider.

1. Is this an apparently isolated malformation and amenable to neonatal surgery? Biochemical and chromosomal analyses may provide important information. Discovery of a chromosomal anomaly means that the malformation observed is only one feature of the syndrome associated with that chromosomal anomaly. Acetylcholinesterase testing will demonstrate a neural tube defect that has gone undetected, as in certain cases of hydrocephaly.

268

2. Once these anomalies have been ruled out, is there prognostic information where support intervention may be considered? In cases of bilateral or low obstructive uropathies, a bladder-to-amniotic sac or pelvis-to-amniotic sac shunt has been proposed since 1982. Data collected by Manning *et al.* (1986) showed that 73 shunts had been performed and 43 children had died *in utero* or at birth, essentially from pulmonary hypoplasia. For the 30 children who survived, pediatric-nephrology follow-up is not known. Considering these poor outcomes, it is reasonable to ask whether the indications for *in utero* shunts were well thought out. Biochemical study of fetal urine (see p. 209) should avoid unnecessary catheterization, as much for more severe lethal forms as for less severe forms with naturally good postnatal prognosis, and may single out those cases leading to a renal insufficiency at birth for whom *in utero* shunt may improve postnatal prognosis of renal function.

Medical therapy

What fetal therapies can be proposed in view of already evaluated methods, as well as those under evaluation for children affected with genetic disease? Bone marrow transplants have been used for treatment of β-thalassaemia and some metabolic disorders such as mucopolysaccaridosis and neurolipidosis. For correction of certain immune deficiencies in the fetus, grafting of stem cells from embryonic liver has been attempted with some success.

Gene therapy on somatic cells, that is insertion of normal genes in somatic cells, is conceptually not much different from organ transplants, in particular of bone marrow. Such methods have been applied for the insertion of genes in circulating cells removed from the patient and returned after ensuring that the technique is functioning. This generally means that the single gene disorders amenable to this gene therapy are limited; it has been considered to correct adenosideminase deficiency and purine nucleosidephosphorylase deficiency in affected children. Techniques are currently being attempted, however, for other genetic conditions.

Support therapy has been proposed for 21-hydroxylase deficiency. In this case, the goal is to avoid the phenotypic effects of virilization during embryonic development; the genetic defect will remain, requiring steroid therapy at birth. With this in mind, daily treatment of the mother with dexamethasone is initiated in the first weeks of pregnancy and certainly prior to 6 weeks beyond the last menstrual period. Treatment will continue throughout pregnancy only if prenatal diagnosis indicates that the expected child is an affected female homozygote. Some success has been reported, as well as failures, and the long-term deleterious effects on healthy children exposed to this treatment during early embryonic development is still unknown.

One must be attentive to high expectations and hopes in fetal therapy. As prenatal diagnosis and termination of pregnancy are often linked, there is tendency to present futuristic progress as a way of avoiding pregnancy termination, and thus permitting oneself to attempt therapeutic or diagnostic methods for which the consequences, and at times deleterious effects, have been inadequately assessed. One should not forget that it is the families who will bear the burden of the failures.

References

David, M. and Forest, M. G. (1984). Prenatal treatment of congenital adrenal hyperplasia resulting from 21 hydroxylase deficiency. *J. Pediat.*, **105**, 799–803.

Dumez, Y., Nathan, C., and Henrion, R. (1984). Diagnostic anténatal et chirurgie foetale. *Rev. Prat.*, **34**, 3345–9.

Elder, J. S. S., Duckett, J. W., and Snyder, H. M. (1987). Intervention for fetal obstructive uropathy: has it been effective. *Lancet*, **ii**, 1007–9.

Gene therapy in man. Recommendations of European Medical Research Councils. (1988). *Lancet*, **i**, 1271–2.

Hirschhorn, R. (1987). Therapy of genetic disorders. *New Engl. J. Med.*, **316**, 623–4.

Krivit, W. and Whitley, C. B. (1987). Bone marrow transplantation for genetic diseases. *New Engl. J. Med.*, **316**, 1085–7.

Liley, A. W. (1963). Intrauterine transfusion of foetus in haemolylic disease. *Br. Med. J.*, **2**, 1107–9.

Manning, F. A., Harrison, M. R., and Rodeck, C., *et al.* (1986). Catheter shunts for fetal hydronephrosis and hydrocephalus. Report of the International Fetal Surgery Registry. *New Engl. J. Med.*, **315**, 336–40.

11 Ethical issues

Applications of fetal medicine bring ethical considerations to the forefront. In this area, the laboratory has a particular responsibility; the result of an analysis will be a determining factor in the parents' decision to pursue or terminate a pregnancy.

The ethical problems of prenatal diagnosis were the subject of a document by the French National Consultative Committee on Ethics (see p. 275). In a number of chapters of this book various issues have already been addressed. A commentary is added here.

When a pregnancy with a predictable risk of abnormality presents, the family must be clearly informed prior to testing of the risk of fetal anomaly, the frequency and severity and the likely therapies available. At the same interview, the possibility of termination of this pregnancy must be addressed in terms of the family's moral values and the physical and psychological trauma for the woman. It is also necessary to weigh on one hand the risk of fetal abnormality and on the other, the miscarriage risk from sampling techniques, as well as the risk of error in laboratory analysis.

This assessment must be made in two ways:

1. *Choosing the cut-off point for the indication of advanced maternal age.* Below 38 years of age the risk of fetal anomaly is smaller than the risk to the fetus of amniocentesis, with variations between one operator and another.

2. *Choosing the sampling technique keeping in mind the diagnosis to be made*: amniocentesis at 16–17 weeks and, if the fetus is affected, interruption of pregnancy at 19–20 weeks, or chorionic villus sampling at 11 weeks with possibility of a result in a few days. Despite remarkable success of chorionic villus sampling for some operators, studies combining data from several centres are not as promising. For transcervical chorionic villus sampling, when the results are normal, 5–8 per cent of pregnancies do not reach term. This explains the move towards transabdominal sampling techniques. Additionally, in 1–2 per cent of cases, cytogenetic analysis presents problems in interpretation of direct analyses: false positives, and sometimes false negatives. In countries where lawsuits are frequent this leads to two methods of analysis (direct and after culture), doubling the work, and, in those doubtful cases, leads to follow-up by amniocentesis or fetal blood sampling. Anxiety brought on by this lack of certainty may lead to a request for an abortion prior to a follow-up test.

Except for some structural chromosomal anomalies, cytogenetic analyses are generally indicated for pregnancies at relatively low risk (1–2 per cent). The question is whether obtaining an early result, with the possibility of early termination (which is in itself laudable), in 2 per cent of at-risk pregnancies (maternal age indications) warrants exposing normal and wanted pregnancies to the risk of sampling and the rate of cytogenetic error.

However, biochemical and molecular analyses on chorionic villus sampling represent tremendous progress and address genetic anomalies where the risk is high (25 per cent in general), therefore justifying the risk of testing.

When the indication for prenatal diagnosis is one determined in a pregnancy where there is an unexpected finding, parents will be confronted first by the detection of an anomaly by ultrasonography and then with confirmation of a diagnosis and the decisions to be made. Detection of a chromosomal anomaly responsible for a malformation syndrome makes the prognosis worse, but in some way simplifies decision-making. In the absence of a chromosomal anomaly, and presented with the possibility of neonatal surgery, one is confronted by a conflict of interest between parents and fetus. In these cases the medical team — obstetrician, ultrasonographer, laboratory, geneticist, neonatologist, and paediatric surgeon — should in each situation present the prognosis so that parents are better placed to make a decision. These are the most difficult situations, and are evolving constantly. For example, neonatal heart surgery has benefited greatly from the possibility of *in utero* diagnosis.

In this book, we have generally dealt mainly with diagnosis of severe conditions manifesting themselves at birth or in the first year of life.

A possible extension of the number of indications raises a number of ethical issues:

- fetal sexing for convenience: the experience of several cytogeneticists demonstrates that this request remains the exception;
- diagnosis of genetic diseases manifesting only in adult life and for which there is *in utero* diagnosis (as in the case of Huntington's disease and polycystic kidney disease);
- diagnosis of certain diseases (for example juvenile insulin-dependent diabetes and certain cancers) where currently only susceptibility can be determined.

In the last 20 years we have seen extraordinary progress in fetal medicine and genetics. Offering prenatal diagnosis today for diseases which may only manifest themselves in adulthood, that is 20–40 years from now, is denying the possibility of further progress in the treatment of these diseases.

An ethical issue which is likely to come to the forefront soon results from the use of serological markers in maternal serum for the selection of pregnancies at risk for a chromosomal anomaly. These techniques are part of a public health policy which includes other tests carried out to monitor pregnancies, tests which, until now, have been done to detect early signs of problems (which may affect fetal development), and may lead to measures minimizing these risks.

In selecting pregnancies at risk for chromosomal anomaly, screening may result in termination of pregnancy. This screening, whose goal is to be praised, will present parents first with an increased risk leading to great anxiety that is difficult to allay (even though in the selected group the risk is 1–2 per cent). They then are faced with the possibility of having to make a decision to terminate, which may be against their moral values. This screening should therefore only be done for informed parents willing to terminate a pregnancy if necessary. This requires counselling of every couple which, already beyond our resources, may become superficial and therefore, from the time of blood sampling, may generate unjustified anxiety in many mothers.

A document by the National Consultative Committee of Ethics on problems incurred by prenatal and perinatal diagnosis

Congenital malformations and hereditary disease represent, in the industrialized world, one of the main causes of morbidity and mortality in childhood. They are unfortunate for the individual, and a psychological and economical burden for the family and society. Medicine has made significant and rapid progress in its understanding of the mechanisms of these disorders. For 10 years now, a number of techniques have permitted prenatal diagnosis of a large and increasing number of anomalies. These techniques hold great hope for the parents who, having had a child affected by anomalies or knowing themselves to be carriers of a disease, have decided not to have children. When it is able to exclude the presence of anomalies, prenatal diagnosis by its nature removes the despair of parents wishing to have children. In contrast, prenatal diagnosis can reveal abnormalities which are presently not amenable to therapy. In fact, progress in medicine still does not allow the cure of a large number of hereditary diseases. At best, it provides a small improvement in lifespan with few improvements in quality of life.

The gap which exists between diagnostic and therapeutic techniques can make one apprehensive that recourse to prenatal diagnosis reinforces the social phenomenon which rejects those considered abnormal, and renders intolerable the slightest anomaly in the fetus or child.

At the level of the individual, prenatal diagnosis presents the parents and physician with the difficult question of termination of pregnancy. Implementation of prenatal diagnosis of genetic abnormalities in the fetus is therefore closely linked to the moral issue brought about by termination of pregnancy.

The decision to be made, that is the choice between voluntary interruption of pregnancy and the birth of a more or less severely handicapped child, puts into question how each one of us perceives life and the value of the individual. The decision to continue or stop the pregnancy belongs to the patient, according to law, and 'in this way avoids any collective eugenics movement'. The decision of the patient must take into consideration their rights as well as what is customary. In terms of rights, according to the [French] law of 17 January 1975, the motive for termination of pregnancy must be the high likelihood that the baby to be born 'will be affected by a severe disorder and recognized as untreatable at the time of diagnosis'. This definition is to be applied to what is going on every day, and in this context four factors must be appreciated: the certainty of the diagnosis, the severity of the disease, the age at the onset of manifestations, and the efficiency of treatment.

In view of the extremely difficult situation in which those who use prenatal diagnosis find themselves, and the ethical nature of the questions which they must confront, the National Ethics Committee considers necessary the formulation of recommendations for the use of and future developments in prenatal diagnosis.

Use of prenatal diagnosis

For some 10 years now development of prenatal diagnosis has been based on very reliable laboratory tests (cytogenetic and biochemical) and their application has been developed by a grouping of diagnostic centres under the appropriate authorities. Within this framework, some tens of thousands of diagnoses have been realized and in each year an increasing number of couples from at-risk groups benefit from these tests.

For several years, visualization by ultrasound has opened new avenues for diagnosis where precision depends on the quality of equipment and the user's expertise. To maintain the good quality of laboratory and ultrasound tests, it is recommended that prenatal diagnosis centres be accredited and that no decision for medical termination of pregnancy be taken without prior consultation with such a centre. This centre must be multidisciplinary and be composed of at least one clinical geneticist, one laboratory geneticist, and one fetal ultrasound specialist; it should be associated with one or more laboratories able to provide the necessary testing.

In practice, the training of physicians and technical staff in this area is a pressing need.

On the legal side, the decision to terminate a pregnancy for reasons of malformation or genetic disease, according to the law of January 17 1975, must include the written authorization of two physicians. It is recommended that at least one of these physicians be competent in the area of law and be associated to an accredited centre. The same regulations must be applied to those terminations occurring earlier than 12 weeks of pregnancy.

The decision to terminate a pregnancy belongs to the parents, who should have been well informed of test results. It is important that the information given is not perceived as a pressure imposed on them. One must not reproach parents who are opposed to prenatal diagnosis or pregnancy termination.

Finally, in order to avoid medically unjustified use as well as the errors which may result from the indiscriminate use of kits permitting diagnosis of sex or of genetic disease from the 9th week of pregnancy, it is recommended that a regulation, similar to that applied to new or dangerous drugs, be applied to the use of kits used for genetic diagnosis.

Developments in prenatal diagnosis

Considering the expectations placed upon prenatal diagnosis, new developments are hoped for and anticipated.

The difficulties discussed above lead one to pursue the extension and expansion of new techniques with some caution. This is why prenatal diagnosis should only be considered where the likelihood of error is low enough to ensure a certainty or quasi-certainty in the diagnosis of an anomaly.

It is recommended that public policy support prenatal diagnosis financially within these parameters. Financing should allow equal access for all to these services, which are often costly.

In cases where diagnosis is reliable and the disease is common and particularly severe, it might be hoped that prenatal diagnosis methods can be developed by general policy: thus, prenuptial or prenatal testing can, if the couple wishes, evaluate risk factors and provide information on carrier status for certain recessive diseases. A public health programme involved in the collecting of data on haemoglobinopathies (sickle cell anaemia and thalassaemia) is possible even now in areas where these diseases are common, and is expected very soon for certain X-linked diseases. Extension of the programme, as soon as possible, to other common severe genetic diseases, still without proper therapy (for example cystic fibrosis), should also take place, taking into consideration the cost of such testing.

Screening for predisposition

Screening for predisposition to certain diseases, some which are frequent and severe, could be done perinatally, postnatally, or in some cases by prenatal diagnosis. In consideration of this, the committee makes the same recommendations, notably concerning its financing and its limitation to diseases for which tests provide a certainty or quasi-certainty in their determination of predisposition, and for which there is an early cure, or treatment. Moreover, the frequency and severity of the disease as well as the cost of the test should be kept in mind. Finally, confidentiality of information collected must be maintained.

Consequences of prenatal diagnosis

Hereditary diseases which today are amenable to prenatal diagnosis usually result in the death of the patient before reproductive age.

Some critics emphasize the dysgenic consequences of medical progress which prevent the playing of 'natural selection' and increase the 'genetic load'; others resist the 'eugenics' which underline the health policies in genetic programs.

All population genetics studies show that although one can in fact reduce the number of births of children affected by genetic disease, medicine today cannot really modify the genetic pool.

New possibilities offered by prenatal diagnosis which is used widely and cautiously, can only be of benefit for the sick, their family, and the entire population.

References

Comité Consultatif National d'Ethique (1985).

Index

abortion
  induced, *see* termination of pregnancy
  spontaneous, *see* spontaneous abortion
acetylcholinesterase
  electrophoresis, *see* cholinesterase electrophoresis
  fetal development 6–7
  neural tube defects 193–8, 268
αN-acetylgalactosaminidase deficiency 126
acidaemias 24, 88–9, 114, 119, 122
acid hydrolases 114
acidurias 24, 89, 120
acquired immune deficiency syndrome 228, 242–6
adenine 63
adenosine deaminase deficiency 187, 269
adrenal hyperplasias, *see* congenital adrenal hyperplasias
adrenocorticotrophic hormone (ACTH) 132
adrenoleucodystrophy 89, 114, 119, 129, 131
Africa and Africans 150, 181, 242–3
agammaglobulinaemia 187
age factors
  fetal, *see* gestational age
  maternal, *see* maternal age, advanced
  paternal 100
AIDS 228, 242–6
  see also HIV
albinism 188
albumin 59, 60, 61
alkaline phosphatase (PAL) 12, 57–9, 61, 145, 209–12
alleles
  α-1-antitrypsin deficiency 185
  cystic fibrosis 144, 209
  DNA analysis 72–3, 76–82
  fragile X 110
  muscular dystrophies 174, 178
allele-specific oligonucleotide (ASO) method 143
alphafetoprotein
  biochemical analysis 56–7, 59, 209
  chorionic villi sampling 34
  fetal development 12–14
  neural tube defects 193–4, 254
  trisomy 21 257, 259, 261–2
alymphocytoses 187
aminoacidopathies 89–90, 113–14, 118, 122

aminoglycans 121
ammonia 63, 211
ammonium 62
amniocentesis 21–7
  chromosome analysis 36, 105–8, 253, 257, 259
  complications/risks 22, 25–7, 262
  congenital adrenal hyperplasia 140
  contraindications 21, 115
  cut-off limits 259, 262, 271
  cystic fibrosis 113, 146–9
  cytomegalovirus 235
  enzyme testing 21, 24, 263
  ethical issues 271
  indications for 113, 115
  laboratory tests 204, 213
  neural tube defects 193–8, 254
  toxoplasmosis 232
amniotic fluid 17–19, 22
  alphafetoprotein in 56–7, 193–8
  biochemical analysis 54–60, 206–9
  bloody **25**, 54–6, 59, 61, 120, 197–8
  brown 25–6, 59
  cell culture 46–50, 184
  cholinesterase electrophoresis 206–9
  chromosome analysis 36, 105–8, 253, 257, 259
  contamination by 38, 61
  cystic fibrosis 113, 146–9
  DNA analysis 65
  herpes virus 239
  leakage of 26
  metabolic disorders 113–18
  mosaicism 102–3
  neural tube defects 193–8, 254
  number of diagnoses on 89
  protein levels 60
  quality of 47, 54–6
  rubella virus 223
  steroid levels 137–9
  volume of 18, 203, 204
  see also anamnios; oligohydramnios; polyhydramnios
anaemia
  and cytomegalovirus 234
  Fanconi's 183–5
  haemolytic 75
  sickle cell, *see* sickle cell anaemia

277

Lightning Source UK Ltd.
Milton Keynes UK
07 October 2009

144621UK00002B/58/A